The Peritoneum

Compliments of

Gere S. diZerega   Kathleen E. Rodgers

The Peritoneum

Foreword by Alan H. DeCherney

With 133 Illustrations

Springer-Verlag

New York   Berlin   Heidelberg   London   Paris
Tokyo   Hong Kong   Barcelona   Budapest

Gere S. diZerega, M.D.
Professor of Obstetrics and Gynecology
University of Southern California
School of Medicine
Livingston Research Center
Los Angeles, CA 90033 USA

Kathleen E. Rodgers, Ph.D.
Assistant Research Professor
University of Southern California
School of Medicine
Livingston Research Center
Los Angeles, CA 90033 USA

Cover illustration: Different modes by which the peritoneum re-epithelializes after surgical injury include contributions from adjacent intact peritoneum, poorly differentiated cells within the connective tissue scaffold, and perivascular connective tissue. The tissue repair cells form "islands" on the surface of damaged peritoneum and then proliferate to re-epithelialize the injured site.

Library of Congress Cataloging-in-Publication Data
diZerega, Gere S.
    The peritoneum / Gere S. diZerega, Kathleen E. Rodgers.
        p. cm.
    Includes bibliographical references and index.
    ISBN 0-387-97830-5. — ISBN 3-540-97830-5
    1. Peritoneum—Physiology. 2. Peritoneum—Surgery. I. Rodgers,
Kathleen E. II. Title.
    [DNLM: 1. Peritoneum—surgery. WI 575 D622p]
    QP 157.D58   1992
    612.3′3—dc20
    DNLM/DLC
    for Library of Congress   92-2221

Printed on acid-free paper.

Production managed by Ellen Seham; manufacturing supervised by Genieve Shaw.
Typeset by Impressions, a division of Edwards Brothers, Inc., Madison, WI
Printed and bound by Edwards Brothers, Inc., Ann Arbor, MI
Printed in the United States of America.

9 8 7 6 5 4 3 2

ISBN 0-387-97830-5 Springer-Verlag New York Berlin Heidelberg
ISBN 3-540-97830-5 Springer-Verlag Berlin Heidelberg New York

Foreword

ENTERING ON A CREATIVE AND ENTERPRISING PROJECT, DRS. DIZEREGA
and Rodgers have taken an innovative look at the peritoneum. They
have provided an interesting, informative, and stimulating text about an
organ that is rarely considered independently—usually being thought of
only as a part of other organs or organ systems.

The peritoneum is an active membrane that serves as both a secretory
organ and a structure that modulates diffusion and osmosis. Both of these
important functions are described in great detail.

The text is divided in classic fashion. The authors first examine the
peritoneal anatomy from both macro and cellular viewpoints, during
which exploration it becomes clear that what appears simply to be a lacy
covering over abdominal organs actually is a complex structure. Furthermore, during the discussion on its embryologic development the authors make comprehensible the complexity confronting the student of
the peritoneum.

The authors then proceed to the practicalities associated with this important organ. To surgeons, for example, the key to the peritoneum is
understanding the organ's repair mechanism, as it is adhesions formed
on the peritoneal surfaces that interfere with the surgeon's hope of success.
Simply stated, adhesions are merely a form of healing. Thus if we could
understand the mechanisms involved in adhesion formation, we might
be able to control them—with the end result of fewer postoperative problems following a surgical procedure. It is in the coverage of such subjects
as this one that diZerega and Rodgers blend their knowledge of proved
concepts with the most current and ongoing research today. Thus information regarding healing is important, and it is only from laboratory and
animal data that such a phenomenon as adhesion formation can become
less problematic.

The peritoneal fluid is another important and dynamic bodily product.
It washes the contents of the peritoneal cavity with various chemical and
cellular modulators on an ongoing basis. This area of interest is another
that the authors have covered in fascinating detail.

The portion of the book concerned with growth factors is probably the most important during this period of our medical development. We have learned from fetal surgery that healing can be complete without scarring. Such healing is probably due to the presence of growth factors, which are perhaps unique to the fetal period. diZerega and Rodgers have paid great attention to these factors, with an eye on understanding the healing and growth process. Fibroblast growth factor, interleukin 1, and tumor necrosis factor are thoroughly discussed—making this section a timely contribution.

Since the early 1980s, macrophages have been known to be the most important cellular element of the peritoneum and peritoneal fluid. During the past few years this cell has attracted more attention than almost any other in biology. Its work as a secretory agent as well as a phagocyte, and its importance in the healing process have been diligently explored and aptly described in this book.

In regard to the clinical aspects of diZerega and Rodgers' treatment of the peritoneum, if we are to arrive at any answers to the problem of how to prevent adhesions postoperatively, for example, it will come from a basic understanding and basic scientific investigation of this organ, including its fluid, cellular components, and chemical matrix (e.g., growth factors).

Although much is known about the peritoneum, far more is to be discovered about this fascinating organ whose surface area is comparable to that of skin. It is a dynamic organ that for too long has been unexplored and dissected. In this text, diZerega and Rodgers have not only answered questions you might not have known you had, they have placed the peritoneum in a context in which it becomes an amazing and stimulating object of study.

Alan H. DeCherney, M.D.
Louis E. Phaneuf, Professor
  and Chairman
Department of Obstetrics and
  Gynecology
Tufts University School of Medicine

Acknowledgments

RESEARCH CONDUCTED ON PERITONEAL REPAIR PERFORMED IN THE AU-thors' laboratory would not have been possible without the support and critical advice of E. Schinagel, J. Campbell, L. Gabel, E. Pines, C. Linsky, D. Johns, T. Cunningham, D. Ellefson, D. Sheffield, R. King, A. Levey, D. Rovee, and M. Brown. The authors would like to acknowledge the contributions made by the research fellows from the Second Department of Surgery, Yamagata University School of Medicine, Yamagata, Japan, especially the following: K. Nishimura, T. Shimanuki, H. Orita, M. Fu-kasawa, H. Abe, and S. Kuraoka. Their contributions were made possible by the continuing fellowship of Professor M. Washio, Chairman of the Second Department of Surgery and Dr. Robert M. Nakamura of the University of Southern California School of Medicine. The authors also want to acknowledge Mr. Charles Morrow for the interpretive artwork created for this book. The authors also wish to acknowledge Ms. Mae Gordon and Ms. Leticia Corona for their diligent preparation of the manuscript and attendance to the correspondence this project required.

A personal acknowledgment is extended to W. Girgis who managed all the animal surgery over the last 7 years and especially to J. Campeau who directed the daily operations of the Livingston Reproductive Biology Laboratory during the entire 11 years of this project.

The authors wish to express their appreciation for the understanding expressed by their families during the completion of this work including Lynn Yonekura and Margaret diZerega as well as Jeremiah, Joshua, and Ronald Rodgers.

Contents

1

Peritoneum

SEROSA IS A TRUNCATION OF THE LATIN *MEMBRANA SEROSA*, WHICH designates a serous membrane lining. Serous is distinguishable from mucinous by the nature of the secretions. Glands that secrete a viscous and slippery secretion are called mucous glands; glands that secrete a relatively clear and watery fluid reminiscent of whey are given the name serous (L. *serum*, whey) glands. The body contains three serous membranes of mesodermal origin: peritoneum, pleura, and pericardium.

Peritoneum is the most extensive serous membrane in the body. The surface area of the peritoneum is generally equal to that of the skin (Gardner, Gray & O'Rahilly, 1969). It forms a closed sac in the male and an open sac in the female as the ends of the fallopian tubes are not covered by peritoneum (Figure 1.1). The peritoneum lines the walls of the abdomen (parietal peritoneum) and is reflected over the viscera (visceral peritoneum). It consists of two layers: a loose connective tissue and a mesothelium. The connective tissue is arranged into loose bundles that interlace in a plane parallel to the surface. There are numerous elastic fibers, especially in the deeper layer of the parietal peritoneum, and comparatively few connective tissue cells. The peritoneum serves to minimize friction and thus facilitate free movement between abdominal viscera; resist or localize infection; and store fat, especially in the greater omentum.

The intra-abdominal surface of the peritoneum is a continuous sheet of mesothelial cells attached to the abdominal wall and viscera by areolar tissue (subserous fascia). Where peritoneum is freely movable, loose connective or "subserous" tissue, rich in elastin and containing varying numbers of fat cells, connects the peritoneum with the underlying tissue. The peritoneum is well supplied with blood vessels and lymphatics, which give rise to a rich capillary network. The mesothelial cells form a continuous layer that rests upon loose mesenchymal connective tissue, a basal lamina, and basement membrane. The mesentery contains a loose network of collagenous and elastic fibers, scattered fibroblasts, macrophages, mast cells, and a varying number of fat cells (Bloom & Fawcett, 1978).

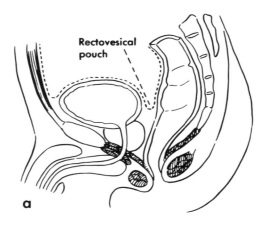

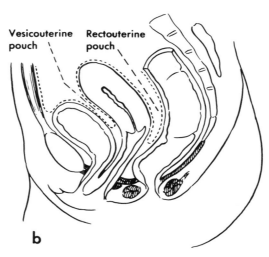

FIGURE 1.1. The peritoneum (broken lines) and the peritoneal pouches or fossae of the pelvis in the male (a), and the female (b), in a median sagittal section. (From Hollinshead, 1971. Reproduced by permission of J.B. Lippincott.)

Histology

Omentum

Omentum is covered by mesothelium on both sides which is folded over the loose connective tissue. The membrane is pierced by numerous holes or fenestrations to form collagenous bundles covered by mesothelial cells that supply the blood vessels. Thicker areas of omentum contain many macrophages, small lymphocytes, plasma cells, a few eosinophils and mast cells. In areas where macrophages accumulate in large numbers the omentum appears grossly to contain "milky spots" (Robbins, 1967).

The mesothelium that covers the peritoneum consists of a single layer of flattened cells with microvilli, peripheral vesicles, and discrete bundles of cytoplasmic microfilaments (Figure 1.2). The cells are attached to one another by desmosomes. The diaphragmatic surface is covered by a single layer of mesothelial cells that contains regional variations. Dome-shaped cells with microvillous projections are arrayed in bands that extended from the musculotendinous junction toward the rib cage. Adjacent cell margins are separated to form mesothelial pores located over lymphatic vessels. Lymphatic endothelial cells form a channel extending from the peritoneal cavity directly into the diaphragmatic lymphatics. The second type of cell that composes the peritoneal covering of the diaphragm is a flat cell that contains numerous microvilli on its apical surfaces and overlays a thin layer of connective tissue instead of lymphatic vessels.

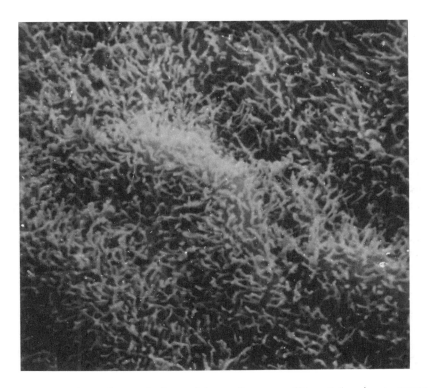

FIGURE 1.2. Normal mesothelium of the peritoneum of the rat showing numerous long microvilli (×5,500.) (Reprinted with permission of Watters & Buck, "Scanning Electron Microscopy of Mesothelial Regeneration in the Rat," *Lab Invest.* 26:604–609, 1972, © by The US and Canadian Academy of Pathology, Inc., Williams & Wilkins, Baltimore, Maryland.)

The cell margins of the flattened cell are in close apposition and do not form pores (Watters & Buck, 1972).

The mesothelial covering of the peritoneum may account for the formation of mesenteric cysts occasionally found in the parietal peritoneum or within supporting structures (mesentary or ligaments). These cysts are thought to arise from embryonic rests of either mesothelium, gut, or urogenital ridge. These cysts can be filled with serous fluid or blood and can range from 1 to 2 cm or 15 to 20 cm in diameter. The cysts occur in either a single cyst or in multiple clusters. Most neoplasms of the peritoneum are metastatic, including ovarian, pancreatic, or other gastrointestinal carcinomas. Primary peritoneal neoplasms are rare and present as mesotheliomas.

Ultrastructure of Peritoneum

Pfeiffer, Pfeiffer, and Misra (1987) described the ultrastructure of the visceral peritoneum covering the stomach, small intestine, and colon of the immature pig using the scanning electron microscope. The peritoneal surface was composed of a single layer of loosely attached squamous epithelial cells that contained scant microvilli. The outer surface contained an undulating surface with a cobblestone appearance.

This monolayer is loosely attached to the underlying connective tissue. At high magnification an abundance of long, widely spaced microvilli cover the apical surface of the mesothelial cells. Adjacent mesothelial cells are joined either by desmosomes or are loosely connected at their peripheral edges. The mesothelium is separated from underlying collagenous bundles by basement membrane. The serosal connective tissue base, upon which the mesothelium of the small intestine rests, is less compacted than that of the stomach.

The apical surface of mesothelial cells contains an abundance of long microvilli, which increase the functional surface area of the peritoneum (Figure 1.3; Watters & Buck, 1972). Microvilli projecting from the mesothelial surfaces dramatically increase the functional surface area of both parietal and visceral peritoneum for both absorption and secretion. A role for mesothelial microvilli in transport function is supported by the absorptive and exudative ability of the mesothelium (Berndt & Gosselin, 1961; Gosselin & Berndt, 1962; Fukata, 1963; Shear, Harvey, & Barry, 1966; Cotran & Karnovsky, 1968). Transport functions of gastrointestinal mesothelium utilize several pathways, including pinocytosis, transmembrane diffusion (Fukata, 1963), and excursion between cell boundaries (Cotran & Karnovsky, 1968).

Basement Membrane

The peritoneum contains a basement membrane supporting both visceral and parietal surfaces. The basement membrane over the stomach is 8 to

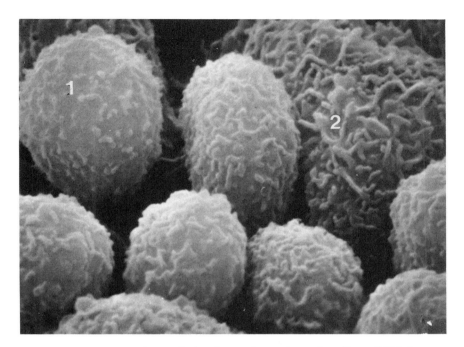

FIGURE 1.3. Features of spherical cells on the peritoneal surface. Cell 1 has numerous microvilli, and cell 2 has thin folds of the membrane (×6,200.) (Reprinted with permission of Watters & Buck, "Scanning Electron Microscopy of Mesothelial Regeneration in the Rat," *Lab Invest.* 26:604–609, 1972, © by The US and Canadian Academy of Pathology, Inc., Williams & Wilkins, Baltimore, Maryland.)

10 μm thick. It consists of a delicate fibrillar plexus and a plexus of reticulum fibers. The orientation of the reticulum and fibroblasts is longitudinal to the plane of expansion appropriate for the anatomical site. Connection with the underlying network of elastin includes collagen and mucopolysaccharides (Figure 1.4; Baron, 1941). The deep longitudinal elastin network is closely connected with an underlying deep latticed collagen by elastin fibers from the lower surface of the longitudinal network that penetrate into the more deeply located collagen.

Blood and Lymphatic Vessels

Blood and lymphatic vessels of the peritoneum are found in the deep collagenous layer. Above this are layers of collagen, mucopolysaccharides, elastin, connective or mesenchymal tissue, superficial collagen, and mesothelial cells. In some areas, for instance intestinal peritoneum, fatty lobules are situated under the elastin within the deep collagen lattice.

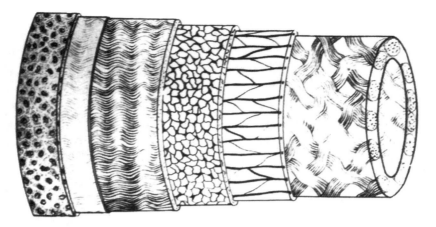

FIGURE 1.4. General scheme of construction of the peritoneum of the small intestine in man, and the fibroarchitecture of the various layers. Innermost layer is a collagen lattice surrounded by a rich microcirculation. A layer of glycosaminoglycans or mucopolysaccharide proteins is covered by elastin. The surface mesothelial cells rest upon a connective tissue matrix of proteins including collagen. (Reprinted by permission of Wiley-Liss, a division of John Wiley & Sons, Inc. from Baron, "Structure of the Intestinal Peritoneum in Man," in *American Journal of Anatomy*, 69:439–497, © 1941 John Wiley.)

Blood vessels of the mesentary or intestinal peritoneum contain adventitial sheaths: elastin for the arteries, collagen for the veins. The sheaths extend onto the capillaries. The deepest vessels of the peritoneum are parallel with the musculature underlying the peritoneum. More superficial vessels, penetrating to the thickness of the deep collagenous layer, are parallel with the spiral arterioles, which prevents overextension of the vessels that may occur by stretching of the peritoneum.

Numerous lymphatic channels lead from the peritoneal cavity, especially from the lower surface of the diaphragm. With each diaphragmatic excursion, relatively large quantities of lymph flow out of the peritoneal cavity into the thoracic duct. If these ducts become occluded (e.g., by cancer, inflammation) the return of protein to the circulation is blocked. As a result, intraperitoneal osmotic pressure rises and ascites ensues (Robbins, 1967).

Free cells including erythrocytes and epithelial cells enter stomata that underlie the accumulated cells (further discussed in Chapter 2). Likewise, fluids, large molecules, and particulate materials are able to enter the diaphragmatic lymphatics through stomata (Leak & Rahil, 1978). This is indicated by the rapid removal of trypan blue dye and colloidal carbon injected intraperitoneally from this cavity into the mediastinal lymphatic vessels and lymph nodes. The importance of the structural integrity of the stoma as a continuous passageway from the peritoneal cavity into the lymphatic lumen is underscored by the loss of this passageway when the diaphragmatic surface is completely occluded by chemical or surgical abrasions that prevent fluid and cellular removal from the peritoneal cavity (Lill, Parsons, & Buchac, 1979).

Mesothelial Histology

The diaphragmatic mesothelium contains two morphologically distinct cell types: flattened and dome-shaped cells (MacCallum, 1903; Allen, 1936; French, Florey, & Morris, 1960). Flattened cells are in close apposition to occluded junctions. In contrast, margins of the dome-shaped cells are often separated by stomata that open into lymphatic vessels (Leak, 1979). Many of the cells migrate over the mesothelial surface, whereas others enter submesothelial lymphatic vessels via stomata (mesothelial pores). These pores may provide a passageway for the removal of fluids as well as large molecules and cells from the peritoneal cavity (Murphy & Morris, 1970; Tsilibury & Wissig, 1977; Leak & Rahil, 1978).

Stomata are present at sites where margins of several lymphatic endothelial cells span the submesothelial connective tissue. This arrangement creates a passageway between the peritoneal cavity and lymphatic lumen. To account for the increased number of stomata observed after peritoneal stimulation, mesothelial cells may respond by retracting their cell margins. Contraction and relaxation of the diaphragmatic muscles during inhalation and exhalation probably leads to widening and narrowing of stomatal orifices. Therefore, a number of passageways would be maintained for a constant removal of fluids and cells by the diaphragmatic lymphatics under normal physiologic conditions.

Embryology

During embryonic and fetal life, the mesentery and visceral ligaments expand or fuse. The greater omentum is an expanded sacculation of the dorsal mesentery of the stomach. During development its surfaces fuse with each other and drape the anterior aspect of the intestine. After 4½ to 5 months of fetal life the peritoneum can be identified as a layer of mesothelium with a thin mesenchymal lining (Baron, 1941). Both lymphatic and blood vessels within these tissues are in close contact due to the absence of intervening fibrous layers. Through months 6 and 7 in utero, the peritoneum develops a deep latticed collagenous layer that forms the basement membrane. Although visceral peritoneum covering the intestine does not contain elastin fibers at this time, the parietal peritoneum of the subdiaphragm is richly endowed with an elastin network. By 6 to 7 months of fetal life the deep collagenous layer begins to appear at the time fetal peritoneum consists primarily of mesothelium and basement membrane. At this time, the elastin fibers are absent. At 8 months of fetal life, fibroblasts align adjacent to the basement membrane and elongate in the axis of greatest physiological tension. The elastin network becomes apparent at about 9 months of fetal life.

Anatomy

Subdivisions of the Greater Sac

The peritoneal cavity is the potential space between the parietal and visceral peritoneum. In general, the parietal and visceral peritoneum are in direct contact with one another (Figure 1.5). The peritoneal cavity is divided into two distinct compartments: (1) the greater sac is the peritoneal cavity per se, and (2) the lesser sac or omental bursa makes up the dorsal surface of the stomach. The two sacs are distinguished by a constriction between the liver and duodenum that is named the epiploic foramen or foramen of Winslow (Hollinshead, 1971).

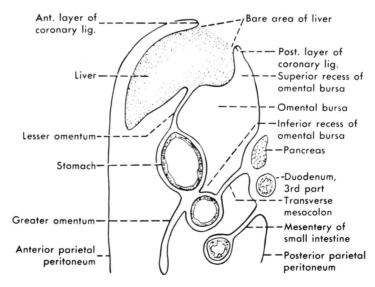

FIGURE 1.5. The disposition of the peritoneum in a sagittal section through the abdominal cavity. (From Hollinshead, 1971. Reproduced by permission of J.B. Lippincott.)

The greater sac is subdivided by the greater omentum, transverse colon, and transverse mesocolon into an upper, anterior part, the supramesocolic compartment, and a lower, posterior part, the inframesocolic compartment. These compartments form channels or recesses that determine how or where peritoneal fluid gravitates or spreads. The supramesocolic compartment is subdivided by the liver into subphrenic and subhepatic spaces. The inframesocolic compartment is further divided by the mesentery of the small intestine into right (upper) and left (lower) parts. The latter drains into the pelvis. The paracolic grooves or gutters are longitudinal depressions lateral to the ascending and descending colon (Garder, 1978).

In some instances the peritoneum can constrict to form bands that lead to abnormal intestinal fixation. These bands are considered to be congenital and are typically attached to the duodenum, jejunum, or transverse colon (Wakefield & Mayo, 1936).

Ligaments or Folds

The term *mesenteries* refers to the peritoneal suspension of the small intestine; "entery" indicating intestine, and the prefix "meso," a general prefix for peritoneum, is used to identify the suspending folds of other organs in the peritoneal cavity, for example mesocolon, mesovarium, etc. When these connective tissues are condensed into a distinct bundle, they are referred to as ligaments. Most ligaments contain blood vessels and nerves. In contrast, viscera more tightly attached to the abdominal wall having only the exposed surface covered by peritoneum are referred to as retroperitoneal viscera. Accordingly, many retroperitoneal structures are also covered at least in part by parietal peritoneum. A large portion of the dorsal aspect of the diaphragmatic surface of the liver is not covered by peritoneum. In the adult human, a 15-cm area of the liver bordered anteriorly by the anterior leaf of the coronary ligament is termed the bare area of the liver. The posterior boundary of this area is the posterior leaf of the coronary ligament where the peritoneum is reflected from the liver to the diaphragm. Although the bare area of the liver is not covered by visceral peritoneum, this site is not directly exposed to the peritoneal cavity due to the communications of the anterior and posterior coronary ligaments with reflections of the adjacent parietal peritoneum.

Innervation

The parietal peritoneum is supplied by nerves from the adjacent body wall, the subdiaphragmatic part by the phrenic nerves, and the remainder by the thoracoabdominal and subcostal nerves and by branches of the lumbosacral plexus (Gardner, Gray & O'Rahilly, 1969). Both sensory and vasomotor nerves supply the peritoneum. Most of the parietal peritoneum is sensitive to pain. Painful stimuli to the anterior and lateral regions are localized to the point of stimulation. By contrast, painful stimuli to the central part of the diaphragmatic peritoneum are referred to the shoulder. Painful stimuli to the peripheral part of the diaphragmatic peritoneum are felt in an intercostal space. The roots of mesenteries contain pain fibers that are sensitive to stretch. Sensory supply to the parietal peritoneum covering the diaphragm involves both the phrenic nerves as well as the intercostals. Thus, diaphragmatic pain may be perceived either at the base of the neck or shoulder (from C_3, C_4, and C_5 via the phrenic nerves) or in the abdominal wall. Since the parietal peritoneum is innervated by branches of the spinal nerves that supply the abdominal wall, peritoneal involvement in visceral disease provides pain sensation through the lower intercostal nerves.

Pain fibers have not been clearly demonstrated for visceral peritoneum. Rather visceral pain is perceived via the viscus itself or stretch or spasm of smooth muscles of the viscus (Garder, 1978; Hollinshead, 1978).

Peritonitis

The most common cause of peritoneal inflammation is bacterial infection, which leads to a neutrophilic infiltrate accompanied by a fibropurulent exudate. Severe bacterial peritonitis leads to abscess and granuloma formation. Sterile peritonitis arises most commonly from the presence of blood, bile, gastrointestinal enzymes, or foreign bodies in the peritoneal cavity. Rarely the peritoneum will undergo a generalized fibrosis on the posterior parietal area. The cause of this unusual problem is unknown. Neutrophils and macrophages commonly adhere to the mesothelium especially during exudative peritonitis (Baradi & Campbel, 1974).

Bacterial toxin not only elicits an increased cellular and fluid infiltrate into the peritoneal cavity, but also causes marked changes in the structure of diaphragmatic mesothelial cells. Many of the peritoneal cells aggregate into mounds at various sites on the mesothelial surface.

The routes by which intraperitoneal effusions spread and the spaces in which they accumulate were studied in surgical patients. Radiographic contrast medium was injected at selected intraperitoneal sites at the conclusion of operations for removal of the gallbladder or appendix. The spread of the contrast medium was followed by roentgenographic examinations taken from 3 to 87 hours after operation (Mitchell, 1941). In roentgenograms taken from 3 to 8 hours after surgery, contrast material was widely disseminated into several of the peritoneal spaces, whether it was introduced into the upper or the lower abdomen. Its movement both from Morison's pouch downward and from the cecal region upward was primarily along the right paracolic gutter and upward from the pelvic space along the left paracolic gutter.

Peritoneal Re-Epithelialization

It was shown in 1919 that peritoneal healing differs from that of skin. Hertzler (1919) observed that when a defect is made in the parietal peritoneum "the entire surface becomes epithelialized simultaneously and not gradually from the borders as in epidermidalization of skin wounds." Although multiplication and migration of mesothelial cells from the margin of the wound may play a small part in the regenerative process it cannot play a major part, since new mesothelium develops in the center of a large wound at the same time as it develops in the center of a smaller one. The granulation and contraction that occur around the edges of skin wounds does not occur during peritoneal healing.

General agreement exists between investigators on the time taken for regeneration of the mesothelial layer. Ellis, Harrison, & Hugh (1965) and Hubbard, Khan, Carag, Albites, & Hricko (1967) reported that healing occurs in 5 to 6 days in the case of parietal peritoneum. Peritoneal defects of 2 × 2 cm and 0.5 × 0.5 cm were both entirely covered by a continuous sheet of mesothelium 3 days after wounding (Ellis, 1962). Glucksman (1966) reported that the visceral mesothelium covering the terminal ileum heals in 5 days, whereas Eskeland & Kjæheim (1966) demonstrated that regeneration of the mesothelial layer of parietal peritoneum is not complete until 8 days. Raftery (1973a,b) confirmed the findings of Eskeland & Kjæheim (1966) that parietal peritoneum of the rat is healed within 8 days.

Mesothelial Regeneration

Eskeland & Kjæheim (1966) and Eskeland (1966a) described the cellular sequence of repair in the parietal peritoneum of rats after either burn or stripping of the peritoneum off of the body wall. Both small and large wounds contained a continuous layer of mesothelial cells by day 8 after injury. Wounds that measured 36 mm in diameter were completely covered with new mesothelium at day 8. The intact peritoneum adjacent to the wound (1 to 3 mm) formed the second day after injury until completion of mesothelial regeneration contained mitotic figures and evidence of migratory activity. Differences between intact mesothelial cells peripheral to the wound and the cytology of the cells on the wound surface were distinct at day 3 after injury. Thereafter, the cytological differences between the cell types became less evident as the cells on the wound surface became more like mature mesothelial cells.

Raftery (1973a) studied the regeneration of parietal and visceral peritoneum using scanning electron microscopic evaluation of healing peritoneal defects in the rat. Twelve hours after injury, numerous polymorphonuclear leukocytes (PMNs) were seen entangled in fibrin strands. Very little cellular infiltrate was found in the depths of the wound compared to the wound surface. At 24 to 36 hours after wounding, the number of cells in the superficial part of the wound was greatly increased; most of the increase in cell number was due to infiltration by macrophages. The macrophages were intertwined with the filaments of fibrin projecting from the wound surface. The base of the wound remained relatively acellular.

At 2 days most of the wound surface was covered with a single layer of macrophages supported by a fibrin scaffold (Figure 1.6). Two additional cell types were also seen on the wound surface: a cell that looked like a primitive mesenchymal cell, which was also seen in small numbers at the base of the wound, and islets of mesothelial cells that were interconnected by desmosomes and tight junctions. No basement membrane was evident beneath these cells.

Three days after injury the number of primitive mesenchymal cells on the wound surface increased although macrophages were still the most prevalent cell type present. The base of the wound contained scattered

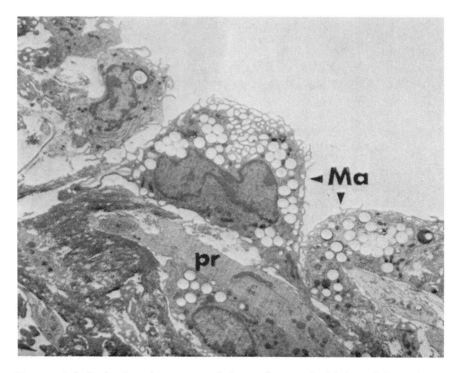

FIGURE 1.6. Parietal peritoneum at 2 days after surgical injury. Macrophages (Ma) containing polystyrene spheres rest on a fibrin base. A process (pr) of a primitive mesenchymal cell extends toward the wound surface (×2,000; From Raftery, 1973a. Reproduced by permission of Butterworth Heinemann.)

mesenchymal cells and some proliferating fibroblasts. The cells on the wound surface at 3 days were similar in appearance to cells in the deeper layers of the wound and were similar to primitive mesenchymal cells.

At 4 days, cells resembling primitive mesenchymal cells or proliferating fibroblasts on the wound surface were in contact with one another. In some areas healing appeared complete at 5 days since a single layer of mesothelial cells was present on the wound surface interconnected by desmosomes and tight junctions. No basement membrane was found beneath the mesothelial cells of parietal peritoneum or cecum at this stage, although one was often present beneath those covering the liver. Thus, peritoneal healing of parietal peritoneum was associated with basement membrane formation at this time in contrast to visceral peritoneum, which, although similar in appearance on the surface, did not contain a basement membrane.

In other areas healing was far less advanced. Primitive mesenchymal cells were present both on the surface and in the base of the wound. At days 5 to 6 the number of macrophages was clearly decreased from the wound surface, whereas most of the wound surface was covered by mesothelial cells (Figure 1.7). At day 7 after surgery the appearance of the wound resembled the appearance on day 6, except that a discontinuous basement membrane was now evident beneath the mesothelial cells lining the parietal peritoneum and covering the cecum. At day 8 a continuous layer of mesothelial cells was present over the wound surface.

A single layer of mesothelial cells resting on a continuous basement membrane was seen at day 10. Fibroblasts in the base of the wound were arranged with their long axis parallel to the wound surface, and bundles of collagen were present between the fibroblasts.

Watters & Buck (1972) studied peritoneal repair after removal of only the surface layer of mesothelium. Special attention was given so as not to damage the underlying connective tissues (Figures 1.8 and 1.9). The denuded areas were examined by scanning electron microscopy through 7 days. Normal parietal mesothelial surface of the rat peritoneal cavity contained a mat of microvilli that obscured the contour of the cells to which they were attached (Figure 1.8). New cells were seen in the surface at 30 minutes after injury (Figure 1.9); at 8 hours most of the surface contained new cells with a variety of morphologies. These authors found a more rapid re-covering of the damaged peritoneal surface than other investigators, perhaps because the depth of the injury was less. These new cells were scattered over the entire surface of the injured site. At 3 days after surgery many of the surface cells contained short microvilli which increased in length by 4 days. A virtually normal appearance via the scanning electron microscope (SEM) was apparent at 7 days.

Visceral versus Parietal Peritoneum

Visceral peritoneum appears to differ little in its healing properties from the parietal peritoneum. Light microscopy (Raftery, 1973a) indicates that

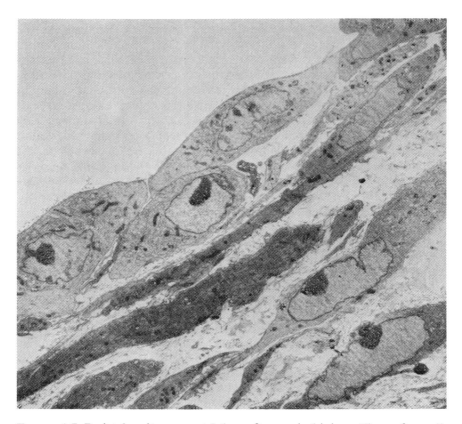

FIGURE 1.7. Parietal peritoneum at 5 days after surgical injury. The surface cells closely resemble the underlying fibroblasts in nuclear and cytoplasmic characteristics (×2,750; From Raftery, 1973a. Reproduced by permission of Butterworth Heinemann.)

the liver acquires a new mesothelial covering 1 day earlier than either cecum or parietal peritoneum. A discontinuous basement membrane is present beneath mesothelial cells covering the liver at 5 days. In contrast, discontinuous basement membrane does not form beneath the mesothelial cells of the parietal peritoneum or cecum until 7 days after surgery. Raftery hypothesized that the liver (viscera) provides a firmer substrate for development of a new mesothelium than either the parietes or the cecum, both of which are subject to greater distention.

By the fifth day after injury, differences between parietal and visceral peritoneal repair are evident. On the surface of wounds in the parietal peritoneum, cells appear to be uniform, containing many microvilli resembling proliferating fibroblasts connected by tight junctions. On the

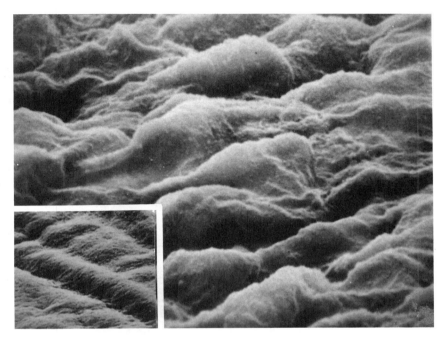

FIGURE 1.8. Surface of wounded area immediately after removal of the mesothelium. An apparently continuous homogeneous material covers numerous fine irregularities. The low magnification shows the irregularities attributed to muscular contraction. (Reprinted with permission of Watters & Buck, "Scanning Electron Microscopy of Mesothelial Regeneration in the Rat," *Lab Invest.* 26:604–609, 1972, © by The US and Canadian Academy of Pathology, Inc., Williams & Wilkins, Baltimore, Maryland.)

surface of the visceral peritoneal wounds, a continuous layer of mesothelial cells forms, joined together by tight junctions or desmosomes. Although a basement membrane is present beneath some of the mesothelial cells covering the liver at this stage, frequent breaks in the basement membrane occur. Basement membrane can be found beneath the mesothelial cells of the new visceral peritoneum, but not beneath the parietal peritoneum.

Seven days after injury, continuous layers of mesothelial cells cover the surface of both the visceral and parietal peritoneum. A basement membrane forms beneath the mesothelial cells in most areas but gaps are still visible. Dense bundles of collagen are present at the basement membrane formed primarily by fibroblasts. By the eighth day, the basement membrane beneath the mesothelial cells of both types of peritoneum is continuous.

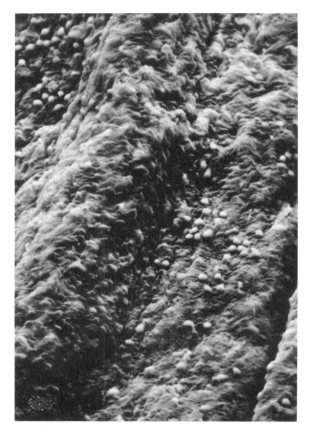

FIGURE 1.9. Wounded area 30 minutes after limited surface injury. Most of the surface is bare. Some cells, mainly rounded in shape, are attached to it (×330.) (Reprinted with permission of Watters & Buck, "Scanning Electron Microscopy of Mesothelial Regeneration in the Rat," *Lab Invest.* 26:604–609, 1972, © by The US and Canadian Academy of Pathology, Inc., Williams & Wilkins, Baltimore, Maryland.)

Neonate

Intestinal obstruction due to adhesion formation was reported to be more prevalent after abdominal surgery in the infant or neonate in comparison to the adult (Devens, 1963; Replogle, Johnson & Gross, 1966). Peritoneal repair occurs more rapidly in the immature rat than in mature animals (Ellis et al., 1965). Accordingly, peritoneal healing in the neonate or pediatric patient manifests a clinically different response to injury in comparison to reperitonealization in the adult.

Raftery (1973b) described the healing of visceral and parietal peritoneum in the immature rat at various times after standardized surgical injury to the liver capsule and parietal peritoneum. Although the wounds looked hemorrhagic and uneven 24 hours after injury, they were smooth and glistening at 3 days, and usually indistinguishable from the normal surrounding parietal peritoneum at 5 days. The cellular changes that accompanied these gross morphological changes were the same as those described for the adult rat except that mesothelial regeneration occurred more rapidly. By 2 days after injury, the acute inflammatory response had subsided leaving primarily macrophages and fibroblasts on the wound surface.

Active fibroblast proliferation occurred at the base of the wound. By 5 days the number of macrophages diminished leaving only fibroblasts. These fibroblasts came together to form the new mesothelium by 7 days, compared with 8 days in the adult. In the case of visceral peritoneum, mesothelial regeneration was complete by 5 days, compared with 7 days in the adult rat. Again, there was no difference in the rate of healing between large and small peritoneal defects.

Source of New Mesothelial Cells

Due to the difficulties of tissue preparation and identification of primitive cell types, as well as availability of vascular, peritoneal fluid and adjacent tissue, the healing of peritoneal defects (i.e., the cytology or histology of peritoneal repair or mesothelial regeneration) remains a controversial subject (Table 1.1). Some investigators suggested that cells detach from the adjacent intact peritoneum and become implanted on the wound surface where they proliferate to a continuous layer of mesothelial cells (mesothelium) (Cameron, Hassan, & De, 1957; Johnson & Whitting, 1962; Bridges & Whitting, 1964). Ellis et al. (1965) assessed the origin of the cells that form the surface of healed peritoneal defects by staining the

---

TABLE 1.1. Five possible methods of mesothelial regeneration.

1. Transformation of underlying undifferentiated mesenchymal cells into a new peritoneal membrane (Robbins, Brunschwig, & Foote, 1949; Brunschwig & Robbins, 1954; Williams, 1955; Ellis, 1962; Bridges & Whitting, 1964; Ellis, Harrison, & Hugh, 1965; Hubbard et al., 1967).
2. Transformation of perivascular cells into a new peritoneal membrane (Johnson & Whitting, 1962; Ellis et al., 1965).
3. Transplantation of cells from peritoneal surfaces of adjacent viscera (Cameron, Hasson & De, 1957; Johnson & Whitting, 1962; Bridges & Whitting, 1964).
4. Transformation of cells from the peritoneal fluid to peritoneal cells (Eskeland, 1966a, 1966b; Eskeland & Kjærheim, 1966).
5. Growth from cells at the periphery of the defect (Cameron et al., 1957; Johnson & Whitting, 1962; Bridges & Whitting, 1964; Ellis et al., 1965; Eskeland, 1966a, 1966b; Hubbard et al., 1967).

cells that remained with trypan blue after excision of parietal peritoneum in rats. On day 3, the entire defect was covered by a sheet of cells. Trypan blue was not detected by microscopy in any of the cells covering the wound. By day 5 the new surface mesothelium achieved continuity with the surrounding edges of the previously undamaged mesothelium. By 7 to 10 days no evidence of mitosis was evident within the wound base or surface nor along the margins of the previous uninjured peritoneum. A similar experiment was performed on another group of rats. A polyethylene sheet was placed over the peritoneal defect after injury and sutured in place. Up to 2 weeks after injury, the surface of the polyethylene was covered by macrophages without appreciable numbers of fibroblastic or mesothelial cells. The cells that did cover the polyethylene were separated by large areas of fibrin. At 3 to 4 weeks after injury the wound surface became covered with mesothelium.

Thus, new peritoneal cells do not arise, to any significant degree, by the centripetal spreading of the mesothelial cells surrounding the wounded area, since they are distributed rather uniformly at an early stage over the wound surface. Cells are scattered over the entire surface as early as 30 minutes after injury. Initially, these cells are morphologically distinct from normal mesothelial cells at the time of their first appearance. After several days they appear to develop the characteristics of mesothelium.

Some investigators consider that metaplasia of fibroblasts within the loose connective tissue beneath the surface of the peritoneum leads to mesothelial regeneration (Robbins, Brunschwig, & Foote, 1949; Williams, 1955; Ellis et al., 1965; Hubbard et al., 1967). Electron microscopic observations identify undifferentiated primitive mesenchymal cells in the perivascular connective tissue, suggesting that these cells may also contribute to the new mesothelial cells. Further experimental evidence for this hypothesis was provided by Ellis et al. (1965), who postulated that peritoneal reformation results from transformation of subperitoneal fibroblasts into an intact mesothelial layer. This supported the work of Robbins et al. (1949) and Williams (1955), who theorized that new peritoneum arose from the transformation of underlying connective tissue cells. Ellis's work was confirmed by Raftery (1973a, 1973b), who further noted that peritoneum appears to arise by metaplasia of subperitoneal fibroblasts. Still others favor the concept that mesothelial regeneration results from differentiation of peritoneal cells; such cells settle on the denuded surface where they spread out and attach to one another.

Evidence also exists that free peritoneal cells provide a source of regenerated mesothelium. Denuded parietal mesothelial surfaces were very quickly (within 4 hours) covered with new cells initially; at 24 hours, flattened cells (with both microvilli and folds) became progressively more plentiful; by 3 days, many cells were extremely flat and were studded with short microvilli that elongated over the next few days (Watters &

Buck, 1972). Cameron et al. (1957) suggested that implantation of free cells from the peritoneal cavity may give rise to new mesothelium. They observed islands of proliferating surface cells on wounds of the liver surface, and concluded that they were mesothelial cells that detached from adjacent areas of peritoneum. This conclusion was supported by Johnson and Whitting (1962).

Summary

New mesothelial cells may have three sources: (1) transformed peritoneal cells, (2) metaplasia of subperitoneal connective tissue cells, or (3) adjacent normal peritoneum (Figure 1.10). Primitive mesenchymal cells identified on the wound surface in the early stages of healing may differentiate into mesothelial cells. Whether these cells are differentiated fibroblast, or undifferentiated multipotential mesenchymal cells is unclear. However, cells that compose the surface of the new peritoneum are probably not macrophages or cells from the peritoneal fluid or adjacent to the surface edge of the injury that have migrated, become adherent to the wound site, and then differentiated into mesothelium. Thus, the origin of new mesothelium remains circumspect because of difficulty in distinguishing between primitive mesenchymal cells and proliferating

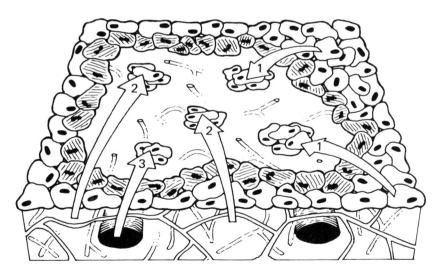

FIGURE 1.10. Possible origins of new mesothelium include (1) primitive mesenchymal cells present at the periphery of the defect; (2) indirectly from primitive mesenchymal cells via differentiation into fibroblast; (3) subperitoneal fibroblasts, which in turn arise from differentiated, but resting, fibroblasts in the perivascular connective tissue.

fibroblasts in the later stages of healing. It is possible that the former give rise to the latter, but definitive evidence for this is lacking.

Injury by Desiccation or Wetting with Isotonic Saline

Prolonged drying of the peritoneum was shown by Ryan, Grobety, and Majno (1973) to also induce significant injury. Immediately after drying, intact mesothelial cells are absent on rat cecum (Figure 1.11; Ryan et al., 1973). Four hours later, no mesothelial cells are present; most of the cecal surface is covered by an irregular thin coating of fibrin without cells. The underlying muscle coat contains gross edema, cellular disintegration and partial occlusion of blood vessels by platelet masses, but no inflammatory cells. At 24 hours after drying, there are many more mononuclear cells in the basal lamina and no fibrin is present on the surface. The underlying tissue, which still shows signs of cell damage and edema, contains some eosinophils and neutrophils, but no macrophages. Continuous wetting of cecal peritoneum with isotonic saline can also produce peritoneal injury resulting in loss of the mesothelium from the surface in large sheets exposing underlying connective tissue. Thus both prolonged drying or wetting with isotonic saline leads to peritoneal injury. Whether a buffered physiological saline would induce injury to the serosa is unknown.

Surgical Injuries

Elkins, Stovall, Warren, Ling, and Meyer (1987) compared the response of rabbit peritoneum to a variety of injuries: excision, abrasion, electrocautery, and linear incision with (2-0 polyglycolic acid) and without suture closure. Through the first 12 hours after injury, all four peritoneal injury sites contained polymorphonuclear leukocytes, surface fibrin deposit, white cell exudate, and both muscle and mesothelial tissue necrosis. Surface fibrin disappeared by 24 hours postsurgery and the other reactions slowly diminished. In contrast, the electrocautery/burn injuries persisted throughout the three week study period.

The area of peritoneal excision without suture closure contained tissue necrosis by 24 hours, and at 48 hours was the first injury site to contain fibroblasts and consistent mesothelial re-epithelialization. Secondary cellular infiltrates of macrophages and plasma cells were noted by 48 hours, and collagen formation was present at 5 days. Gross healing was present at 5 days. By 7 days, tissue necrosis was resolved, and at 21 days postsurgery this injury site was the only one with abundant fibroblasts and subepithelial collagen. Healing appeared to occur by proliferation and metaplasia of mesothelial cells. The peritoneal excision site showed less inflammatory reaction and more prompt re-epithelialization than the other peritoneal injury sites.

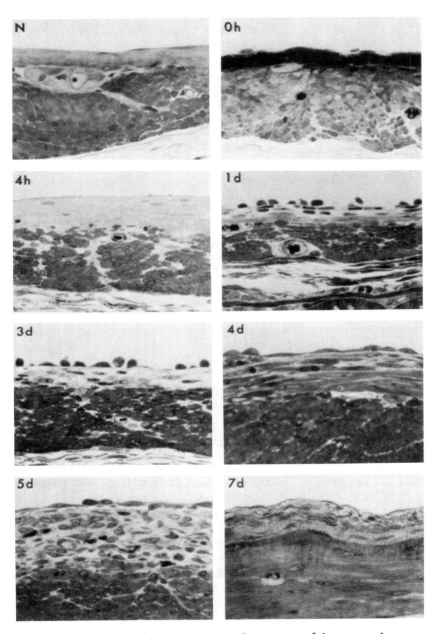

FIGURE 1.11. Histology of cecum shows various stages of damage and recovery after drying injury of surface: normal cecum (**N**); immediately after drying (0h); 4 hours (4h); 1 day (1d); 3 days (3d); 4 days (4d); 5 days (5d); and 7 days (7d) (×400; Ryan et al., 1973). Reproduced with the permission of J.B. Lippincott Company, Philadelphia, PA.

Where sutures were used to close the peritoneal incision, early inflammatory changes were similar to those observed after other peritoneal injuries. At 24 hours after surgery, there were some early signs of reestablished mesothelial integrity, although this was not a consistent finding until 48 hours after surgery. Collagen formation became apparent at 5 days postsurgery. The major difference between this site and the peritoneal excision site without repair was the presence of an intense foreign body reaction surrounding the sutures. This ongoing tissue reaction persisted at 5 days, as evidenced by a foreign body granuloma, and at 3 weeks postoperatively, as seen by the presence of fat necrosis. Gross healing was present at 2 to 3 weeks.

Elkins et al. (1987) and Bellina, Hemmings, Voros, and Ross (1984) both noted at the sites of peritoneal cautery and suture repair deep submesothelial hemorrhage and necrosis, which prolonged the duration of inflammation and associated delay in collagen deposition. The sites of cauterization contained tissue necrosis and inflammation three weeks after surgery. Cauterization of peritoneal injury induced more tissue damage than other types of wounding. Early collagen deposition was noted at 5 days after surgery. However, at 3 weeks these lesions contained PMNs, tissue necrosis, and granulation tissue, with no fibroblasts and minimal collagen formation. Thus, healing at the cauterized site was not completed by 3 weeks postoperatively. Elkins et al. found that mesothelial regeneration did not occur after peritoneal damage to a 2×2 cm area with electrocautery.

Filmar, Jeta, McComb, and Gomel (1989) compared the histology of uterine horn repair in rats after incision with the carbon dioxide laser or microcautery. Incisions were reapproximated with 10-0 nylon sutures. Although the general appearance of the scars and the amount of collagen that accumulated over a 21-day observation period were similar, foreign body reaction as measured by histiocyte and giant cell infiltration was significantly greater in the electrocautery group. Carbon particles that formed in response to cautery may lead to formation of foreign body granulomas. Cutting with the carbon dioxide laser caused significantly more necrosis and foreign body reaction than cutting with microscissors. Sharp mechanical transection was followed by the least amount of tissue reaction and necrosis, and an absence of particulate carbon. Montgomery, Sharp, Bellina, and Ross (1983) compared the healing patterns of canine uterine peritoneum and myometrium after injury by CO_2 laser, scalpel or electric knife standardized to a 3 cm incision. Their observations confirmed those of other investigators in that necrosis was less with the scalpel than with either CO_2 laser or electric knife.

Conclusion

The special complexity of peritoneal morphology including surface covering by mesothelial cells, a vascularized connective tissue underpining laced by extracellular matrix proteins, leads to a unique response to injury

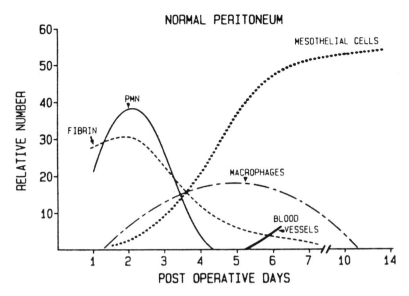

FIGURE 1.12. Change in the relative number of cellular elements and fibrinolysis (fibrin) at the site of peritoneal injury in mature rats during the course of re-epithelialization. (Summarized from Johnson & Whitting, 1962; Bridges & Whitting, 1964; Ellis et al., 1965; Eskeland & Kjærheim, 1966; Raftery 1973a, 1973b; diZerega, 1990).

(Figure 1.12; diZerega, 1990). Large peritoneal injuries re-epithelialize as quickly as small peritoneal injuries. Virtually all types of surgical injury including cutting, coagulation, drying, and abrasion induce an inflammatory reaction that may lead to adhesion formation. Clean excision of peritoneal tissue without suture placement to reapproximate edges provides the best opportunity for rapid reperitonealization. Peritoneal repair is not accelerated with reapproximation of incised peritoneal edges. Reapproximation of peritoneal edges increases tissue necrosis and foreign body reactions that may slow the healing process. The prolonged presence of an acute inflammatory reaction in areas of extensive thermal injury disrupt healing.

References

Allen L. (1936). The peritoneal stomata. *Anat Rec.* 67:89–99.

Baradi AF, Campbel WG. (1974). Exudative peritonitis induced in mice by bovine serum albumin. *Arch Pathol.* 97:2–12.

Baron MA. (1941). Structure of the intestinal peritoneum in man. *Am J Anat.* 69:439–497.

Bellina JH, Hemmings R, Voros JI, Ross LF. (1984). Carbon dioxide laser and electrosurgical wound study with an animal model: a comparison of tissue damage and healing patterns in peritoneal tissue. *Am J Obstet Gynecol.* 148:327–334.

Berndt WO, Gosselin RE. (1961). Rubidium and creatinine transport across isolated mesentery. *Biochem Pharmacol.* 8:359–366.

Bloom W, Fawcett DW. (1978). *A Textbook of Histology.* 9th ed. Philadelphia: WB Saunders; 186–187.

Bridges JB, Whitting HW. (1964). Parietal peritoneal healing in the rat. *J Pathol Bact.* 87:123–130.

Brunschwig A, Robbins GF. (1954). Regeneration of peritoneum: experimental observations and clinical experience in radical resections of intra-abdominal cancer. In: *XV Congr Soc Internat Chir, Lisbonne 1953.* Bruxelles: Henri de Smedt; 756–765.

Cameron GR, Hassan SM, De SN. (1957). Repair of Glisson's capsule after tangential wound of the liver. *J Pathol Bact.* 73:1–10.

Cotran RS, Karnovsky JJ. (1968). Ultrastructural studies on the permeability of the mesothelium to horseradish peroxidase. *J Cell Biol.* 37:123–137.

Devens K. (1963). Recurrent intestinal obstruction in the neonatal period. *Arch Dis Child.* 38:118–119.

diZerega GS. (1990). The peritoneum and its response to surgical injury. In: diZerega GS, Malinak LR, Diamond MP, Linsky CB, eds. *Treatment of Post Surgical Adhesions.* New York: Wiley-Liss: 358:1–11.

Elkins TE, Stovall TG, Warren J, Ling FW, Meyer NL. (1987). A histologic evaluation of peritoneal injury and repair: implications for adhesion formation. *Obstet Gynecol.* 70:225–228.

Ellis H. (1962). The aetiology of post-operative abdominal adhesions. An experimental study. *Br J Surg* 50:10–16.

Ellis H, Harrison W, Hugh TB. (1965). The healing of peritoneum under normal and pathological conditions. *Br J Surg.* 52:471–476.

Eskeland G, Kjærheim Å. (1966a). Regeneration of parietal peritoneum in rats. I. A light microscopical study. *Acta Pathol Microbiol Scand.* 68:353–378.

Eskeland G. (1966b). Growth of autologous peritoneal cells in intraperitoneal diffusion chambers in rats. I. A light microscopical study. *Acta Pathol Microbiol Scand.* 68:481–500.

Filmar S, Jeta N, McComb P, Gomel V. (1989). A comparative histologic study on the healing process following tissue transection: Part I. CO_2 laser and electromicrosurgery. *Am J Obstet Gynecol.* 160:1068–1072.

French JE, Florey HW, Morris B. (1960). The absorption of particles by the lymphatics of the diaphragm. *J Exp Physiol.* 45:88–93.

Fukata H. (1963). Electron microscopic study on normal rat peritoneal mesothelium and its changes in absorption of particulate iron dextran complex. *Acta Pathol Jpn.* 13:309–325.

Gardner E, Gray DJ, O'Rahilly R. (1969). *Anatomy: A Regional Study of Human Structure.* 3rd ed. Philadelphia: WB Saunders; 387–395.

Glucksman D. (1966). Serosal integrity and intestinal adhesions. *Surgery.* 60:1009–1011.

Gosselin RE, Berndt WO. (1962). Diffusional transport of solute through mesentery and peritoneum. *J Theor Biol.* 3:487–495.

Hertzler AE. (1919). *The peritoneum.* St. Louis: CV Mosby.

Hollinshead WH. (1971). The thorax, abdomen, and pelvis. In: *Anatomy for Surgeons.* New York: Harper & Row; 2:78–161,305,307,632.

Hubbard TB, Khan MZ, Carag VR, Albites VE, Hricko GM. (1967). The pathology of peritoneal repair: its relation to the formation of adhesions. *Ann Surg.* 165:908–916.

Johnson FR, Whitting HW. (1962). Repair of parietal peritoneum. *Br J Surg.* 49:653–660.

Leak LV, Rahil K. (1978). Permeability of the diaphragmatic mesothelium: the ultrastructural bases for "stomata." *Am J Anat.* 151:557–569.

Leak LV. (1979). The adhesion of peritoneal cells to the diaphragmatic mesothelium. *Bibl Anat* 17:115–124.

Lill SR, Parsons RH, Buchac I. (1979). Permeability of the diaphragm and fluid resorption from the peritoneal cavity in the rat. *Gastroenterology.* 76:997–1002.

MacCallum WG. (1903). On the mechanism of absorption of granular material from the peritoneum. *Johns Hopkins Hosp Bull.* 14:105–112.

Mitchell GAG. (1941). The spread of acute intraperitoneal effusions. *Br J Surg.* 28:291–296.

Montgomery TC, Sharp JB, Bellina H, Ross LF. (1983). Comparative gross and histological study of the effects of scalpel, electric knife and carbon dioxide laser on skin and uterine incisions in dogs. *Lasers Surg Med.* 3:9–22.

Pfeiffer CJ, Pfeiffer DC, Misra HP. (1987). Enteric serosal surface in the piglet. A scanning and transmission electron microscopic study of the mesothelium. *J Submicrosc Cytol.* 19:237–246.

Raftery AT. (1973a). Regeneration of parietal and visceral peritoneum: an electron microscopical study. *J Anat.* 115:375–392.

Raftery AT. (1973b). Regeneration of parietal and visceral peritoneum. A light microscopical study. *Br J Surg.* 60:293–299.

Replogle RL, Johnson R, Gross RE. (1966). Prevention of postoperative intestinal adhesions with combined promethazine and dexamethazone therapy: experimental and clinical studies. *Ann Surg.* 163:580–588.

Robbins GF, Brunschwig A, Foote FW. (1949). Deperitonealization: clinical and experimental observations. *Ann Surg.* 130:466–479.

Robbins SL. (1967). *A Textbook of Histology.* 3rd ed. Philadelphia: WB Saunders; 891–896.

Ryan GB, Grobety J, Majno G. (1973). Mesothelial injury and recovery. *Am J Pathol.* 71:93–112.

Shear J, Harvey JD, Barry KG. (1966). Peritoneal sodium transport: enhancement by pharmacologic and physical agents. *J Lab Clin Med.* 67:181–188.

Tsilibury EC, Wissig SL. (1977). Absorption from the peritoneal cavity: SEM study of the mesothelium covering the peritoneal surface of the muscular portion of the diaphragm. *Am J Anat.* 149:127–133.

Wakefield EG, Mayo CW. (1936). Intestinal obstruction produced by mesenteric bands in association with failure of intestinal rotation. *Arch Surg.* 33:47–67.

Watters WB, Buck RC. (1972). Scanning electron microscopy of mesothelial regeneration in the rat. *Lab Invest.* 26:604–609.

Williams DC. (1955). The peritoneum. A plea for a change in attitude towards this membrane. *Br J Surg.* 42:401–405.

2

Peritoneal Fluid

THE PERITONEAL CAVITY OF THE HUMAN USUALLY CONTAINS 5 TO 20 ml of serous exudate which varies widely depending on the physiological condition. In the female, this volume changes during the menstrual cycle to reach maximal levels after ovulation (Figure 2.1; Alfonsin & Leiderman, 1980). When pressure in the hepatic sinusoids rises more than 5 to 10 mm Hg, fluid containing large amounts of protein transudes through

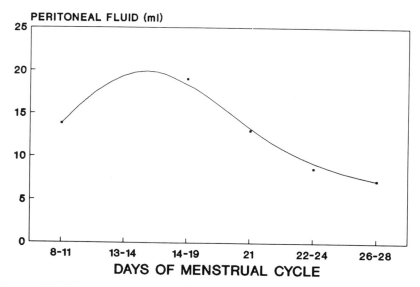

FIGURE 2.1. The volume of fluid harvested from the peritoneal cavity of patients undergoing laparoscopy at various days of the menstrual cycle is shown. The volume of peritoneal fluid peaks around the time of ovulation and declines to approximately 7 ml at the end of the menstrual cycle. These data are the mean volume harvested from three to six patients per time point (Alfonsin & Leiderman, 1980).

the liver surface into the abdominal cavity. Excess fluid in the peritoneal cavity is either a transudate (specific gravity <1.010), which accumulates (ascites) from peritoneal obstruction or circulatory differences (failure, portal cardiac hypertension, hypofibrinogenemia, etc.), or an exudate (specific gravity >1.020), which arises from inflammation. The hepatic resistance to portal blood flow induces a capillary pressure in the visceral peritoneum that is higher than elsewhere in the body (Guyton, 1973). The pH of peritoneal fluid ranges between 7.5 and 8.0 and contains significant buffering capacity (Greenwalt, Nakamura, & diZerega, 1988). The pH of peritoneal fluid in aspirates from 59 patients with perforated peptic ulcer was 7.0 to 7.8 (Howard & Singh, 1963). Due to the hydrostatic pressure gradient between plasma and the peritoneal compartment, normal peritoneal fluid also contains many of the plasma proteins in about 50% of the plasma concentration (Aune, 1970a, 1970b, 1970c, 1970d).

Plasma that accumulates in the peritoneal cavity provides a source of fibrinogen. The resultant fibrin may play an important role in the aggregation of peritoneal cells on the diaphragmatic surface and over the visceral or parietal surfaces (Zinsser & Pryde, 1952). The amounts of peritoneal fluid and plasma greatly increase in the peritoneal cavity during postsurgical repair or following an inflammatory insult (Felix & Dalton, 1955).

Volume

The volume of fluid in the peritoneal cavity may influence the sequelae of pathologic conditions. Dunn, Barke, Ahrenholz, Humphrey, & Simmons (1984) reported that increasing the volume of an *Escherichia coli* inoculum from 1 to 30 ml in the rat peritoneal cavity converted a nonlethal into a lethal injection (Figure 2.2). Increasing the intraperitoneal volume with saline significantly facilitated the proliferation of *E. coli*. Further, clearance of *E. coli* from the peritoneal cavity was retarded when the organisms were injected in 30 ml compared to 1 ml. In vitro studies of opsonization and phagocytosis demonstrated that either diluting the opsonin source or decreasing the ratio of phagocytes to bacteria results in diminished phagocytosis (Cohn & Morse, 1959; Hirsch & Church, 1960; Jenkins & Benacerref, 1960; Roberts, 1967). In larger volumes, fewer phagocyte-microbe interactions may occur.

Cells of the Serous Exudate

Peritoneal fluid contains a variety of free floating cells, including (1) macrophages; (2) desquamated mesothelial cells; (3) small lymphocytes; (4) eosinophils; (5) mast cells; and (6) in inflammatory exudates, large

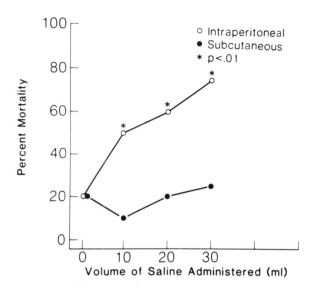

FIGURE 2.2. The effect of peritoneal fluid on growth of *E. coli* in the peritoneal cavity. Each point represents the mean ± SD from six experiments in which two animals per group were studied. Bacterial growth was significantly greater at 1 through 6 hours in animals receiving the bacterial inoculum in 30 ml saline IP ($p < .01$). (From Dunn et al., 1984. Reproduced by permission of J.B. Lippincott.)

numbers of polymorphonuclear cells. Free macrophages originate in the milky spots of the omentum and migrate into the abdominal cavity. They are similar to the mononuclear cells in the inflammatory exudate derived from local macrophages. Desquamated mesothelial cells keep their squamous form or become spherical-like in tissue culture. In situ, these mesothelial cells become fibroblasts in the presence of inflammation. The vast majority of small lymphocytes in peritoneal fluid migrate from the omental vasculature. In inflammatory exudates there are large numbers of polymorphonuclear cells derived from the peripheral circulation. In some animals (guinea pig) eosinophilic leukocytes of hematogenous origin are found in normal peritoneal fluid. Relatively large numbers of free floating mast cells occur in the rat and mouse peritoneal fluid. Normal peritoneal fluid of the rat consists of 51% lymphocytes, 40% macrophages and 9% other cells such as mast cells and plasma cells (Eskeland, 1969). Essentially no mesothelial cells were found in a differential count of 27,000 cells from rat peritoneal fluid (Shelton & Rice, 1959).

Studies analyzing endometrial cells in peritoneal fluid report incidences varying from 0% to 59% (Koninckx, Ide, Vandenbroncke, & Brosens, 1980; Badawy et al., 1984; Willemsen et al., 1985; Bartosik, Jacobs, & Kelly, 1986; Mungyer et al., 1987; Kulenthran & Jeyalakshmi, 1989). All reports in which endometrial tissue was identified in peritoneal fluid used cytological and/or cell block analyses (Table 2.1; Koninckx et al., 1980; Badawy et al., 1984; Bartosik et al., 1986). Whereas Koninckx et al. (1980), Bartosik et al. (1986), and Kruitwagen et al. (1991) observed endometrial tissue in peritoneal fluid as frequently in women with endometriosis as in those without, Badawy et al. (1984) identified endometrial tissue more frequently in women with endometriosis. Kruitwagen et al. (1991) identified endometrial epithelial cells in 79% of peritoneal aspirates obtained during the early follicular phase based upon colony formation by these cells in vitro and utilization of a monoclonal antibody. These data indicate that retrograde transport of viable endometrial cells during menstruation occurs in women with patent tubes. No correlation between viable endometrial cells and endometriosis was reported.

Several studies examined the level of macrophage activation associated with endometriosis and infertility. In 1983, Halme, Becker, Hammond, Raj, and Raj showed that macrophages harvested from the peritoneal cavity of infertile women with endometriosis were more active than macrophages from fertile women. A higher proportion of macrophages from

TABLE 2.1. Incidence of endometrial cells in peritoneal fluid.

Authors (year)	Analyzing method used	Cycle phase	Endometriosis	Incidence of endometrial cells in PF[a]
Blumenkrantz et al. (1981)	Not specified	Menstruation	Not specified	0 (3)
Koninckx et al. (1980)	Cytology	Proliferative	Present	75 (4)
			Absent	54 (13)
		Luteal (days 14 to 20)	Present	53 (17)
			Absent	53 (17)
		Luteal (days 21 to 25)	Present	25 (16)
			Absent	31 (16)
Badawy et al. (1984)	Cytology	Not specified	Present	31 (45)
			Absent	10 (57)[b]
Willemsen et al. (1985)	Culture	Late proliferative	Not specified	0 (115)
Bartosik et al. (1986)	Cytology cell block	Not specified	Present	19 (32)
			Absent	11 (9)
Kulenthran et al. (1989)	Cytology	Days 8 to 20	Not specified	0 (21)
Kruitwagen et al. (1991)	Culture	Days 1 to 7	Present	69 (12)
			Absent	92 (12)

From Kruitwagen et al., 1991.
PF, peritoneal fluid.
[a]Values are percents with no. of samples in parentheses.
[b]Including women with occluded tubes.

women with endometriosis (46% versus 15%) exhibited positive staining for acid phosphatase (Figure 2.3, Halme et al., 1983). In addition, the samples from patients with endometriosis tended to have macrophages larger in size (another measure of macrophage differentiation). Peritoneal fluid from fertile and infertile patients with endometriosis was also characterized. In peritoneal fluid from patients with endometriosis, there were higher levels of acid phosphatase and neutral protease, but no change in the level of prostaglandins E_2 and $F_{2\alpha}$ (Halme et al., 1983) suggesting that the macrophages secrete active products into the peritoneal fluid. These authors suggested that the increased activity of the macrophages was secondary to the endometrial implants and could contribute to infertility. Further studies by this group identified an increased number of large, mature macrophages in the peritoneal cavity of women with endometriosis, with increased ability to phagocytose opsonized zymosan (Halme, Hammond, Hulka, Raj, & Talbert, 1984a; Halme, Becker, & Haskill, 1987). These observations were confirmed and extended by Dunselman, Hendrix, Bouckaert, and Evers (1988). In this study, peritoneal fluid macrophages from patients with endometriosis showed significantly increased erythrophagocytosis and lowered chemoluminescence than macrophages from controls. These data also suggest that macrophages from patients with endometriosis are more differentiated than controls.

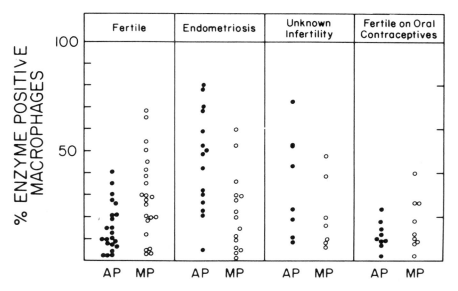

FIGURE 2.3. The percentage of positive macrophages for acid phosphatase (AP) and myeloperoxidase (MP) in pelvic fluid cell pellets. The solid circles = AP and the open circles = MP. (From Halme et al., 1983. Reproduced by permission of C.V. Mosby.)

Further studies were conducted to determine if these activated macrophages could support the proliferation of endometrial tissue and thereby contribute to the disease. As is discussed further in Chapters 3 and 4, macrophages can induce the proliferation of cells, such as fibroblasts and endothelial cells, involved in inflammation, tissue repair, and neovascularization through the secretion of factors such as interleukin-1, tumor necrosis factor (TNF), and macrophage-derived growth factor (MDGF). Studies show increased levels of these factors associated with endometriosis. Fakih et al. (1987) reported the presence of interleukin-1 in the peritoneal fluid of patients with endometriosis but not controls. In a study of 55 patients, macrophages from 23 women released significant amounts of MDGF activity in vitro (Halme, White, Kauma, Estes, & Haskill, 1988). Macrophages from 10 of 36 women (28%) with normal pelvic anatomy or tubal occlusion/pelvic adhesions released significant MDGF activity. Alternatively, macrophages from 13 of 19 (68%) women with endometriosis secreted MDGF. In a study of the release of TNF in vitro in response to the exotoxin associated with toxic shock syndrome toxin 1 (TSST-1) or to lipopolysaccharides (LPS), enhanced release of TNF by peritoneal macrophages from women with endometriosis com-

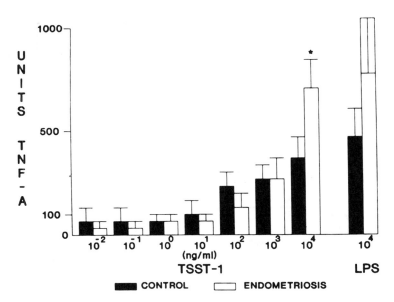

FIGURE 2.4. Tumor necrosis factor-α release by peritoneal macrophages in vitro in response to increasing concentrations of TSST-1 in 12 subjects with endometriosis and 10 without endometriosis. Bars represent mean values ± SEM of each group. TNF-A, tumor necrosis factor-α; TSST-1, toxic shock syndrome toxin 1; LPS, lipopolysaccharide. (From Buyalos et al., 1991. Reproduced by permission of Elsevier Science.)

pared with those without endometriosis was observed (Figure 2.4; Halme, 1989; Buyalos, Rutanen, Tsui, & Halme, 1991). These studies implicate macrophages in the peritoneal cavity with a possible contribution to the infertility associated with endometriosis (perhaps through phagocytosis of sperm or damage to the ova after ovulation) and to the progression of endometriosis through the release of growth factors to support the growth of endometrial tissue.

Peritoneal Surface Area

Peritoneum is the most extensive serous membrane in the body. It is generally accepted that the peritoneal surface area is approximately the same as the surface area of the skin (Esperanca & Collins, 1966). Traditionally, the surface area of the adult peritoneum is considered to be approximately 22,000 cm^2 (Odel, Ferris, & Power, 1948). This datum was derived from the personal communication from the Russian investigator of a study that made peritoneal measurements using premeasured paper to cover the peritoneal surfaces (as reported by Esperanca & Collins, 1966). His calculations were 1,500 cm^2 for a 2,900-gm neonate and 20,780 cm^2 for a 70-kg adult. Accordingly, the neonate has twice the peritoneal area of the adult based on body weight (522 versus 284 cm^2/kg). Similar results (17,000 cm^2) were reported by Wegner (1877) using similar techniques. Subsequently, Esperanca and Collins (1966) utilized tracings made on oiled paper of unfixed peritoneum from six adult and six infant postmortem specimens (Table 2.2). Their reported areas ranged from 8,800 to 12,000 cm^2 for adults with an average of 177 cm^2/kg body weight. Peritoneal surface area of infants ranged between 475 and 1,400 cm^2 with an average of 383 cm^2/kg body weight.

TABLE 2.2. Peritoneal surface area (cm^2).

	Adult	Infant
Intestine	4,815	665
Liver	624	139
Anterior abdominal wall	411	79
Diaphragm	424	35
Stomach	631	32
Omentum	1,581	29
Mesentery	1,469	32
Spleen	149	25
Pelvic organs	275	29
Total peritoneal area	10,379	1,065
Weight (kg)	59.3	2.743
Peritoneal area (cm^2)/body weight (kg)	177	383

From Esperanca & Collins, 1966.

More recently, Cromack, Cromack, Pretorius, and DeMeules (1985) determined the minimum volume sufficient to coat the peritoneal surface of rats and then extrapolated using the following equation for generalized coating volumes: peritoneal coating volume minimum = body surface area $(cm^2) \times 9.27 \times 10^{-3}$ ml/cm². For a 2.5-kg rabbit this equals 16 ml; for a 75-kg human this equals 178 ml.

The intraperitoneal circulation follows the pattern shown in Figure 2.5 (Levison & Pontzer, 1979). This was determined by the movement of water-soluble contrast material selectively injected into various intraperitoneal spaces (Mitchell, 1941; Levison & Pontzer, 1979). In general, the distance a material spreads depends upon its volume, viscosity, and specific gravity. The mobility of the small bowel tends to limit the accumulation of fluid in the central portion of the peritoneal cavity under normal circumstances (Ahrenholz & Simmons, 1988). The most depen-

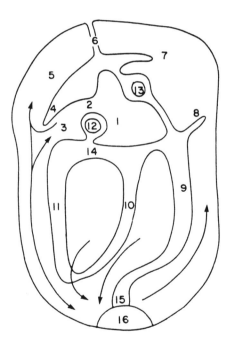

FIGURE 2.5. Circulation of fluid in the peritoneal cavity. Solid arrows indicate the flow generated by diaphragmatic movement and absorption of material from the diaphragmatic lymphatics. 1. Lesser sac. 2. Foramen of Winslow. 3. Morison's pouch. 4. Right triangular ligament. 5. Right subphrenic space. 6. Falciform ligament. 7. Left subphrenic space. 8. Phrenocolic ligament. 9. Bare area of the descending colon. 10. Root of the small bowel mesentery. 11. Bare area of ascending colon. 12. Duodenum. 13. Esophagus. 14. Root of the transverse mesocolon. 15. Bare area of rectum. 16. Bladder. (From Levison & Pontzer, 1979. Reproduced by permission of John Wiley and Churchill Livingstone, Inc.)

dent recess is the pelvis where the pouch of Douglas lies between the rectum and the body of the uterus. The perirectal and perivesical fossae lie lateral to the rectum and bladder. The peritoneal circulation favors unilateral spread of exudate because the phrenocolic ligament, which spans the diaphragm, spleen, and splenic flexure of the colon, interrupts the flow into the left subphrenic space during respiration (Ahrenholz & Simmons, 1988). As a result, left subphrenic abscesses are commonly associated with retrogastric (lesser sac) lesions. Bilateral subphrenic abscesses are uncommon, since the right and left subhepatic spaces are separated by the falciform ligament. The left subhepatic space is divided by the gastrohepatic omentum into an anterior space and a lesser sac (Ahrenholz & Simmons, 1988). However, truly massive abscesses may extend down one gutter to the pelvis and up the opposite side (Altemeier, Culbertson, & Fidler, 1975).

Peritoneal Fluid Transport

Clinical Studies

Fluid is both filtered into and absorbed from the peritoneal space through the peritoneum. Numerous large lymphatic channels lead from the peritoneal surface of the diaphragm (Figure 2.6). With each diaphragmatic excursion significant quantities of lymph flow out of the peritoneal cavity into the thoracic duct. Absorption of colloid and larger particles from the pleural and peritoneal spaces occurs almost exclusively by way of the parietal lymphatics (Figure 2.7). The absorption rate is dependent upon the material absorbed. Smaller substances, such as ions, are equilibrated almost immediately between capillary blood and the lumen of mesothelium-lined spaces. The diaphragm contains a specialized anatomical system that transports 60% to 80% of the peritoneal fluid taken up by lymphatics (Yoffey and Courtice, 1970). Particles and cells (up to 1 μm diameter) are removed through stomata that communicate with lymphatic lacunae under the mesothelium (Casley-Smith, 1964).

Absorption of water and electrolytes from the peritoneal cavity actively occurs in human beings (Pappenheimer, 1953; Courtice & Simmonds, 1954; Crone, 1963). Dehydrated children absorb up to 500 ml of physiologic saline in less than 24 hours (Courtice & Simmonds, 1954; Crone, 1963). Since this volume is large in relation to total body water in infants, intraperitoneal infusions can be used for hydration. Isotonic saline solutions are absorbed while solute concentrations become equilibrated between blood and peritoneal fluid (Shear, Swartz, Shinaberger, & Barry, 1965). The rate of absorption during equilibration is primarily dependent upon crystalloid osmotic pressure gradients across the peritoneal membrane and is most rapid when serum osmolality exceeds osmolality in

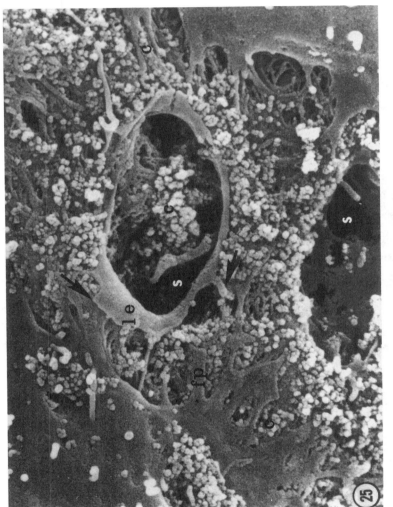

FIGURE 2.6. A scanning electron micrograph from the lacunar roof showing stomata (s). The lymphatic endothelium (le) extends onto the diaphragmatic surface and makes contact with the cell margins and processes of the mesothelial cell (arrows). Numerous carbon particles (c) are localized within gaps between filamentous cell processes (fp) and within the stomata (×14,500). (From Leak & Rahil, 1978. Reproduced by permission of Wiley-Liss.)

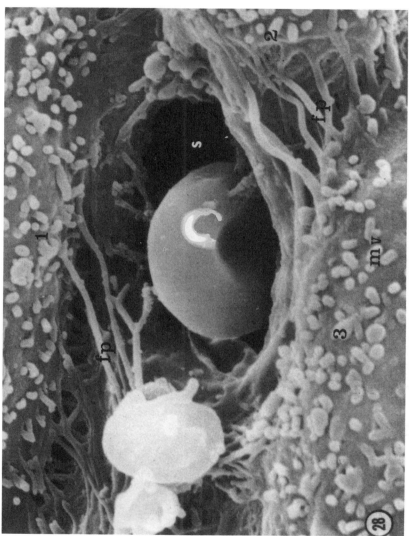

FIGURE 2.7. A stoma (s) is located at the junction of several cells (numbered 1 to 3). A red blood cell was caught in the process of entering the stoma. Numerous filamentous processes (fp) and microvilli (mv) are also shown (×13,600). (From Leak & Rahil, 1978. Reproduced by permission of Wiley-Liss.)

the peritoneal fluid. Hypotonic saline solutions are absorbed more rapidly than isotonic saline solutions because the osmotic pressure gradient across the peritoneum is greater. By contrast, when hypertonic saline solutions are instilled into the peritoneal cavity, intraperitoneal fluid volume increases as water moves out of the vascular space.

Shear et al. (1965) measured the rate of fluid and electrolyte absorption from the peritoneal cavity in adults. Equilibrium of an albumin dialysate occurred within 2 hours after peritoneal infusion at a rate of 0.5 ml per minute. Despite wide variations in body weight, the peritoneal absorption rate varies little (Figure 2.8). Rate of absorption after osmotic equilibration in the four study subjects was 30 to 37 ml per hour. In patients with cirrhosis and ascites, however, effective serum oncotic pressure and hydrostatic portal pressure are major determinants of rate and direction of fluid movement (Atkinson, 1959; Atkinson & Losowsky, 1961, 1962; Carter, 1953; Blackfan & Maxcy, 1918; Losowsky, Jones, Lieber, & Davidson, 1963).

Animal Studies

Quantitative data are available regarding the rate of absorption of water and electrolytes from the peritoneal cavity utilizing small volumes of fluid in laboratory animals. The data show that 25 ml of 0.9% saline or an isotonic solution containing sodium chloride, sodium bicarbonate and

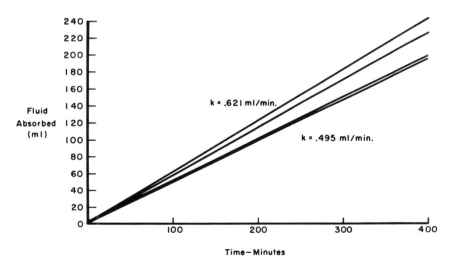

FIGURE 2.8. Rate of absorption of fluid after osmotic equilibration (absorption phase) in four patients. Fluid absorbed after 2 hours was set at zero, and lines for each patient were drawn from calculated slopes. (From Shear et al., 1965. Reproduced by permission of New England Journal of Medicine.)

potassium chloride was completely absorbed within 22 hours of intraperitoneal injection in guinea pigs weighing 490 to 620 gm (Schechter, Cary, Carpentieri, & Darrow, 1933). Mice weighing between 25 and 30 gm absorbed 30% to 50% of the administered volume when 5 ml of an isotonic, balanced electrolyte mixture was infused into the peritoneal cavity (Kruger, Greve, & Schueler, 1962). In a similar study, 100 ml of 0.95% saline solution was placed intraperitoneally in rabbits; 11 to 30 ml was absorbed in 1 hour. Thereafter, the rate of absorption markedly decreased (Atkinson & Losowsky, 1961).

Zinsser and Pryde (1952) evaluated the rate and distribution of fluid administered into the peritoneal cavity of dogs. A variety of radiopaque materials was followed after intraperitoneal injection by roentgenography with and without peritonitis. Although the rate of intraperitoneal distribution was relatively slower with more viscous solutions, all preparations were distributed within a few hours. Large quantities of fluid exudates enhanced the rate of intraperitoneal distribution. However, when paralytic ileus was induced, radiopaque material did not spread beyond the midline before 6 hours or above the midabdomen before 12 hours. Thus, bowel motility is required for normal intraperitoneal circulation.

The presence of fibrinogen and or "fibrin gel" in the peritoneal cavity also impedes fluid distribution. Conversely, fluid distribution and even bacterial proliferation may be enhanced in the presence of sufficient heparin to reduce coagulation. Thus, the presence of prior inflammation, low viscosity or anticoagulation enhances the rate of intraperitoneal circulation, which ileus and especially fibrin appear to impede.

Red blood cells are rapidly removed from the peritoneal cavity (Mengert, Cobb, & Brown, 1951). Intraperitoneal blood transfusion results in 70% of the Cr^{51}-labeled erythrocytes in the peripheral circulation 48 to 96 hours after intraperitoneal injection in animal studies. These parameters are not different from those that occur after intravenous injection of Cr^{51}-labeled erythrocytes.

Blood in Peritoneal Fluid

Polishuk and Sharf (1965), performing culdoscopy during the menstrual period, found blood-stained peritoneal fluid (PF) in 50% of the patients. Blumenkrantz, Gallagher, Bashore, & Tenckhoff (1981) observed the occurrence of blood contaminated dialysate in 9 out of 11 patients undergoing peritoneal dialysis during their menstrual period. Recently, a systematic study by Halme et al. (1984b) indicated that retrograde menstruation is a common and physiological event in menstruating women with patent tubes.

Transperitoneal Exchange

Attempts were made to determine peritoneal permeability by the appearance rate of different size solutes from the intravascular pace into the peritoneal cavity (Aune, 1970a, 1970b, 1970c, 1970d). The peritoneal blood supply is abundant and can be disregarded as a limiting factor for the transperitoneal transport of substances such as urea, para-aminohippuric acid (PAH), inulin, and serum albumin (Aune, 1970d). The relative rate of net influx into the peritoneal cavity is generally not related to molecular weight since the peritoneum does not function as a molecular weight sieve, per se.

Flessner, Dedrick, & Schultz (1985a) evaluated the effects of molecular weight on peritoneal transport in the rat. Plasma and peritoneal samples were collected for 3 to 4 hours after either (1) an intraperitoneal injection of dialysis fluid with tracer or (2) an intravenous injection of tracer material simultaneously with an intraperitoneal injection of dialysis solution without tracer (Flessner et al., 1985a). The exchange of dextrans ranging in molecular weight from 19,400 to 160,000 and ^{125}I-bovine serum albumin (BSA) between dialysis fluid (5% BSA in Krebs-Ringer solution) in the peritoneal cavity and plasma suggests a functional asymmetry in transport of large molecules across the blood capillary wall (Figure 2.9). Substances injected intravenously moved from the blood capillaries into the peritoneal cavity. Flessner et al. concluded that filtration and/or unidirectional pinocytosis accounts for plasma-to-peritoneal transport of solutes with a molecular weight greater than 20,000 (Flessner et al., 1985a; Flessner, Dedrick, & Schultz, 1985b). Substances of molecular weight greater than or equal to 39,000 move from the peritoneal cavity to the plasma via peritoneal lymphatics; transportation of 19,000 molecular-weight dextran from the cavity to the plasma occurs primarily via lymphatics with some blood capillary uptake (Table 2.3). Higher intraperitoneal osmotic pressure causes a small reverse flux of water from the tissue to the peritoneal cavity. However, lymphatic transport is not important for low molecular weight (<1,000) substances.

Macromolecules (720,000 molecular weight) injected into the peritoneal cavity will be preferentially transported to the blood via the two major lymphatic systems draining the peritoneal cavity (subdiaphragmatic and mesenteric). The visceral tissues (except the layers close to the peritoneal surface, <1 mm) are not exposed to high concentrations during intraperitoneal delivery of macromolecules. Convection dominates over diffusion in the transport of macromolecules into the tissue. Thus, the abdominal wall and diaphragm tend to accumulate these substances if they are not taken up by lymphatics (Flessner, Dedrick, Fenstermacher, Blasberg, & Sieber, 1986).

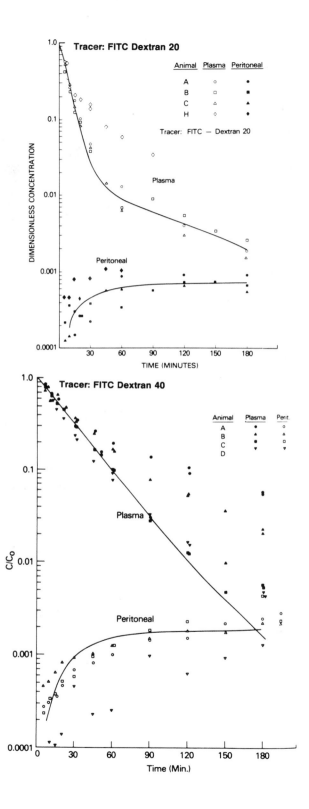

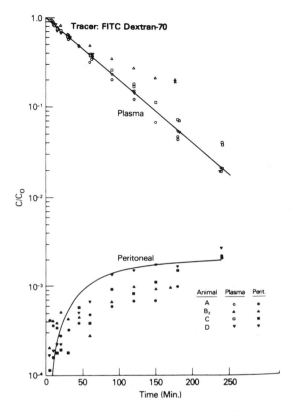

FIGURE 2.9. Plasma-to-peritoneal transport of Dextran 20, 40 (facing page) and 70 (above). All dextrans are metabolized from larger sizes to smaller ones that can more easily be excreted. The excretion loss as well as the distribution to other compartments, including the peritoneal cavity accounts for much of the rapid decrease in plasma concentations (From Flessner et al., 1985a). Reproduced by permission of American Psychological Society.

Summary

Filtration and/or unidirectional pinocytosis is responsible for plasma-to-peritoneal transport of large solutes (molecular weight greater than 20,000), whereas the lymphatics are responsible for peritoneal-to-plasma transport. Aune (1970a, 1970c, 1970d) demonstrated the filtration of large molecular weight substances including protein from the plasma to the peritoneal cavity and the return of these proteins to the plasma primarily via the lymphatics. Molecular weight has relatively minor effects on the transfer of large substances between the peritoneal cavity and the plasma (Flessner et al., 1985a, 1985b). Peritoneal-to-plasma transport of substances with molecular weight greater than 20,000 is governed by the

TABLE 2.3. Transportation of dextran, by molecular weight, from the peritoneal cavity to the plasma.

Substance	Direction of transport	P_p, mm Hg	$V_p(t_f)/V_p(0)$ Mean ± SD	Model output
Dextran 20	1	2.8 ± 0.3	0.85 ± 0.02	0.85
Dextran 20	2	3.5 ± 0.4	0.80 ± 0.03	0.83
Dextran 40	1	3.8 ± 0.3	0.86 ± 0.01	0.82
Dextran 40	2	4.0 ± 0.2	0.78 ± 0.04	0.82
Dextran 70/BSA	1	4.4 ± 0.4	0.82 ± 0.00	0.81
Dextran 70/BSA	2	3.6 ± 0.3	0.80 ± 0.02	0.83
Dextran 150	1	3.1 ± 0.6	0.86 ± 0.03	0.84
Dextran 150	2	2.8 ± 0.1	0.85 ± 0.01	0.85

Values are means ± SD. P_p, peritoneal hydrostatic pressure; BSA, bovine serum albumin. Direction of transport: 1, peritoneal to plasma; 2, plasma to peritoneal. $V_p(t_f)$, measured volume at end of experiment; $V_p(0)$, volume at time 0. (From Flessner et al., 1985d).

lymph flow rate. These solutes exhibit a relatively constant rate of capillary mass transfer with increasing molecular weight and a decreasing effective tissue distribution (Flessner, Fenstermacher, Blasberg, & Dedrick, 1985c; Flessner et al., 1986).

Peritoneal Absorption

The actual tissue concentration of macromolecules in the abdominal wall is much higher than the concentration in visceral tissue. This may be due to either the availability of a large extracellular space or an enhanced rate of convection (Flessner et al., 1985b). When fluid is instilled into the cavity, pressure (2 to 5 mm Hg) is exerted on all surfaces. For the small intestine, the pressure is symmetrically imposed radially around its surface, which compresses the lumen. As a result, the pressure difference across the tissue is less than the peritoneal pressure. The abdominal wall, because it is bordered on one side by subcutaneous tissue that is at (or below) atmospheric pressure, experiences the entire intraperitoneal hydrostatic pressure which not only stretches the muscle but induces a change in the extracellular space (Reed & Wiig, 1981).

The diaphragm is also exposed to a significant but fluctuating pressure. It is equal to the pressure in the peritoneal cavity minus the pressure in the pleural space, which depends on the state of respiration. In addition, the diaphragm is the major site of lymphatic uptake from the peritoneal cavity (Yoffey & Courtice, 1970; Flessner, Parker, & Sieber, 1983). The anatomic mechanism of particle uptake in mice and rats occurs through stomata that communicate with lymphatic lacunae under the diaphragmatic mesothelium and employs intracellular uptake by both small (0.05 μm) and large (0.1 to 1μm) vesicles (Casley-Smith 1964; Leak & Rahil, 1978; Bettendorf, 1979).

The decreasing concentration profiles in the viscera (liver, stomach, intestines) are due to well-developed lymphatic systems within the tissue. In the stomach and intestines there are lymphatics in each of the layers (mucosa, submucosa, and muscularis) that communicate from one plexus to the next through short vessels perpendicular to the gut axis (Barrowman, 1978). Lymph flows from the mucosa outward toward the muscularis and from there to mesenteric nodes.

Distribution Models

A simplified distributed model of peritoneal solute transport was described by Dedrick, Flessner, Collins and Schultz (1986) that enables prediction of peritoneal transport from measurements of tissue diffusion, capillary permeability, and capillary surface area. The shell-and-tube model is an idealization of the actual peritoneal cavity that provides an anatomical perspective of the peritoneal mass exchange (Figure 2.10). The tube represents the gut and the shell represents the parietal tissue

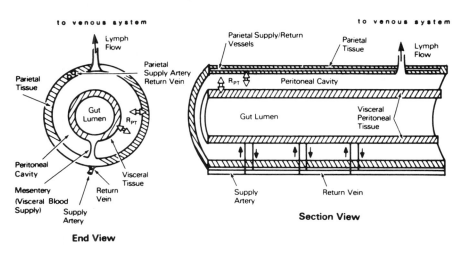

FIGURE 2.10. Conceptual model of peritoneal shell-and-tube mass exchanger. Transverse and sagittal views of an idealized peritoneal cavity. Shell (parietal tissue) and tube (viscera) each have their own blood supplies. Mass transfer occurs between fluid in the cavity and tissue through which blood flows. Lymphatic flow returns peritoneal fluid directly to venous system. R_{PT} is the rate of mass transfer from peritoneal cavity to tissue. (From Flessner et al., 1985a. Reproduced by permission of American Physiological Society.)

surrounding the cavity. Separate blood flow supplies the visceral and the parietal tissue. The mesentery contains the visceral blood supply, whereas the parietal blood supply is separate from the visceral supply. Lymph flow occurs through diaphragmatic stomata (Bettendorf, 1978). These are represented by an opening in the parietal wall. Solutes leave the peritoneal cavity either via the lymphatics by bulk flow or via the tissue by convection and diffusion. Transport from the plasma to the cavity occurs via the tissue space only.

Figure 2.11 depicts a compartmental representation of the peritoneal transfer system in relation to the rest of the body. The body has been divided into two compartments. One is the distribution compartment, which consists primarily of plasma and the interstitial fluid that rapidly equilibrates with plasma. The mass transfer between the cavity and surrounding tissues is represented as R_{PT}. The more slowly equilibrating tissues are grouped together as body-exchange compartment.

Figure 2.12 displays the peritoneal and plasma concentration versus time for both directions of transport. Equilibration of the two spaces occurs during transport from the plasma to the peritoneal cavity when the plasma concentration of solute drops below the peritoneal concentration and the solute begins to be reabsorbed back into the plasma (Flessner et al., 1985b). This phenomenon is reflected in the tissue concentration profiles of Figure 2.12 in which the shape of the profile changes over the course of dialysis. As a result, the peak tissue concentrations lag

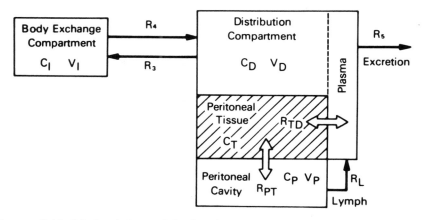

FIGURE 2.11. Mechanistic model of peritoneal transport. C_I, concentration in compartment I; V_I, volume in compartment I; R_3, R_4, and R_5, rates of mass transfer; R_{TD}, rate of mass transfer from peritoneal tissue to distribution compartment; R_{PT}, rate of mass transfer from peritoneal cavity to tissue; R_L, rate of mass transfer from peritoneal cavity to distribution compartment via lymph. (From Flessner et al., 1985a. Reproduced by permission of American Physiological Society.)

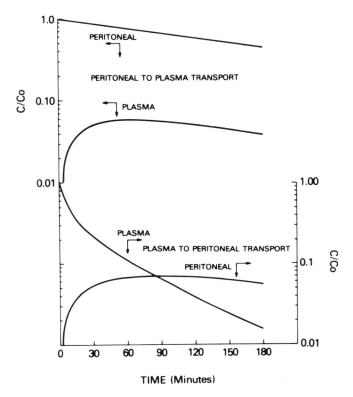

FIGURE 2.12. Peritoneal transport simulation for sucrose: dimensionless concentration (C/Co) versus time (min) for characteristic parameters. (From Flessner et al., 1985a. Reproduced with permission of American Physiological Society.)

behind the plasma concentrations by 3 to 4 minutes. In the case of peritoneal-to-plasma transport, the tissue profiles in Figure 2.13 illustrate how rapidly the "pseudo–steady state" is attained.

A larger peritoneal surface area enhances both fluid transfer and mass transfer from the peritoneal cavity. However, with the larger area, the transfer from the plasma to the peritoneal cavity is increased early in the dialysis but then decreases as the plasma concentration decreases. In contrast, a decrease in peritoneal surface area reduces mass transfer in both directions. This explains the rationale for intraperitoneal rather than intravenous placement of medicaments to act in the peritoneal space.

Tissue Concentration Gradients

Flessner et al. (1985c) measured concentration gradients resulting from passive transport between the peritoneal cavity and the plasma. All tissues surrounding the cavity maintained concentration gradients and therefore

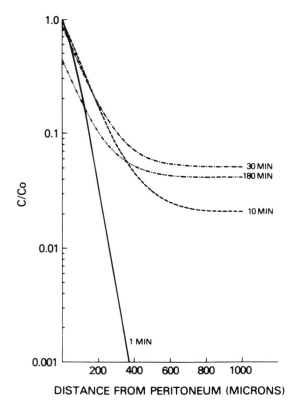

FIGURE 2.13. Peritoneal tissue void concentration gradients for sucrose: perito-neal-to-plasma transport. Dimensionless concentration (C/Co) versus distance (μm) from peritoneum versus time (min) of dialysis for characteristic parameters. (From Flessner et al., 1985a. Reproduced with permission of American Physiological Society.)

are probable routes of transport. Figure 2.14 shows how the tissue concentration of a drug may decrease over a given distance, 90% in about 300 μm. From these studies Flessner et al. estimated tissue compliances based on pressures recorded in the peritoneal dialysis experiments. This pressure is exerted against the entire peritoneal surface. Local pressure gradients (change in pressure versus distance) are established in each tissue dependent upon its location. The abdominal wall has the intra-peritoneal pressure imposed across it (thickness—2 to 2.5 mm). In contrast, the small intestine is surrounded by fluid as well as by the large intestine, and because it is supported by other tissues, it will have pressure gradients different from those in the abdominal wall. Compliances for tissue close to the peritoneum, where pressures are 2 to 5 mm Hg, will be high (Guyton, 1965; Wiederhielm, 1972; Reed & Wiig, 1981; Wiig &

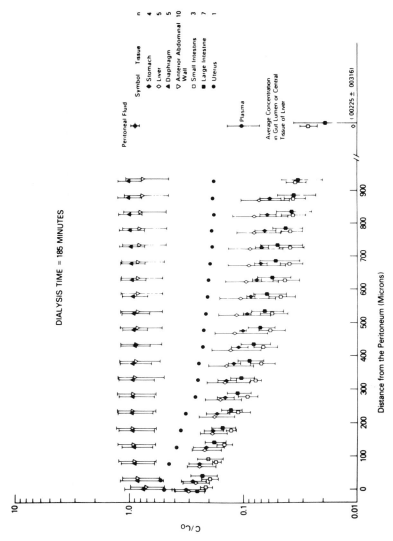

FIGURE 2.14. Peritoneal-to-plasma transport of ^{125}I-human serum albumin. Tissue concentration (based on wet tissue weight) divided by initial peritoneal concentration versus distance in microns from peritoneum. Duration of dialysis: 185 min. (From Flessner et al., 1985c. Reproduced with permission of American Physiological Society.)

Reed, 1981), 4 to 100 ml/100 g tissue, whereas the compliance deeper in the tissue will depend on the actual interstitial pressure, which will usually be lower.

Interspecies Scaling

The intrinsic permeability of the peritoneum is similar among mammalian species (Figure 2.15; Dedrick et al., 1986). The rate constant for the concentration change during absorption of solutes from the peritoneal cavity can be expressed as clearance/V_p, where V_p is the volume of fluid in the peritoneal cavity. If the relative volume (ml/kg) is held the same between two species, the concentration would be expected to decrease more slowly in the larger species. Duration for peritoneal clearance of solvent is comparable between species; the volumes vary as the ⅔ power of body weight. For example, the concentration in a peritoneal volume

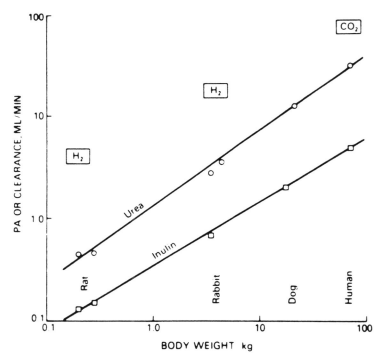

FIGURE 2.15. Mass transfer coefficient or clearance for urea and inulin in the rat, rabbit, dog, and human. Clearance of dissolved hydrogen is also shown in the rat and rabbit, and carbon dioxide is also shown in the human. (From Dedrick et al., 1986. Reproduced by permission of Field, Rich.)

of 50 ml in a 250-g rat should follow approximately the same time course as the concentration in 2,000 ml in a 60-kg human subject.

Hypertonic or hypotonic dialysate, peritonitis, hydrostatic pressure, and a variety of pharmacologic manipulations can influence peritoneal transport. The net change may be a result of more than one underlying mechanism. Consideration of the spatially distributed character of peritoneal transport can serve conceptually to integrate a variety of diverse mechanisms.

Intraperitoneal Pharmacokinetics

In general, the permeability area product decreases as approximately the square root of molecular weight (Dedrick, Myers, Bungay, & De Vita, 1978). Large difference in the pharmacokinetic advantage of intraperitoneal drug administration results from two factors. First, because of metabolism in the liver, much of the drug never reaches the systemic circulation. Second, the total body clearance of one drug may be much larger than the total body clearance of another drug.

Intraperitoneal drugs also penetrate through the peritoneum into the adjacent viscera. Flessner et al. (1985c) determined the depth of penetration radiolabeled tracers made into the peritoneum after intraperitoneal (IP) administration. Both parietal and visceral peritoneum contained concentration gradients and, as such, serve as routes of transport.

The tissue penetration of many drugs is quite different from that of small molecular weight molecules (Dedrick, Zahorko & Binder, 1975). The qualitative nature of the concentration profiles within parietal and visceral surfaces may be partly explained by the fact that peritoneal pressure is expressed across the entire abdominal wall. Thus, the transabdominal wall pressure difference represents the peritoneal pressure minus atmospheric pressure (Dedrick, 1985). Since the visceral surfaces that are submerged within the peritoneal cavity probably support relatively little transmural pressure, the driving force for convection is much smaller; therefore, movement into the visceral surfaces may well be a diffusive process.

Summary Model

The general pharmacokinetic features of drugs administered intraperitoneally to mammals are illustrated in Figure 2.16 (Dedrick et al., 1978; Flessner, Fenstermacher, Dedrick & Blasberg, 1985d). In this figure, the body is represented by a single compartment with volume of distribution (V_D) and drug concentration (C_P). The body communicates with fluid in the peritoneal cavity with volume (V) and concentration area (A) by a diffusive process characterized by permeability (P). The drug may also

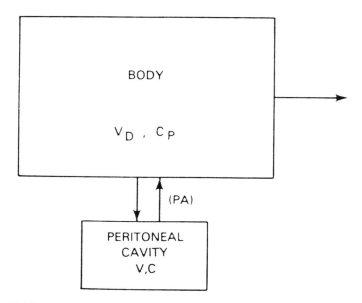

FIGURE 2.16. Two-compartment open model for peritoneal pharmacokinetics. V_D, volume of distribution; C_P, drug concentration; V, volume; C, concentration; A, area; P, permeability (Dedrick et al., 1978).

be carried by convective transport with transperitoneal fluid movement or lymph flow. The permeability-area product (PA) expresses the drug clearance (ml/minute). The magnitude may be usefully compared with blood flows and clearance by various organs in assessing the relative quantitative significance of concurrent kinetic processes. When k greatly exceeds PA, the concentration at steady state in the peritoneal cavity substantially exceeds the body's concentration (Dedrick, 1985).

If the volumes of distribution are constant the mass balance equations for each compartment are as follows:

$$V_D \frac{dC_P}{dt} = PA[C - RC_P] - kC_P \qquad [2.1]$$

$$V \frac{dC}{dt} = PA[RC_P - C] \qquad [2.2]$$

where k is the whole-body clearance by all processes and R represents the equilibrium dialysate to plasma C ratio (required to account for plasma protein binding). Equation 2.1 must be modified if significant metabolism occurs in the liver because this would produce an effect similar to the first-pass phenomenon following oral drug administration. Since most drugs are absorbed from the peritoneum via the portal system

(Equation 2.1), "bioavailability" may be considerably reduced for drugs that undergo hepatic clearance (Dedrick et al., 1978).

Figure 2.17 shows PA as a function of molecular weight. P is inversely proportional to the square root of molecular weight over the range of interest. Values are considerably less than whole-body clearances of many anticancer drugs. Figure 2.17 should not be used to estimate PA for a molecule with any significant lipid solubility because transcellular transport mechanisms may greatly increase the rate of diffusion compared with the expected value if permeability is limited by capillary junctions. The peritoneal permeability is variable, is affected by drugs, and may be altered in disease states (Dedrick et al., 1978).

This simple model does not take into account the possibility of extensive metabolism of a drug during its first pass through the liver. Drugs are absorbed from the peritoneal cavity both into the liver, through the portal system, and directly into the systemic circulation, by capillary beds that bypass the portal system. The amount of "first-pass" metabolism increases the pharmacokinetic advantage of interperitoneal administration.

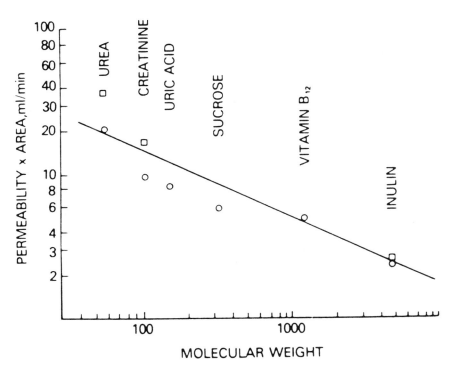

FIGURE 2.17. Peritoneal permeability × area versus molecular weight. This shows that peritoneal permeability is a function of the molecular weight (Dedrick et al., 1978).

Summary

From considerations of intraperitoneal pharmacokinetics, those properties that make a drug appropriate for intraperitoneal administration become apparent. First, the drug should be capable of inducing its pharmacologic action locally. For example, a drug such as cyclophosphamide, which requires hepatic activation, would not likely be of unique benefit when administered into the peritoneal cavity. The drug should possess a low peritoneal permeability-area product and should be rapidly cleared from the plasma. Finally, it would be advantageous if antidotal agents were available for IV use that also possessed poor peritoneal permeability.

References

Ahrenholz DH, Simmons RL. (1988). Peritonitis and other intra-abdominal infections. In: Howard RJ, Simmons RL, eds. *Surgical Infectious Diseases.* 2nd ed. Connecticut: Appleton & Lange, 605–646.

Alfonsin AE, Leiderman S. (1980). Peritoneal fluid throughout the cycle. *Obstet y Gin Lat Amer.* 38:53–56.

Altemeier WA, Culbertson WR, Fidler JP. (1975). Giant horseshoe intra-abdominal abscess. *Ann Surg.* 181:716–725.

Atkinson M. (1959). Effect of diuretics on portal venous pressure. *Lancet.* 2:819–823.

Atkinson M, Losowsky MS. (1961). Mechanism of ascites formation in chronic liver disease. *Q J Med.* 30:153–166.

Atkinson M, Losowsky MS. (1962). Plasma colloid osmotic pressure in relation to formation of ascites and oedema in liver disease. *Clin. Sci.* 22:383–389.

Aune S. (1970a). Transperitoneal exchange. I. Peritoneal permeability studied by transperitoneal plasma clearance of urea, PAH, inulin, and serum albumin in rabbits. *Scand J Gastroenterol.* 5:85–97.

Aune S. (1970b). Transperitoneal exchange II. Peritoneal blood flow estimated by hydrogen gas clearance. *Scand J Gastroenterol.* 5:99–104.

Aune S. (1970c). Transperitoneal exchange. III. The influence of transperitoneal fluid flux in the peritoneal plasma clearance of serum albumin in rabbits. *Scand J Gastroenterol.* 5:161–168.

Aune S. (1970d). Transperitoneal exchange IV. The effect of transperitoneal fluid transport on the transfer of solutes. *Scand J Gastroenterol* 5:241–252.

Badawy SZ, Cuenca V, Marshall L, Munchback R, Rinas AC, Coble DA. (1984). Cellular components in peritoneal fluid in infertile patients with and without endometriosis. *Fertil Steril.* 42:704–08.

Barrowman JA. (1978). *Physiology of the gastrointestinal lymphatic system.* Cambridge: Cambridge University Press; 3–30.

Bartosik D, Jacobs SL, Kelly LJ. (1986). Endometrial tissue in peritoneal fluid. *Fertil Steril.* 46:796–802.

Bettendorf U. (1979). Electron microscopic studies on the peritoneal resorption of intraperitoneally injected latex particles via the diaphragmatic lymphatics. *Lymphology.* 12:66–70.

Blackfan KD, Maxcy KF. (1918). Intraperitoneal injection of saline solution. *Am J Dis Child* 15:19–28.

Blumenkrantz MJ, Gallagher N, Bashore RA, Tenckhoff H. (1981). Retrograde menstruation in women undergoing chronic peritoneal dialysis. *Obstet Gynecol.* 57:667–673.

Buyalos RP, Rutanen E-M, Tsui E, Halme J. (1991). Release of tumor necrosis factor alpha by human peritoneal macrophages in response to toxic shock syndrome toxin-1. *Obstet Gynecol.* 78:182–186.

Carter FS. (1953). Intraperitoneal transfusions as method of rehydration in African child. *East Afr Med J.* 30:499–505.

Casley-Smith JR. (1964). Endothelial permeability—the passage of particles into and out of diaphragmatic lymphatics. *J Exp Physiol.* 49:365–383.

Cohn ZA, Morse SI. (1959). Interactions between rabbit polymorphonuclear leukocytes and staphylcocci. *J Exp Med.* 110:419–443.

Courtice FC, Simmonds WJ. (1954). Physiological significations of lymph drainage of the serous cavities and lungs. *Physiol Rev.* 34:419–447.

Cromack DT, Cromack TR, Pretorius G, DeMeules JE. (1985). Development of a predictive value equation for the minimum fluid volume to completely coat the intraperitoneal surface of rodents. *Surg Forum.* 36:477–478.

Crone C. (1963). Does 'restricted diffusion' occur in muscle capillaries? *Proc Soc Exp Biol Med.* 112:435–455.

Dedrick RL, Zahorko DS, Binder RA. (1975). Pharmacokinetic considerations on resistance to anticancer drugs. *Cancer Chemother Rep.* 59:795–804.

Dedrick RL, Myers CE, Bungay PM, De Vita VT Jr. (1978). Pharmacokinetic rationale for peritoneal drug administration in the treatment of ovarian cancer. *Cancer Treat Rep.* 62:1–11.

Dedrick RL. (1985). Theoretical and experimental bases of intraperitoneal chemotherapy. *Semin Oncol.* 12:1–6.

Dedrick RL, Flessner MF, Collins JM, Schultz JS. (1986). A distributed model of peritoneal transport. In: Maher JF, Winchester JF, eds. *Frontiers in Peritoneal Dialysis.* New York: Field, Rich; 31–35.

Dunn DL, Barke RA, Ahrenholz DH, Humphrey EW, Simmons RL. (1984). The adjuvant effect of peritoneal fluid in experimental peritonitis. *Ann Surg.* 199:37–43.

Dunselman GAJ, Hendrix MGR, Bouckaert PXJM, Evers JLH. (1988). Functional aspects of peritoneal macrophages in endometriosis of women. *J Reprod Fertil.* 82:707–710.

Eskeland G. (1969). Growth of autologous peritoneal cells in intraperitoneal diffusion chambers in rats. I. A light microscopical study. *Acta Pathol Microbiol Scand.* 68:481–500.

Esperanca MJ, Collins DL. (1966). Peritoneal dialysis efficiency in relation to body weight. *J Ped Surg.* 1:162–169.

Fakih H, Baggett B, Holtz G, Tsang K-Y, Lee JC, Williamson HO. (1987). Interleukin-1: a possible role in the infertility associated with endometriosis. *Fertil Steril.* 47:213–217.

Felix M, Dalton AJ. (1955). A phase contrast microscope study of free cells native to the peritoneal fluid of DBA/a mice. *J Natl Cancer Inst.* 16:415–455.

Flessner MF, Parker RJ, Sieber SM. (1983). Peritoneal lymphatic uptake of fibrinogen and erythrocytes in the rat. *Am J Physiol.* 244 (Heart Circ Physiol 13):H89–H96.

Flessner MF, Dedrick RL, Schultz JS. (1985a). A distributed model of peritoneal-plasma transport: analysis of experimental data in the rat. *Am J Physiol.* 248 (Renal Fluid Electrolyte Physiol 17):F413–F424.

Flessner MF, Dedrick RL, Schultz JS. (1985b). Exchange of macromolecules between peritoneal cavity and plasma. *Am J Physiol.* 248 (Heart Circ Physiol 17):H15–H25.

Flessner MF, Fenstermacher JD, Blasberg RG, Dedrick RL. (1985c). Peritoneal absorption of macromolecules studied by quantitative autoradiography. *Am J Physiol.* 248 (Heart Circ Physiol 17):H26–H32.

Flessner MF, Fenstermacher JD, Dedrick RL, Blasberg RG. (1985d). A distributed model of peritoneal-plasma transport: tissue concentration gradients. *Am J Physiol.* 248 (Renal Fluid Electrolyte Physiol 17):F425–F435.

Flessner MR, Dedrick RL, Fenstermacher JD, Blasberg RG, Sieber SM. (1986). Peritoneal absorption of macromolecules. In: JF Maher, JF Winchester, eds. *Frontiers in Peritoneal Dialysis.* New York: Field, Rich; 41–46.

Greenwalt D, Nakamura RM, diZerega G. (1988). Determination of pH and pKa in human peritoneal fluid. *Curr Surg.* 45:217–218.

Guyton AC. (1965). Interstitial fluid pressure: II. Pressure-volume curves of interstitial space. *Circ Res.* 16:452–460.

Guyton AR. (1973). The special fluids systems of the body. In: Guyton AR, ed. *Textbook of Medical Physiology.* 4th ed. Philadelphia: WB Saunders; 29–50.

Halme J, Becker S, Hammond MG, Raj MHG, Raj S. (1983). Increase activation of pelvic macrophages in infertile women with endometriosis. *Am J Obstet Gynecol.* 145:333–337.

Halme J, Becker S, Wing R. (1984a). Accentuated cyclic activation of peritoneal macrophages in patients with endometriosis. *Am J Obstet Gynecol.* 148:85–90.

Halme J, Hammond MG, Hulka JF, Raj SG, Talbert LM. (1984b). Retrograde menstruation in healthy women and in patients with endometriosis. *Obstet Gynecol.* 64:151–154.

Halme J, Becker S, Haskill S. (1987). Altered maturation and function of peritoneal macropahges: possible role in pathogenesis of endometriosis. Am J Obstet Gynecol. 156:783–789.

Halme J, White C, Kauma S, Estes J, Haskill S. (1988). Peritoneal macrophages from patients with endometriosis release growth factor activity in vitro. *J Clin Endocrinol Metab.* 66:1044–1048.

Halme J. (1989). Release of tumor necrosis factor alpha by human peritoneal macrophages in vivo and in vitro. *Am J Obstet Gynecol.* 161:1718–1725.

Hirsch JG, Church AB. (1960). Studies of phagocytosis of group A streptococci by polymorphonuclear leukocytes in vitro. *J Exp Med.* 111:309–322.

Howard JM, Singh CM. (1963). Peritoneal fluid pH after perforation of peptic ulcers. *Arch Surg.* 81:141–142.

Jenkins C, Benacerref B. (1960). In vitro studies on the interaction between mouse peritoneal macrophages and strains of *Salmonella* and *Escherichia coli. J Exp Med.* 112:403–417.

Koninckx PR, Ide P, Vandenbroucke W, Brosens IA. (1980). New aspects of the pathophysiology of endometriosis and associated infertility. *J Reprod Med.* 24:257–263.

Kruger S, Greve DW, Schueler FW. (1962). Absorption of fluid from peritoneal cavity. *Arch Int Pharmacodyn Ther.* 137:173–178.

Kruitwagen RFPM, Poels LG, Willemsen WNP, de Ronde IJY, Jap PHK, Rolland R. (1991). Endometrial epithelial cells in peritoneal fluid during the early follicular phase. *Fertil Steril.* 55:297–303.

Kulenthran A, Jeyalakshmi N. (1989). Dissemination of endometrial cells at laparoscopy and chromotubation—a preliminary report. *Int J Fertil.* 34:256–258.

Leak LV, Rahil K. (1978). Permeability of the diaphragmatic mesothelium: the ultrastructural basis for 'stomata.' *Am J Anat.* 151:557–594.

Levison ME, Pontzer RE. (1979). Peritonitis and other intra-abdominal infections. In: Mandell GL, Douglas RG Jr, Bennett JE, eds. *Principles and Practice of Infectious Diseases.* 2nd ed. New York: Wiley; 476–503.

Losowsky MS, Jones DP, Lieber CS, Davidson CS. (1963). Local factors in ascites formation during sodium retention in cirrhosis. *N Engl J Med.* 268:651–653.

Mengert WF, Cobb SW, Brown WW Jr. (1951). Introduction of blood into peritoneal cavity: experimental study. *JAMA.* 147:34–37.

Mitchell GAG. (1941). The spread of acute intraperitoneal effusions. *Br J Surg.* 28:291–313.

Mungyer G, Willemsen WNP, Rolland R, Vemer HM, Ramaekers FCS, Jap PHK, Poels LG. (1987). Cells of the mucous membrane of the female genital tract in culture: a comparative study with regard to the histogenesis of endometriosis. *In Vitro Cell Dev Biol* 23:111–117.

Odel HM, Ferris DO, Power MH. (1948). Clinical considerations of the problem of extra renal excretion: peritoneal lavage. *Med Clin North Am.* 32:989–1076.

Pappenheimer JR. (1953). Passage of molecules through capillary walls. *Physiol Rev.* 33:387–423.

Polishuk WZ, Sharf M. (1965). Culposcopic findings in primary dysmenorrhoea. *Obstet Gynecol* 26:746–748.

Reed RK, Wiig H. (1981). Compliance of the interstitial space in rats. I. Studies on hindlimb skeletal muscle. *Acta Physiol Scand.* 113:297–303.

Roberts R. (1967). The interaction in vitro between group B meningococci and rabbit polymorphonuclear leukocytes. Demonstration of type specific opsonins and bactericidins. *J Exp Med.* 126:795–817.

Schechter AJ, Cary MK, Carpentieri AL, Darrow DC. (1933). Changes in composition of fluids injected into peritoneal cavity. *Am J Dis Child.* 46:1015–1026.

Shear L, Swartz C, Shinaberger JA, Barry KG. (1965). Kinetics of peritoneal fluid absorption in adult man. *N Engl J Med.* 272:123–127.

Shelton E, Rice ME. (1959). Growth of normal peritoneal cells in diffusion chambers: a study of cell modulation. *Am J Anat.* 105:281–341.

Wegner G. (1877). Chirurgische Bemerkungen über die peritoneal Höhle, mit besonderer Berücksichtigung der Ovariotomie. *Arch Klin Chir* 20:51–57.

Wiederhielm CA. (1972). The interstitial space. In: Fung YC, ed. *Biomechanics: Its Foundations and Objectives.* Englewood Cliffs; NJ: Prentice Hall, 273–286.

Wiig H, Reed RK. (1981). Compliance of the interstitial space in rats II. Studies on skin. *Acta Physiol Scand.* 113:307–315.

Willemsen WNP, Mungyer G, Smets H, Rolland R, Vemer H, Jap P. (1985). Behavior of cultured glandular cells obtained by flushing of the uterine cavity. *Fertil Steril.* 44:92–95.

Yoffey JM, Courtice FC. (1970). *Lymphatics, Lymph, and the Lymphomyeloid Complex.* London: Academic Press; 206–213.

Zinsser HH, Pryde AW. (1952). Experimental study of physical factors; including fibrin formation, influencing the spread of fluids and small particles within and from the peritoneal cavity of the dog. *Ann Surg.* 136:818–827.

3

Growth Factors

GROWTH FACTORS ARE PROTEINS THAT WORK AS PARACRINE OR AU-
tocrine modulators of cell proliferation. Many growth factors have been
isolated that were originally purified on the basis of a specific biological
effect and subsequently named for this effect. Once the factor was isolated
to homogeneity, the amino acid sequence was determined and recombinant proteins developed. Upon testing of recombinant proteins in a
variety of systems it was found that many factors not only have overlapping functions but also act on a wide range of cell types to produce a
variety of actions. In addition to the effects of individual factors on cells
involved in the wound healing process, many of these factors interact
with other substances to antagonize or synergize their effects, perhaps
through the use of similar second-messenger systems or modulation of
receptor-ligand affinity. The susceptibility of tissues to modulation by
growth factors may change as wound healing progresses.

Due to the ease of application and observation, most of the studies
described below examined the effects of growth factors in the healing of
skin wounds (Figure 3.1). At the end of this section studies examining
the effects of growth factors on peritoneal healing will be considered.

The cells involved in peritoneal repair, including fibroblasts, macrophages, and endothelial cells, secrete a variety of factors that mediate not
only the proliferation of their target cell (such as fibroblast growth factor
[FGF] or epidermal growth factor [EGF]), but also regulate inflammatory
responses and the formation of extracellular matrices. However, these
factors are involved in a wide range of actions including stimulation of
cell growth, inhibition of cellular proliferation, and alterations of cell
functions unrelated to proliferation.

This chapter summarizes the actions and mechanisms of action of the
various growth factors postulated to be involved in peritoneal healing,
what is known about their modulation of skin repair, and data on the
effects of these factors on peritoneal repair processes (Table 3.1).

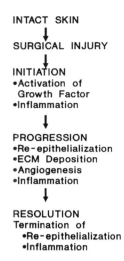

INTACT SKIN

SURGICAL INJURY

INITIATION
•Activation of
 Growth Factor
•Inflammation

PROGRESSION
•Re-epithelialization
•ECM Deposition
•Angiogenesis
•Inflammation

RESOLUTION
Termination of
 •Re-epithelialization
 •Inflammation

FIGURE 3.1. A schematic for dermal wound healing. Stages that can be modulated by growth factors are highlighted.

TABLE 3.1. Summary of results derived from a rabbit model on the modulation by growth factors of cells derived from the site of peritoneal injury (TRC).

Postsurgical day	Growth Factor						
	EGF	PDGF	FGF	TGF-β	IL-2	IL-1	IGF-I
Proliferation							
d_2	↑	↑	↑↑↑	↓↓↓	N.C.	N.C.	N.C.
d_5	↑	↑	↑↑↑	↓↓↓	N.C.	N.C.	N.C.
d_7	↑↑	↑	↑↑↑	↓↓↓	N.C.	N.C.	N.C.
d_{10}	↑↑↑	↑	↑↑↑	↓↓↓	N.C.	N.C.	N.C.
Protein synthesis							
d_{10}	N.D.	N.D.	N.D.	↑↑	N.D.	↑	N.D.

Stimulation of tissue repair cells (TRC) function, derived from the postsurgical site of peritoneal repair, is indicated by ↑. Suppression of TRC function is denoted by ↓. If the TRC function was not changed by the growth factor, this is indicated by N.C. If the effect of the growth factor was not assessed, this is indicated by N.D. (Fukasawa et al., 1989; Rodgers KE & diZerega GS, in press).

Epidermal Growth Factor

Epidermal growth factor (EGF) was originally identified as a peptide that stimulated the growth of basal epithelial cells. EGF is a single polypeptide chain of 53 amino acids, containing a molecular weight of 6,045 d and an isoelectric point of pH 4.6 (Carpenter & Cohen, 1979). Originally isolated from mouse submaxillary glands (Cohen, 1962), urogastrone is a factor that was isolated from human urine and has all the properties of murine EGF (Gregory, 1975; Hollenberg & Gregory, 1976).

Biological Activity

EGF stimulates proliferation of cultured cells of ecto-, meso-, and endodermal origin (Carpenter & Cohen, 1979). EGF stimulates the proliferation and keratinization of keratinocytes and production of cells of squamous, conjunctival and pharyngeal tissue (Figure 3.2; Sun & Green, 1977). Single-cell preparations of epidermal keratinocytes can fuse and form an epithelium in culture (Green, Kehinde, & Thomas, 1979). Granulosa cells, corneal endothelial cells, vascular smooth muscle, chondrocytes, and fibroblasts are some of the cell types of mesodermal origin that respond to EGF (Gospodarowicz, Greenburg, Bialecki, & Zetter, 1978b). Although of endodermal origin, liver cells and thyroid cells respond to EGF (Richman, Claus, Pilkis, & Friedman, 1976; Bucher, 1978; Koch & Leffert, 1979; McGowan, Strain, & Bucher, 1981; Leffert & Koch, 1982; Roger & Dumont, 1982; Westermark, Karlsson, & Westermark, 1983). EGF also has antiproliferative effects on hair follicle cells and squamous carcinoma cells (Panaretto, Leish, Moore, & Robertson, 1984; Kamata et al. 1986). One of the effects of EGF unrelated to proliferation is the suppression of gastric acid secretion (Gregory, 1975).

EGF was shown to stimulate the proliferation of many cells involved in skin repair. The stimulation of keratinocyte proliferation and keratinization could be instrumental in the enhancement of skin repair. EGF also stimulates the proliferation of cells of mesodermal origin such as fibroblasts and endothelial cells. This action of EGF may also allow the acceleration of both skin and peritoneal repair.

EGF promotes proliferation of the basal cell layer of various epithelia

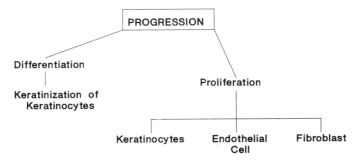

FIGURE 3.2. The activities involved in wound healing that are modulated by epidermal growth factor.

from fetal, neonate, or adult origin and requires cell attachment to the basement membrane (Cohen & Elliott, 1963; Cohen, 1965; Cohen & Taylor, 1974). EGF regulates the proliferation and development of fetal tissues. For example, infusion of EGF into fetal lambs or rabbits accelerates the maturation of the lung (Sundell et al., 1975; Catterton et al., 1979; Sundell, Gray, Serenlus, Scobedo, & Stahlman, 1980). Further studies showed that the administration of EGF to the fetus altered many developmental processes and was either teratogenic (causing cleft palate or softening of the skull) or it simply accelerated normal processes. In addition, in vivo administration of antibodies to EGF did not modify normal development. Therefore, the role of EGF in fetal development remains elusive.

Mechanism of Action

EGF stimulates the proliferation of many types of quiescent cells. To accomplish this, a complex series of events occurs at the cellular level (Figure 3.3). First, EGF complexes with its receptor on the cell surface. Following this, the protein kinase activity intrinsic to the receptor is activated leading to self-phosphorylation and phosphorylation of other cellular substrates (Carpenter, King, & Cohen, 1979; Ushiro & Cohen, 1980). This tyrosine-specific kinase activity is part of the cytoplasmic domain of the EGF receptor (Ullrich, et al., 1984; Hunter & Cooper, 1985; Yarden & Ullrich, 1988). Mutations of the EGF receptor that abolish the protein kinase activity are unable to stimulate various cellular responses to EGF, even though there is normal ligand binding by these receptors (Honegger et al., 1987a, 1987b; Chen et al., 1987; Schlessinger, 1987). These studies also show that kinase activity involves intracellular trafficking of the EGF receptor (Honegger et al., 1987a, 1987b).

After binding, an increase in membrane fluidity and pinocytosis occurs, which allows the formation of clusters of receptor-ligand complexes in coated pits and their endocytic internalization into lysosomes for degradation (Carpenter & Cohen, 1976a; Haigler, McKanna, & Cohen, 1979b; Carpenter 1985). These changes correlate with rapid morphological alterations, such as membrane ruffling followed by the cell becoming more rounded (Chinkers, McKanna, & Cohen, 1979). After 30 minutes, EGF is found in cytosolic endocytic vesicles (Schlessinger, Schechter, Willingham, & Pastan, 1978; Haigler, McKanna, & Cohen, 1979a), which then form multivesicular bodies (secondary lysosomes [Gorden, Carpentier, Cohen, & Orci, 1978; Haigler et al., McKanna, & Cohen, 1979a]). Concurrent with this, many metabolic alterations occur in the cells, such as increased nutrient uptake (Carpenter & Cohen, 1979; Haigler et al., 1979b), ion fluxes (Rozengurt & Heppel, 1975), and cytoskeletal organization (Schlessinger & Geiger, 1981). Activation of cytoplasmic enzymes and stimulation of protein and DNA synthesis are some of the

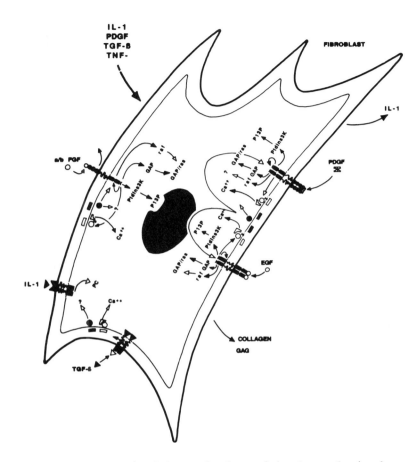

FIGURE 3.3. A schematic of the mechanisms of signal transduction by growth factors. Changes in calcium levels is designated by Ca^{2+}. Inositol phosphate metabolism is designated by PtdIns3K and P13P. (Modified from a schematic representation created by John B. Macauley for the Genzyme Corporation. Used with permission.)

delayed effects of EGF binding to its receptor. Approximately 6 to 8 hours after binding of EGF to its receptor, DNA synthesis is stimulated (Carpenter & Cohen, 1976b; Shechter, Hernaez, & Cuatrecasas, 1978; Haigler & Carpenter, 1980).

Wound Healing

The possibility that EGF could accelerate wound healing due to its ability to promote the proliferation of fibroblasts was examined. EGF was shown to enhance the epithelialization of skin defects in male but not female mice. This effect was observed between 1 and 10 μg/dose (applied topically every 8 hours) (Niall, Ryan, & O'Brien, 1982). These studies were repeated and confirmed using partial thickness cutaneous burns in pigs (Brown et al., 1985). In the study, human epidermal growth factor (hEGF) was applied in a lanolin cream. Fifty percent of the treated wounds were healed prior to any of the control wounds. Other studies showed improved healing in wounds to rabbit ears (Franklin & Lynch, 1979). Additional studies showed an increase in fibroblast organization, collagen production, and neovascularization following EGF treatment (Buckley, Davidson, Kamerath, Wolt, & Woodward, 1985). Most recently, studies by Cooper, Hansbrough, Foreman, Sakabu, & Laxer (1991) demonstrated that EGF slowly released from a polyacrylamide vehicle increased the epithelialization of wounds in a nude mouse model using grafted human tissue. In a model in which the Achilles tendon was transected, injection of urogastrone twice daily increased the dry weight, collagen content and DNA content of the lesion (Franklin, Gregory, & Morris, 1986). Laato, Ninikoshi, Gerdin, & Lebel (1985) reported an increase in granulation tissue with topical EGF. Further studies showed that local application of EGF to sponge implants in rats promoted the development of granulation tissue, extracellular matrix (collagen and glycosaminoglycan), as well as fibroblast and capillary infiltration (Laato, Ninikoshi, Gerdin, & Lebel, 1986; Davidson et al., 1988). One study showed that EGF increased epithelial and hair growth and reduced inflammation following administration to skin wounds in pigs (Eisinger, Sadan, Soehnchen, & Silver, 1988). In another wound chamber model of tissue repair, a slight increase in collagen deposition was noted at later time points with the addition of EGF (Grotendorst, Martin, Penceu, Sodek, & Harvey, 1985).

More recent studies using full-thickness skin wounds in pigs showed that EGF had a minimal benefit on wound healing compared with lactated Ringer's solution (Jijon & Gallup, 1989). In contrast, Chvapil, Gaines, and Gilman (1988) reported that a vehicle, i.e., lanolin cream, had a greater effect on wound healing than EGF. Most recently, experiments in a model using full-thickness wounds in a rabbit ear indicate that although EGF accelerated re-epithelialization of the wound, there is no concomitant increase in the deposition of extracellular matrix (Pierce, Yanagihara, Thomason, & Fox, 1990). Therefore, the benefit of EGF to skin healing is controversial. Most studies showed that EGF is of the greatest benefit when used in conjunction with other growth factors (described below).

EGF was also tested in 12 patients undergoing skin grafting for burns or reconstructive surgery. When EGF was applied topically in lanolin cream every 12 hours it reduced the healing time by 1 to 1.5 days. Histologic examination of the wounds showed completely regenerated and stratified epithelium (Brown et al., 1988).

Peritoneum

This section on peritoneal healing discusses the effects of growth factors on the function of tissue repair cells (TRCs, as reviewed in Chapter 4) harvested from the site of intraperitoneal trauma in rabbits (summarized in Table 3.1). Since EGF may directly modulate the growth of TRCs, which may consist of fibroblasts and/or mesothelial cells, during post-surgical healing, TRCs were harvested at various days after surgery and cultured, and the proliferation in response to EGF was measured. Five days after surgery, TRCs incorporated the greatest amount of thymidine in basal conditions. EGF further stimulated the incorporation of thymidine (a measure of proliferation) into TRCs (Figure 3.4). However, the response of postsurgical days 7 and 10 TRCs to EGF was significantly greater than that of postsurgical days 2 and 5. EGF, as shown above in the section on dermal wound healing, can accelerate re-epithelialization in vivo. However, there is not a concomitant increase in extracellular matrix production. EGF, which stimulates proliferation of TRCs, may function as a competence factor involved in the transition of cells from the G_0 to S phase.

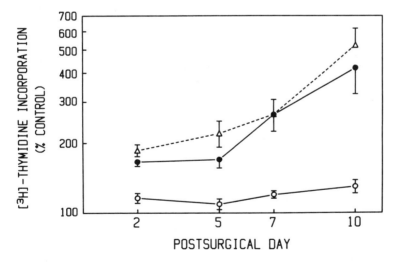

FIGURE 3.4. [³H]-Thymidine incorporation into postsurgical tissue repair cells (TRCs). Tissue repair cells were recovered from abraded peritoneum at various days after surgery and incubated for 4 days. TRCs were then plated into 96-well plates. At 24 hours after plating, growth factors were added. After 48 hours of incubation, TRCs were pulsed with 0.1 μCi [³H]thymidine for 24 hours. Data represent means ± SEM. (△), 100 ng/ml FGF; (●), 1 ng/ml EGF; (○), 10 ng/ml PDGF. (From Fukasawa et al., 1989. Reproduced by permission of Academic Press.)

Summary

EGF may be beneficial in the acceleration of wound healing due to its mitogenic effects on epidermal cells, fibroblasts, and endothelial cells. Some studies on the effects of EGF on skin wound healing suggest re-epithelialization is accelerated by EGF administration, whereas extra-cellular matrix deposition is not.

Fibroblast Growth Factor

Fibroblast growth factors (FGFs) are closely related molecules with a similar range of biologic activities that interact with the same receptor, but differ in some of their physical properties (Bohlen, Esch, Baird, & Gospodarowicz, 1985; Neufeld & Gospodarowicz, 1986; Gospodarowicz, 1985). Basic FGF (bFGF) has a molecular weight of 15,000 d and an isoelectric point (pI) of pH 9.6 and has been purified from various organs including brain, pituitary, adrenal gland, kidney, corpus luteum, retina, placenta, prostate, thymus, bone and macrophages (Gospodarowicz, 1986; Esch et al., 1985; Gospodarowicz, Neufeld, & Schweigerer, 1986; Baird et al., 1986; Lobb et al., 1986). Basic bFGF was identified by its ability to stimulate fibroblast proliferation (Gospodarowicz, 1974; Gospodarowicz & Moran, 1974). Acidic FGF (aFGF), pI of 5.6, was isolated only from neural tissue (brain and retina) and was identified by its ability to stimulate myoblast proliferation and differentiation (Gospodarowicz, Weseman, & Moran, 1975; Gospodarowicz, Mescher, & Moran, 1978c). Although aFGF can stimulate endothelial cell proliferation, it is 30- to 100-fold less potent than bFGF (Macaig, Cerundolo, Isley, Kelley, & Forand, 1979; Lemmon et al., 1982; Bohlen et al., 1985).

Biological Activity

In Vitro Effects

Basic bFGF has both short- and long-term effects on the growth and morphology of responsive cells. Human skin fibroblasts, Balb/c 3T3 fibroblasts, and vascular endothelial and smooth muscle cells maintained in culture with bFGF become elongated and increase locomotory activity (Gospodarowicz & Moran, 1974, 1975; Gospodarowicz, Cheng, Lui, & Bohlen, 1984). FGF also induces membrane ruffling and reduces cell-substratum adhesion, which are indications of transformation in most responsive cell types (Figure 3.5; Gospodarowicz, 1984). bFGF was shown to be a potent mitogen for cells of mesodermal origin including mesothelial cells, fibroblasts, and vascular smooth muscle cells (Gospodarowicz, Massaglia, Cheng, Lui, & Bohlen, 1985; Gospodarowicz, 1986). Addition of bFGF to cultures of most cell types of mesodermal origin

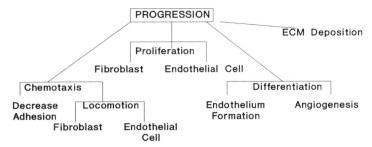

FIGURE 3.5. The activities involved in wound healing that are modulated by fibroblast growth factor.

greatly reduces the average doubling time through shortening of the G_1 phase (Gospodarowicz et al., 1985). bFGF also affects cell differentiation. Addition of bFGF to cultures of endothelial cells allows these cells to exhibit functional and morphological characteristics of endothelium in vivo (Vlodavsky & Gospodarowicz, 1979; Vlodavsky, Johnson, Greenburg, & Gospodarowicz, 1979; Greenburg, Vlodavsky, Foidart, & Gospodarowicz, 1980; Tseng, Savion, Stern, & Gospodarowicz, 1982). bFGF also delays the senescence of cultured cells, such as granulosa and adrenal cortical cells (Gospodarowicz & Bialicki, 1978; Simonian, Hornsby, Ill, O'Hare, & Gill, 1979).

Basic bFGF can control the synthesis and deposition of various components of the extracellular matrix (ECM) such as collagen, fibronectin and proteoglycans by chondrocytes and other cells (Gospodarowicz & Tauber, 1980; Gospodarowicz, Vlodavsky, & Savion, 1981; Gospodarowicz, 1983a; Kato & Gospodarowicz, 1985). Deposition of these matrices at the appropriate time following initiation of wound repair is essential to tissue integrity. bFGF can stimulate the production of plasminogen activator, a fibrinolytic enzyme, and collagenase by endothelial and carcinoma cells (further discussed in Chapters 7 and 8, respectively; (Mira, Lopez, Joseph-Silverstein, Rifkin, & Ossowski, 1986; Montesano, Vassalli, Baird, Guillemin, & Orci, 1986; Moscatelli, Presta, & Rifkin, 1986). Plasminogen activator catalyzes the cleavage of plasminogen to the active enzyme plasmin. Early production of plasmin and collagenase would be beneficial in the removal of fibrin and thereby allow more effective clearance of debris and tissue remodeling. bFGF may be instrumental in promoting wound repair through its effects on extracellular matrix production and protease secretion.

Besides stimulating cell proliferation and differentiation, bFGF was shown to have other regulatory effects. These include modulation of prolactin and growth hormone production as well as modulation of granulosa cell response to follicle-stimulating hormone (Johnson, Baxter, Vlodav-

sky, & Gospodarowicz, 1980; Schonbrunn, Krashoff, Westerdorf, & Tashyan, 1980; Mondschein & Schomberg, 1981; Adashi, Resnick, Bergeman,
& Gospodarowicz, 1987).

In Vivo Effects

Basic bFGF may be instrumental in the induction of mesoderm during
embryonic development, in limb regeneration, in the early development
of the nervous system, in wound healing, and in angiogenesis.

During embryonic development, the mesoderm is induced from the
animal hemisphere by signals or morphogens from the vegetal region of
the zygote (Nieuwkoop 1969; Smith, Dale, & Slack, 1985). Exposure of
explants from the animal pole of stage 8 *Xenopus* blastulae to bFGF
facilitated differentiation of mesodermal structures (Slack, Darlington,
Heath, & Godsave, 1987). Therefore, bFGF may act as an early embryologic differentiation factor to induce mesoderm formation. In am-
phibian models of amputation and regeneration it was shown that the
administration of bFGF promoted the formation of heteromorphic limb
regeneration through the recruitment (Gospodarowicz & Mescher, 1981)
and mitogenesis of blastoma cells (Gospodarowicz et al., 1978c; Mescher,
Gospodarowicz, & Moran, 1979).

Basic bFGF may also be involved in the early development of the
nervous system. It initiates neurite outgrowth, promotes the growth and
survival of nerve cells, and leads to the expression of cholinergic differentiation in culture (Togari, Dickens, Huzuya, & Guroff, 1985; Morrison,
Sharma, DeVeillis, & Bradshaw, 1986; Wagner & D'Amore, 1986; Walicke, Cowan, Ueno, Baird, & Guillemin, 1986). In addition, FGF-like
activity is present in the mesencephalic and telencephalic regions of the
brain in the embryo during the time when neural mass is increasing
(Risau, 1986).

Mechanism of Action

All cells that respond to FGF bear specific FGF cell surface receptors
(Figure 3.3); aFGF and bFGF share the same receptor and can displace
one another from their binding sites (Neufeld & Gospodarowicz, 1986).
Cell surface–bound FGF is slowly internalized and does not appear to
be degraded after internalization (Neufeld & Gospodarowicz, 1985; Olwin
& Hauschka, 1986). In contrast to other growth factors, tyrosine phosphorylation of the receptor cannot be readily detected following FGF
binding (Neufeld & Gospodarowicz, 1985), suggesting that the FGF receptor may lack tyrosine kinase activity. Following binding of FGF to
its receptor, diacylglycerol formation, protein kinase C activation, and
Ca^{2+} mobilization are induced within minutes (Tsuda, Kaibuchi, Kawahara, Fukuzaki, & Takai, 1985; Kaibuchi, et al., 1986). Within 3 hours

after binding, FGF increases lectin receptor mobility (which may be associated with increased locomotion observed with FGF), membrane fluidity and ruffling (Gospodarowicz, Brown, Birdwell, & Zetter, 1978a; Gospodarowicz et al., 1978b; 1979a). The pleiotropic responses that occur following addition of FGF to 3T3 fibroblasts includes stimulation of cellular transport systems, polyribosome formation, ribosomal and transfer RNA synthesis, DNA synthesis, and oncogene expression. FGF stimulates the synthesis and release of the glycoprotein proliferin as well as many other proteins including the so-called superinducible protein (Nilsen-Hamilton, Shapiro, Massoglia, & Hamilton, 1980; Nilsen-Hamilton, Hamilton, Allen, & Massoglia, 1981; Hamilton, Nilsen-Hamilton, & Adams, 1985; Parfett et al., 1985). Together with these changes, FGF stimulates DNA synthesis and cell division. Like other growth factors, FGF appears to be a competence factor that allows responsiveness of cells to transferrin and high-density lipoproteins (progression factors) (Jiminez de Asua, O'Farrell, Clinigan, & Rudland, 1977; Stiles et al., 1979; Gospodarowicz, 1983b). bFGF induces the rapid appearance of c-*fos* and c-*myc*, cellular oncogenes associated with cell differentiation (Armelin et al., 1984; Mueller, Bravo, Burkshardt, & Curran, 1984).

Wound Healing

A few studies on the effects of bFGF on wound healing have been conducted. One study showed that bFGF increased incisional tensile strength in rats (McGee et al., 1988). After a single injection of bFGF into a sponge implanted subcutaneously in rats, fibroblasts and dilated capillaries were present at earlier time points than in control rats (Davidson et al., 1988). In a nude mouse model using grafted human skin, bFGF was actually deleterious to epithelialization (Cooper et al., 1991).

Peritoneum

The effect of FGF on the proliferation of peritoneal TRCs has also been examined (Table 3.1). From the biologic actions described above, it was conceivable that FGF could elevate the proliferation of TRCs directly. TRCs were harvested at various days after surgery and placed in culture, and the incorporation of thymidine was quantified. FGF stimulated the incorporation of thymidine into TRCs (Figure 3.4). As with EGF, the response of postsurgical days 7 and 10 TRCs to FGF was greater than that of postsurgical days 2 and 5. Again FGF, may function as a competence factor participating in the transition of cells from G_0 to S phase.

Summary

FGF may modulate wound healing through increasing the proliferation of cell types involved in the wound healing process, such as endothelial cells and fibroblasts, and the induction of new blood vessel formation, i.e., angiogenesis and modulation of the production of extracellular matrix and proteases.

Platelet-Derived Growth Factor

Platelet-derived growth factor (PDGF) was identified in 1975 as a mitogenic factor present in whole blood–derived serum but absent in plasma-derived serum (Kohler & Lipton, 1974; Ross, Glomset, Kariya, & Harker, 1974). The sources of PDGF-dependent mitogenic activity include platelets, neoplastic cells, activated vascular endothelial cells, and monocyte-macrophages (Ross, Raines, & Bowen-Pope, 1986; Libby, Warner, Salomon, & Birinyi, 1988). The molecular weight of PDGF is approximately 30,000 d. PDGF has an isoelectric point of pH 9.8 to 10 and is a hydrophobic molecule. The protein is a heterodimer of two highly disulfide-linked peptides (A-chain and B chain), which are approximately 60% homologous to one another (Deuel & Huang, 1983; Heldin & Westermark, 1984; Ross et al., 1986; Deuel, 1987; Ross, 1986). The amino acid sequence of the PDGF B-chain has a 96% homology with p28 sis, the protein product of the oncogene v-*sis* (Doolittle et al., 1983; Waterfield, et al., 1985).

Biological Activity

PDGF is a potent mitogen for mesenchymally derived connective-tissue–forming cells, such as fibroblasts or smooth muscle cells. PDGF inhibits the binding of some growth factors on some cell types, i.e., EGF to fibroblasts (Figure 3.6; Wrann, Fox, & Ross, 1980; Collins, Sinnett-Smith, & Rozengurt, 1983; Decker & Harris, 1989). PDGF is also chemotactic for the same cells in which it induces proliferation (Grotendorst, Chang, Seppa, Kleinman, & Martin, 1982). When it binds to cells, PDGF induces

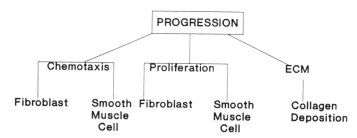

FIGURE 3.6. The activities involved in wound healing that are modulated by platelet-derived growth factor.

increased expression of several genes including c-*fos*, c-*myc*, and β-interferon genes (Stiles, 1983; Zullo, Cochran, Huang, & Stiles, 1985). PDGF also induces reorganization of actin and cell shape changes that may be involved in mitogenesis.

In addition to inducing proliferation and chemotaxis, PDGF stimulates the synthesis of cholesterol and expression of low-density lipoprotein receptors. PDGF also increases prostaglandin (PG) PGE_2 synthesis through two separate mechanisms: increased arachidonic acid production and cyclooxygenase synthesis (Habernicht et al., 1986). PDGF is also a potent vasoconstrictive agent through induction of smooth muscle contraction (Berk, Alexander, Brock, Gimbrone, & Webb, 1986).

Sources of PDGF

Although PDGF was originally isolated from the alpha granule of platelets, PDGF can be isolated from a variety of cell types and its production can be induced by a variety of stimuli. PDGF is released with a variety of other constituents as a result of platelet aggregation. Nonactivated monocytes do not express the gene for PDGF. However, when monocytes are stimulated to differentiate into macrophages, such as in inflammatory events like healing, they secrete PDGF (Shimokado et al., 1985). When monocytes are activated by various stimuli such as lipopolysaccharide, concanavalin A, zymosan, or attachment to plastic, they secrete PDGF. Messenger ribonucleic acid (mRNA) levels in these cells correspond with their ability to secrete PDGF (Martinet et al., 1986). A number of diploid cells are able to secrete PDGF. Arterial endothelial cells can release PDGF when stimulated with coagulation factors (DiCorleto & Bowen-Pope, 1983; Gajusek, Carbon, Ross, Nawroth, & Stern, 1986). PDGF is secreted upon culture of vascular endothelium (Barrett, Gajdusek, Schwartz, McDougall, & Benditt, 1984). Cultured smooth muscle cells from atherosclerotic lesions also secrete PDGF (Libby et al., 1988). Interleukin-1 (IL-1) can induce gene expression for PDGF-A in fibroblasts, which in turn causes the secretion of a homodimer of PDGF-A that stimulates proliferation in an autocrine fashion. Using in situ hybridization, Goustin, Betscholtz, Pfeiffer-Ohlsson, Persson, & Ryndert (1985) were able to show expression of a PDGF-like molecule by cytotrophoblast in developing placenta.

Mechanism of Action

PDGF induces its biological effects through binding to cell-surface receptors (Figure 3.3; Bowen-Pope & Ross, 1985). Through cross linking experiments, the PDGF receptor was identified as a 180 kd membrane glycoprotein with an intracellular domain containing a tyrosine kinase. The receptor consists of two subunits (α and β) that are brought together by the chains of the PDGF dimer (Seifert et al., 1989). The configuration of the receptor depends upon the chains that make up the protein. That is, the α-subunit of the receptor can bind to either the A- or B-chain, whereas the β-subunit can only bind the B-chain. In addition, various cell types have different levels of the receptor subunits and therefore the type of PDGF that can bind varies from cell to cell.

There are immunoglobulin-like domains that bind PDGF on the extracellular portion of the receptor. On the intracellular domain, there is a tyrosine kinase that phosphorylates the receptor upon PDGF binding (Ek, Westermark, Wasteson, & Heldin, 1982). After binding, the receptors aggregate and internalize into endosomes and lysosomes where both the receptor and PDGF are degraded. PDGF initiates a series of intracellular events that leads to DNA synthesis. Cells traverse the cell cycle from the G_0/G_1 phase to the S phase (Ross et al., 1986). One of the first events that occurs is the hydrolysis of membrane phospholipids (phosphotidylinositol). Phospholipid breakdown leads to the formation of diglycerides, which in turn activate protein kinase C. PDGF binding also induces an increase in intracellular calcium ions (Westermark, Heldin, Ek, & Westermark, 1983).

Wound Healing

Initial studies of PDGF on wound healing examined subcutaneously implanted wound chambers. These studies show that PDGF enhances the rate of new tissue formation as measured by an influx of connective tissue cells, an increase in DNA synthesis, and an increase in collagen deposition (Figure 3.6; Grotendorst et al., 1985). Further studies demonstrated that addition of partially purified PDGF to skin injuries (0.5 mm thick, which removes epidermis and superficial dermis) accelerated wound healing. In this study, the wounds were treated 7 days after injury. Application of purified PDGF did not affect the amount of new tissue that occurred but slightly increased cell density. However, when PDGF was applied in combination with EGF and insulin-like growth factor (IGF-I) an increase occurred in the width of new epidermis, and connective tissue and thicker epidermis formed. Addition of partially purified PDGF to day-4 wounds increased the cellular and extracellular components of the wound (Lynch, Nixon, Colvin, & Antoniades, 1987). These studies indicate that synergistic interactions between growth factors may be more beneficial in the promotion of wound healing.

Studies using recombinant PDGF showed that a single application of PDGF-BB increased the strength of skin incisions and increased the number of macrophages and fibroblasts (Pierce et al., 1988b, 1989a). In rats treated with depo-type steroids to inhibit wound healing, PDGF-BB (homodimer) did not affect the breaking strength of skin incisions (Pierce et al., 1989b). In contrast, PDGF-BB did improve skin closure of full-thickness skin excisions in rats treated with cortisone acetate (Engrav, Richey, Kao, & Murray, 1989). Treatment of full-thickness skin wounds in diabetic mice was accelerated following repeated administration of PDGF-AB or PDGF-BB (Sprugel, Greenhalgh, Murray, & Ross, 1991).

Peritoneum

The effect of PDGF on the proliferation of cultured TRC harvested at various postsurgical days was also studied (Table 3.1). PDGF stimulated the proliferation of day 10 TRCs but to a lesser extent than EGF and FGF (Figure 3.4). PDGF is known to stimulate the proliferation of fibroblasts (130% of control levels) especially under conditions of confluent cultures. The effect of PDGF on proliferation is thought to induce the entry of G_0-arrested cells into the proliferative phase of the cell cycle. TRCs may be undergoing a mitotic cycle and therefore do not manifest as great a response to the addition of PDGF.

Summary

Wound healing involves the coordinated interaction of several types of cells. PDGF is chemotactic and mitogenic for fibroblasts and smooth muscles cells. Since replacement of these cells on the traumatized surface is essential to wound healing, through promoting these activities PDGF may aid in the wound closure processes.

Interleukin-1

Several different laboratories isolated interleukin-1 (IL-1) over a period of 20 years using a variety of bioassays. Due to the pleiotropic nature of these bioassays and the variety of organ systems affected (i.e., induction of fever [brain], hepatic acute phase protein synthesis [liver], neutrophilia [bone marrow], and activation of lymphocyte proliferation [immune system]), there was a great deal of controversy as to whether or not this molecule was the same or a family of proteins that were co-purified (Murphy, Chesney, & Wood, 1974; Dinarello, Renfer, & Wolff, 1977; Rosenwasser, Dinarello, & Rosenthal, 1979; McAdam & Dinarello, 1980; Murphy, Simon, & Willoughby, 1980; Saklatvala, Sarsfield, & Townsend, 1985; Matsushima, Kimball, Durum, & Oppenheim, 1985). It was not until 1984 when the molecular cloning of IL-1 was accomplished (Auron et al., 1984, Lomedico et al., 1984) and these activities produced by the recombinant molecule that the controversy was resolved. Two forms of IL-1 were identified by molecular cloning: IL-1α (pI 5) and IL-1β (pI 7) (March et al., 1985). The two forms of IL-1 are initially synthesized as 31-kd precursor polypeptides and share only small sequences of homology. Despite the lack of homology, both forms of IL-1 have structural similarities, such as similar precursor sizes, potential glycosylation sites, and polybasic regions. In addition, they bind the same receptor on all cell types thus far examined (Dower et al., 1985; Furutani et al., 1985; Van Damme, DeLey, Opdenakker, Biliau, & DeSomer, 1985; Dower & Urdal, 1987). These IL-1s are processed from their precursor molecules to their 17-kd mature forms (Giri, Lomedico, & Mizel, 1985; Limjuco et al., 1986). IL-1 has significant sequence homology with aFGF and bFGF, another set of molecules that share function and receptors and exist in both an acidic (pI 5) and basic (pI 7) form.

By examining the relative mRNA levels for IL-1α and IL-1β in human macrophages using Northern blot analyses, it was determined that there are two independent mechanisms regulating expression of mRNA. IL-1β is expressed constitutively, and much more IL-1β than IL-1α is produced upon polyclonal stimulation (March et al., 1985; Matsushima, Taguchi, Kovacs, Young, & Oppenheim, 1986a; Demczuk, Baumberger, Mach, & Dayer, 1987; Fenton et al., 1987). However, in murine peritoneal exudate cells stimulated by adherence to lipopolysaccharide, expression of IL-1α and IL-1β is concurrent and transient (Fulbrigge, Chaplin, Kiely, & Unanue, 1987). IL-1β gene expression can be induced simply by adherence of the macrophages to plastic, further stimulated by interferon and lipopolysaccharide or superinduced by the addition of cycloheximide to culture of macrophage-like lines (Mizel & Mizel, 1981; Arenzana-Seisdedos & Virelizier, 1983; Arend, D'Angelo, Massoni, & Joslin, 1985a; Arenzana-Seisdedos, Virelizier, & Fiers, 1985; Newton, 1985; Burchett et al., 1988; Haskill, Johnson, Eierman, Becker, & Warren, 1988; Arend et al., 1989).

The secretion of IL-1 is also highly regulated. First, neither form of IL-1 contains a signal peptide sequence and unlike most secretory proteins, IL-1 accumulates within the cell (Luger, Stadler, Katz, & Oppenheim, 1981; March et al., 1985; Auron et al., 1987). Both forms of IL-1 (precursor and mature) are secreted simultaneously and secretion is delayed compared to that of peptides with a signal sequence, such as tumor necrosis factor (Hazuda, Lee, & Young, 1988). IL-1 may leak out of monocytes following activation due to compromised cell viability (Giri & Lepe-Zuniya, 1983). However, pulse-chase experiments indicate this is not the case (Hazuda et al., 1988). Incubation of the precursor form of IL-1β with membranes from human monocytes or purified proteases cleaves the protein to the mature, biologically active forms of 17 to 19 kD (Black et al., 1988). In addition, treatment of IL-1–producing cells with trypsin or plasmin will release biologically active IL-1 presumably from the exposed outer surface of the cell (Matsushima et al., 1986a; Conlon et al., 1987). Therefore, secretion of IL-1 may require cleavage of membrane-bound IL-1 by proteases.

Biological Activity

IL-1 is a pleiotropic molecule; a multiplicity of factors isolated by a number of bioassays are now known to be IL-1. Both forms of IL-1 affect a variety of organ systems. They augment T cell responses, induce fever, induce hepatic acute phase protein synthesis, induce sleep, and enhance histamine release from basophils or eosinophil degranulation (reviewed by Dinarello et al., 1986a; Pincus, Whitcomb, & Dinarello, 1986). IL-1s are secreted from a variety of cell types including monocytes and macrophages, dendritic cells, Langerhans cells, B cells, endothelial cells, mesangial cells, astrocytes, neutrophils, fibroblasts, and epithelial cells, and they affect a variety of cell types and organ systems (Gery & Waksman, 1972; Chuo, Francis, & Atkins, 1977; Farr, Dorf, & Unanue, 1977; Luger et al., 1981; Fontana, Kristinsen, Pub, Gemsa, & Weber, 1982; Iribe, Koga, Kotani, Kusumoto, & Shiba, 1983; Lovett, Ryan, & Sterzel, 1983; Gahring, Baltz, Pepys, & Daynes, 1984; Gilman, Rosenberg, & Feldman, 1984; Goto, Nakamura, Goto, & Myoshinagu, 1984; Durum, Higuchi, & Ron, 1984; Sauder, Dinarello, & Morhenn, 1984a; Arend et al., 1985a; Duff et al., 1984). The secretion of IL-1, along with several other cytokines, is elevated during acute or chronic inflammatory events, such as bacterial infection, and may account for many of the acute symptoms of infection.

Effects on Hepatic and Central Nervous System Function

Alterations in hepatic protein synthesis occur following exposure of hepatocytes to IL-1. IL-1 induces the synthesis of acute phase proteins, such as serum amyloid A (SAA), C-reactive proteins (CRP), complement components, and some clotting factors and protease inhibitors. In contrast, IL-1 decreases the synthesis of albumin and transferrin by hepatocytes (Perlmutter, Goldberger, Dinarello, Mizel, & Colten, 1986a; Perlmutter, Dinarello, Punsal, & Colten, 1986b). Recombinant IL-1 was shown to regulate the synthesis of these proteins through alterations in the rate of mRNA transcription (Ramadori, Sipes, Dinarello, Mizel, & Colter, 1985). IL-1 also suppresses the activity of liver cytochrome P-450 mixed function oxidases and increases the synthesis of metalloproteins (Ghezzi et al., 1986).

IL-1 also affects the central nervous system through the induction of monophasic fever and the release of ACTH (Dinarello, 1985; Matsushima, Kimball, Durum, & Oppenheim, 1985a; Bernton, Beach, Holaday, Smallbridge, & Fein, 1987). In addition, IL-1 stimulates the secretion of corticotropin releasing factor from hypothalamic neurons (Sapolsky, Rivier, Yamamoto, Plotsky, & Vale, 1987). IL-1 also induces an increase in slow wave sleep in rabbits (Kreuger, Walter, Dinarello, Wolff, & Chedid, 1984).

Effects on Endothelial Cells and Fibroblasts

IL-1 induces changes in cells central to the progress of wound repair (i.e., endothelial cells and fibroblasts; Figure 3.7). The alterations in endothelial cell function may be correlated with the development of pathological lesions in vascular tissue. IL-1 may alter fibroblast function in such a way as to contribute to the development of fibrosis. IL-1 stimulates the proliferation of fibroblasts either through direct stimulation of DNA synthesis or through the induction of receptors for growth factors such as EGF and TGF-α (Schmidt, Mizel, Cohen, & Green, 1982; Estes, Pledger, & Gillespie, 1984). Alternatively, other studies found that addition of PDGF or prostaglandins to cultures of quiescent fibroblasts enhanced IL-1 receptor expression (Akahoshi, Oppenheim, & Matsushima, 1988; Bonin & Singh, 1988). Through the stimulation of fibroblast and endothelial cell proliferation, IL-1 could promote more rapid repair of healing wounds.

Arachidonic acid metabolism by both endothelial cells and fibroblasts is also modulated by IL-1. The synthesis and release of prostaglandin PGI_2 and PGE_2, both potent vasodilators, by endothelial cells is elevated following exposure to IL-1 (Rossi, Breviario, Ghezzi, Dejana, & Montovani, 1985; Dejana et al., 1987). IL-1α and IL-1β augment the synthesis and elaboration of PG, in particular PGE_2, from confluent fibroblasts in culture (Bernheim & Dinarello, 1985; Wood et al., 1985; Zucali et al., 1986; Elias, Gustilo, Baeder, & Freundlich, 1987). PGs are thought to mediate many of the inflammatory events observed following in vivo administration of IL-1. PGs, in addition to causing vasodilation, can modulate leukocyte chemotaxis and function, and induce edema formation and platelet aggregation. Therefore, PGs, and in turn IL-1 indirectly, can affect wound repair at several different stages. PGs can also inhibit cell proliferation, thereby providing a feedback loop for the regulation of enhanced cell proliferation from IL-1 exposure.

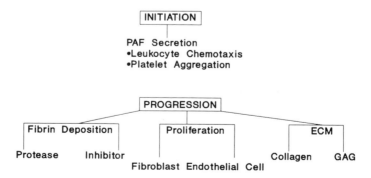

FIGURE 3.7. The activities involved in wound healing that are modulated by interleukin-1.

IL-1 also contributes to the mediation of inflammatory events through stimulating the release of platelet activating factor (PAF) by endothelial cells (Figure 3.7; Dejana et al., 1988). PAF is a lipid that induces aggregatory and secretory responses in platelets (Demopoulos, Pinckard, & Hanahan, 1979, McManus, Fitzpatrick, Hanahan, & Pinckard, 1983). PAF can also induce acute allergic and inflammatory reactions. In vivo PAF induces rapid neutropenia and in vitro studies show that PAF induces PMN chemotaxis, aggregation, secretion and respiratory burst (McManus, Hanahan, Demopoulos, & Pinckard, 1980; Pinckard et al., 1980; Shaw, Pinckard, Ferrigni, McManus, & Hanahan, 1981; Smith, Bowman, & Iden, 1984). PAF also initiates a dose-dependent aggregation of human peripheral blood monocytes (Yasaka, Boxer, & Baehner, 1982). In contrast to the effects of PAF on PMN function, it has little, if any, effect on monocyte respiratory burst and chemotaxis (Yasaka et al., 1982; Czarnetzki, 1983). On the other hand, PAF does enhance respiratory burst and arachidonic acid metabolism of differentiated macrophages (Hartung, 1983; Hartung, Parnham, Winkelmann, Engleberger, & Hadding, 1983; Bachelet, Masliah, Vargeftig, Bereziat, & Colard, 1986). IL-1 induces adherence of endothelial cells for both neutrophils and lymphocytes and causes the expression of endothelial activation antigens (Bevilacqua, Pober, Wheeler, Cotran, Gimbrone, 1985; Cavender, Haskard, Joseph, & Ziff, 1986; Pohlman, Stanness, Beatty, Ochs, & Harlon, 1986; Pober et al., 1986a). The increase in neutrophil adherance for endothelial cells following exposure to IL-1 may be instrumental in modulating the wound healing process. Therefore endothelial cell activation by IL-1 may be requisite to an inflammatory response.

IL-1 also modulates the secretion of components of the extracellular matrix and proteases that degrade and remodel these matrices by several types of cells. IL-1 directly increases the transcription of mRNAs for types I, III, and IV collagens by fibroblasts and epithelial cells (Krane, Dayer, Simon, & Byrne, 1985; Matsushima, Bano, Kidwell, & Oppenheim, 1985b; Canalis, 1986). In addition, IL-1 stimulates the synthesis of glycosaminoglycans, especially hyaluronate, by fibroblasts (Bronson, Bentilami, & Siebert, 1987). These data indicate that IL-1 may be essential in the remodeling of repaired tissue.

IL-1 also modulates protease and protease inhibitor synthesis by endothelial cells and fibroblasts in such a way as to increase fibrin deposition. That is, IL-1 will increase the secretion of plasminogen activator (PA) inhibitors by both fibroblasts and endothelial cells. IL-1 induces procoagulant activity on the surface of endothelial cells and increases the production of PA inhibitor (PAI), which inhibits formation of plasmin from plasminogen, by endothelial cells (Bevilacqua, Pober, Majeau, Contran, & Gimbrone, 1984; Bevilacqua et al., 1985; Bevilacqua, Schleef, Gimbrone, & Laskutoff, 1986a; Emeis & Kooestra, 1986; Nachman, Hajjar, Silverstein, & Dinarello, 1986; Nawroth, Handley, Esmon, &

Stern, 1986a; Dejana et al., 1987). IL-1 also increases the production of PA and PAI secretion by fibroblast synoviocytes and chondrocytes (Bunning et al., 1987; Leizer et al., 1987; Medcalf & Hamilton, 1986; Michel & Quertermous, 1989) and decreases the production of PA. IL-1 was shown to induce collagenase secretion by synovial cells and fibroblasts and metalloproteinases from chondrocytes (Postlethwaite, Lachman, Mainardi, & Kang, 1983; Krane et al., 1985; McCroskery, Arai, Amento, & Krane, 1985; Balavoine et al., 1986; Schnyder, Payne, & Dinarello, 1987; Stephenson et al., 1987). IL-1 modulates the fibrinolytic system in such a way as to reduce fibrin clearance. Prolonged fibrin deposition may allow the organization of fibrin by fibroblasts and mesothelial cells and hence increase the possibility of adhesion formation (Herschlag et al., 1991).

Effects of IL-1 on Host Immune System

IL-1 was isolated by recombinant DNA technology using T-cell activation as a bioassay and was subsequently found to have all the functions described above. IL-1 is central to the generation of an immune response. IL-1, along with other stimuli, can activate T cells, as measured by proliferation, IL-2 production, and IL-2 receptor expression, and B cells, as measured by proliferation, IL-6 production, and antibody synthesis (Kaye et al., 1984; Muraguchi, Kehrl, Butler, & Fauci, 1984; Herman, Dinarello, Kew, & Rabson, 1985; Davis & Lipsky, 1986; Libby et al., 1986a; Lowenthal, Cerrottini, & MacDonald, 1986; Matsushima et al., 1985a; Van Damme & Billiau, 1987; Jelink & Lipsky, 1987). IL-1 also increases natural killer cell function (Hirano et al., 1986).

IL-1 induces secretion of many other cytokines involved in the immune response (Bagby et al., 1986; Broudy, Kaushansky, Harlan, & Adamson, 1987; Zucali et al., 1986; Zucali, Elfenbein, Barth, & Dinarello, 1987). In addition, IL-1 exerts effects on cells of myeloid lineage. IL-1 is a potent inducer of PMN infiltration in vivo and causes chemotaxis of PMNs in vitro (Luger, Charon, Colot, Micksche, & Oppenheim, 1983; Sauder, Mounessa, Katz, Dinarello, & Gallin, 1984b; Granstein, Margolis, Mizel, & Sauder, 1985; Beck, Habicht, Benach, & Miller, 1986; Sayers et al., 1988). IL-1 also stimulates basophil histamine release and neutrophil and eosinophil degranulation (Smith, Bowman, & Speziale, 1986; Subramanian & Bray, 1987). IL-1 can stimulate the release of PGE_2 from monocytes (Bonney & Humes, 1984; Boraschi & Tagliabue, 1984). Lastly, IL-1 induces the differentiation of macrophages (Hanazawa et al., 1988).

Systemic Effects

Most of the effects described above occur at the cellular level. Systemic administration, either through intraperitoneal or intravenous injection, mimics the introduction of endotoxin, including fever, and increasing levels of ACTH, cortisol, and acute phase proteins as well as blood neutrophils. Many of these responses may be beneficial in aiding the host in defense against a microbial infection. Acute changes, such as fever and neutrophilia, may help to defend against bacterial infection through slowing of microbial replication and enhancement of immune function. Subsequently, IL-1 also stimulates an immune response to the microbe through generalized humoral and cell-mediated immune responses.

Mechanism of Action

An 80-kd receptor for IL-1 was observed on a variety of cell lines (Dower et al., 1985; Kilian et al., 1986; Lowenthal & MacDonald, 1986; Matsushima, Akahoshi, Yamada, Furutani, & Oppenheim, 1986b; Bird & Saklatvala, 1987; Bron & MacDonald, 1987), and was subsequently purified and cloned using in situ hybridization (Sims et al., 1988; Urdal, Call, Jackson, & Dower, 1988). There is a second class of IL-1 receptor with a higher affinity than the 80-kd receptor. Since other IL-1 specific binding proteins were observed in cross-linking experiments, investigators are proposing a two polypeptide receptor complex similar to the IL-2 receptor, which has a high, intermediate, and low affinity configuration depending upon the combination of the polypeptides (Bird & Saklatvala, 1987; Kroggel, Martin, Pingoud, Dayer, & Resch, 1988).

Following binding of IL-1 to its receptor, a variety of biological responses rapidly occur (Figure 3.3). IL-1 may transduce the signal for ligand binding via a novel mechanism of phospholipid hydrolysis (Rosoff, Savage, & Dinarello, 1988). IL-1 binding to Jurkat cells stimulates the rapid release of diacylglycerol without increases in phosphatidylinositol turnover or inositol phosphate levels (Abraham, Ho, Barna, & McKean, 1987). However, phosphatidylcholine cleavage and release is elevated upon binding of IL-1 to its receptor. Once IL-1 has bound to its receptor, it is rapidly internalized and recycled. Following internalization of IL-1, the IL-1 receptor complex is shuttled to the lysosome where the IL-1 is degraded. It is still unknown if internalized IL-1 effects the cell activation required for some of the biological processes (Bird & Saklatvala, 1987).

Inhibitors of IL-1

The function of IL-1 could be inhibited at several sites. Receptor binding antagonists or factors that interfere with the intracellular pathways used by IL-1 could inhibit IL-1 function. A competitive inhibitor of IL-1 binding to cells was purified from the urine of patients with monocytic leukemia (Seckinger, Lowenthal, Williamson, Dayer, & MacDonald, 1987). Uromodulin is an immunosuppressive protein isolated from the urine of pregnant women that inhibits IL-1 activity through binding to the IL-

1 (Muchmore & Decker, 1985, 1986; Brown, 1986). Inhibitors of IL-1 activity have also been purified from the culture medium of a myelomonocytic cell line and stimulated human peripheral blood monocytes or macrophages (Arend, Joslin, & Massoni, 1985b; Rodgers, Scott, Mundin, & Sissons, 1985; Balavoine et al., 1986; Barak et al., 1986; Roberts, Prill, & Mann, 1986a; Berman, Sandberg, Calabia, Andrews, & Friou, 1987). A punitive IL-1 inhibitor was found constitutively in culture medium from PMNs (Tiku, Tiku, Liu, & Skosey, 1986). Secretory products from keratinocytes and submandibular glands were also shown to block IL-1 function (Kemp, Mellow, & Sabbadini, 1986; Schwartz, Urbanska, Gschnait, & Luger, 1987; Walsh, Lander, Seymour, & Powell, 1987).

Wound Healing

There are no data published on the effects of IL-1 on dermal wound healing.

Peritoneum

The effects of IL-1 on the proliferation and level of protein synthesis of TRCs harvested at various postsurgical days has been examined (Fukasawa, Yanagihara, Rodgers, & diZerega, 1989). In this study of TRC, IL-1α did not stimulate proliferation, but did stimulate protein synthesis (Table 3.1). Thus IL-1 may function as an initiation factor similar to PDGF.

More recent studies showed that in vitro exposure to IL-1 can enhance the secretion of PA and PAI from rabbit peritoneal macrophages harvested following peritoneal surgery (Figures 3.8 and 3.9; Kuraoka, Campeau, Rodgers, Nakamura, & diZerega, 1992). At early postoperative times, higher levels of IL-1 were necessary to elevate these activities. However, at later times after surgery, IL-1 modulated PA and PAI activity in a dose-dependent manner with as little as 3 U/ml, which is within the range of spontaneous secretion of IL-1 by postsurgical macrophages.

IL-1 was implicated in adhesion formation. As can be seen in Table 3.2, administration of IL-1α in conjunction with 16 Gy of total abdominal irradiation, which caused adhesion in 57% of the mice when given alone, resulted in adhesion formation in 100% of the mice (McBride, Mason, Withers, & Davis, 1989). In addition, it was shown that administration of IL-1 can potentiate adhesions resulting from cecal abrasion, but injection of IL-1 into nonsurgical rats did not lead to adhesion formation (Herschlag et al., 1991).

Summary

IL-1 is a pleiotropic cytokine that can modulate wound repair at a variety of levels. IL-1 modulates the production of PG, collagenase, PA, and PAI

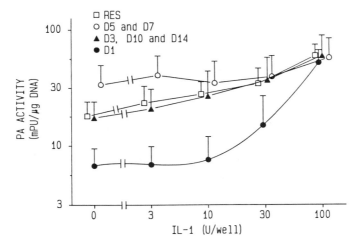

FIGURE 3.8. Composite graph of the plasminogen activator (PA) activity of macrophages recovered from the peritoneal cavity of rabbits after surgery, as a function of varying concentrations of IL-1. The units are defined by a thymocyte comitogen assay. Each point (□, day 0 or resident; ●, day 1; ○, days 5 and 7; △, days 3, 10, and 14 after peritoneal surgery) represents the geometric mean ± SD of four or five replicate experiments. (From Kuraoka et al., 1992. Reproduced by permission of Academic Press.)

by a number of cells and induces proliferation in many of these cells. IL-1 also mediates many of the acute inflammatory events that occur after trauma and stimulates host defense mechanisms against microbial infection. There are no published studies that show that IL-1 accelerates the healing of skin wounds. Although, IL-1 did not stimulate TRC proliferation, it did modulate protease and protease inhibitor secretion of postsurgical macrophages.

Tumor Necrosis Factor

Tumor necrosis factor (TNF) is another polypeptide that is pleiotropic and shares many functions with IL-1. TNF is also thought to be a primary mediator in the pathogenesis of infection, inflammation, and host defense. When TNF was cloned it was found to be identical with cachectin, a molecule important in the pathogenesis of cachexia (Carswell et al., 1975; Beutler et al., 1985a, 1985b; Pennica, Hayflick, Bringham, Palladino, & Goeddal, 1985; Caput et al., 1986). TNF is produced as a prohormone of 233 amino acids and processed to a mature peptide of 157 residues and a molecular weight of 17 kd (Shirai, Yamaguchi, Ito, Todd, & Wallace, 1985; Beutler & Cerami, 1986). TNF shares 28% homology

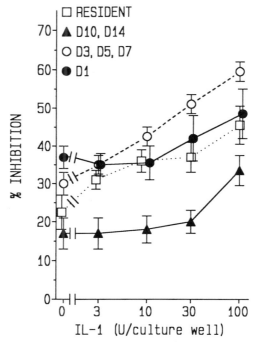

FIGURE 3.9. Composite graph of the percentage inhibition of PA activity (% PAI) in macrophage-spent media cultured with varying concentrations of IL-1. Macrophages were recovered from the peritoneal cavity of rabbits at different days after peritoneal surgery. Each point (□, day 0 or resident; ●, day 1; ○, days 3, 5, and 7; △, days 10 and 14) represents means ± SEM of four or five replicate experiments. (From Kuraoka et al., 1992. Reproduced by permission of Academic Press.)

at the protein level with lymphotoxin (Gray et al., 1984; Pennica et al., 1984; Aggarwal, Eessalu, & Hass, 1985). TNF and lymphotoxin share some biological activities and a common receptor (Aggarwal et al., 1985). The benefit or detriment of TNF to the host depends upon the concentration of the peptide. At low concentration TNF may mediate some tissue remodeling and inflammatory events but at high concentrations TNF will cause irreversible shock and tissue damage.

Biological Activity

As stated, TNF is a pleiotropic hormone with many of the same functions as IL-1 (Figure 3.10). Early studies identified TNF as an agent that is released during bacterial infection leading to tumor necrosis (Coley, 1893; Shear, 1944; O'Malley, Achinstein, & Shear, 1962; Naut, 1980). Intra-

TABLE 3.2. Effect of timing of IL-1α administration on survival and adhesion formation after total body irradiation.

Treatment	No surviving (%)	Median time to death (days)[a]	Incidence of adhesions (%)[b]
TAI + saline IP, −1 h[c]	70	54	57.1
TAI + IL-1α, −3 days[c]	60	53	83.3
TAI + IL-1α, −20 h	30	15	66.7
TAI + IL-1α, −4 h	10	8	100
TAI + IL-1α, +4 h	70	41	85.7
TAI + IL-1α, +1 day	30	54	100
TAI + IL-1α, +4 days	90	54	33.3

TAI, total abdominal irradiation; +, time after irradiation; −, time before irradiation.
[a]Groups of 10 mice received 16 Gy of total body irradiation and the stated treatments. The number surviving (%) on day 88 is shown along with the median time to death.
[b]The incidence of adhesions in the survivors 88 days after irradiation.
[c]IL-1α (10^3 units) was given IP in 0.2-ml volumes of saline diluent at the stated times (McBride et al., 1989).

venous injection of endotoxin, which leads to secretion of TNF, produces fever, myalgia, headache, and nausea coincident with a peak in serum TNF levels (Hesse et al., 1988). Administration of larger quantities of endotoxin or endotoxin-free recombinant TNF leads to lethal tissue injury and fatal shock (Tracey et al., 1986, 1987). Many of the biologic effects of TNF at the cellular level described below correlate with the systemic effects of TNF.

Source of TNF

TNF is synthesized by a variety of activated phagocytic and nonphagocytic cells, including macrophages, natural killer cells, astrocytes, and microglial cells. A wide variety of infectious or inflammatory stimuli, i.e., endotoxin, complement protein 5a, IL-1, etc., will trigger TNF syn-

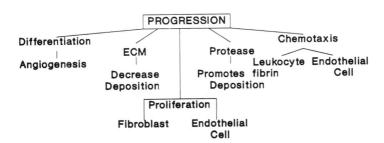

FIGURE 3.10. The activities involved in wound healing that are modulated by tumor necrosis factor.

thesis. Alternatively, the anti-inflammatory agent dexamethasone inhibits the synthesis of TNF if given concurrently with other stimuli (Beutler, Tkacenko, Milsark, Krockin, & Cerami, 1986). In addition, the secreted form of TNF can be found cell-associated in a transmembrane form or through binding to a TNF receptor (Bakouche, Ichinose, Heicappell, Fidler, & Lachman, 1989; Kriegler, Perez, DeFay, Albert, & Lu, 1988).

Modulation of Hemostasis by TNF

TNF was shown to alter the hemostatic properties of vascular endothelium (Pober, 1987). This occurs through many avenues including production of procoagulant activity and inhibition of cell-surface thrombomodulin (Bevilacqua et al., 1986b; Nawroth & Stern, 1986). This may enhance coagulation and lead to disseminated intravascular coagulation. Exposure of endothelial cells to TNF also alters expression of adhesion molecules and IL-1 production (Collins, Lapierre, Riers, Strominger, & Prober, 1986; Libby et al., 1986a, 1986b; Nawroth et al., 1986a, 1986b; Pober et al., 1986a, 1986b; Pohlman et al., 1986). This increase in coagulation potential for endothelial cells following exposure to TNF may contribute to hemorrhagic necrosis of tumors.

Cachexia

As stated above, TNF was shown to be identical to the molecule cachectin, which induces cachexia. Studies of cellular energy balance showed that adipocytes and skeletal myocytes become very catabolic, i.e., net lipolysis and glycogenolysis, respectively, when incubated with TNF (Guy, 1975; Torti, Dieckmann, Beutler, Cerami, & Ringold, 1987; Lee, Zentella, Pekala, & Cerami, 1987). Hepatocytes produce increased levels of acute-phase proteins and take up elevated levels of amino acids in response to TNF (Warren, Donner, Starnes, & Brennan, 1987). Animals chronically exposed to TNF become anorexic, lose weight, and become depleted in whole-body protein and lipid (Oliff et al., 1987; Tracey et al., 1988). These metabolic alterations may be beneficial during the acute phase of an infection to mobilize energy stores that meet the increased synthetic demands of the host defense systems, but may be detrimental when the stimulation becomes chronic.

TNF as an Inflammatory Mediator

TNF is an endogenous pyrogen capable of inducing fever both through a direct effect on the hypothalamus and through the induction of IL-1 production (Dinarello, Cannon, & Wolff, 1986b). TNF, like IL-1, is able to act as an osteoclast-activating factor and to induce PGE_2 and collagenase secretion by synovial cells (Dayer, Beutler, & Cerami, 1985; Bertolini, Nedwin, Bringman, Smith, & Mundy, 1986). TNF also activates

PMNs and induces differentiation of certain myeloid cell lines (Gamble, Harlan, Klebanoff, & Vadas, 1985; Shalaby et al., 1985; Takeda et al., 1986; Trinchieri et al., 1986; Nathan, 1987).

TNF has opposing activities on hematopoiesis. TNF can induce the production of granulocyte-macrophage colony-stimulating factor by a variety of cell types (Munker, Gasson, Ogawa, & Koeffler, 1986). However, TNF can inhibit the expression of a variety of bone marrow progenitors including granulocyte-macrophage, erythroid and erythroid-macrophage-megakaryocyte-granulocyte forming units (Degliantoni et al., 1985; Broxmeyer et al., 1986).

Like IL-1, TNF also modulates protease secretion. TNF suppresses the secretion of PA from endothelial cells while enhancing the secretion of PA from synoviocytes (Chapman & Stone, 1985; Leizer, & Hamilton, 1989). In addition, TNF enhances the secretion of PAI from endothelial cells and collagenase from synoviocytes (Chapman & Stone, 1985; Kunkumian et al., 1989).

Evidence is mounting that TNF is important in viral infection and the pathogenesis of immune-mediated disease. TNF may also act as an antiviral mediator (Mestan et al., 1986). Preliminary evidence indicates that TNF may also participate in several clinical disorders including rheumatoid arthritis, autoimmune disease, graft versus host disease, and renal allograft rejection (Maury & Teppo, 1987; Piguet, Grau, Allet, & Vasalli, 1987; Jacob & McDevitt, 1988).

Tissue Remodeling

As a growth factor, TNF can stimulate the proliferation of fibroblast and mesenchymal cells and induce the biosynthesis of other growth factor (Sugarman et al., 1985; Fransen, Van Der Heyden, Ruysschaert, & Fiers, 1986; Vilcek et al., 1986). TNF is also angiogenic and is chemotactic for endothelial cells (Leibovich et al., 1987). Angiogenesis is induced in vivo in a rabbit corneal eye model following injection of TNF. This may be partially due to the activation of endothelial cells by TNF. However, in vitro studies showed that TNF, like IL-1, is also chemotactic. TNF was also shown to inhibit collagen production by embryonic bone cells and cultured human fibroblasts at the transcriptional level (Solis-Herruzo, Brenner, & Chojkier, 1988). TNF stimulates resorption and inhibits proteoglycan synthesis by explants of cartilage (Saklatvala, 1986).

Mechanism of Action

A variety of normal and tumor cell lines express high-affinity receptors for TNF (Figure 3.3), but no correlation is found between the number of receptors and the sensitivity of the cell to cytostasis or cytotoxicity by TNF (Williamson, Carswell, Rubin, Prendergast, & Old, 1983; Baglioni,

McCandless, Tavernier, & Fiers, 1985; Kull, Jacobs, & Cuatrecasas, 1985; Sugarman et al., 1985; Tsujimoto, Kip, & Vilcek, 1985; Ruggiero, Latham, & Baglioni, 1987). Very little is known about the postreceptor binding events of TNF. Treatment of cells with chemicals that stimulate protein kinase C inhibit TNF binding to cells. This may result from changes in the affinity of the receptor for TNF rather than through increased internalization of the receptor (Johnson & Baglioni, 1988).

Studies of the postreceptor binding events of TNF were conducted with a breast adenocarcinoma cell line (MC-7). In contrast to the degradation of TNF by other cell lines, TNF accumulates in this adenocarcinoma (Ruggiero, Tavernier, Fiers, & Baglioni, 1986; Imamura, Spriggs, & Kufe, 1987; Vuk-Pavlovic & Kovach, 1989). In this same study, it was shown that the TNF receptors are recycled following TNF degradation. Other studies indicate that TNF has a direct effect at the nuclear level (Alexander, Nelson, & Coffey, 1987; Vuk-Pavlovic, Svingen, Vroman, & Kovach, 1987; Elias, Moore, & Rose, 1988).

Wound Healing

One study tested the effect of TNF on skin wound healing. TNF-α was tested in a rat model through injection into wound cylinders composed of a stainless steel wire mesh. In this model, TNF-α had little effect on protein DNA and hydroxyproline accumulation in the chambers (Steenfos, Hunt, Scheuenstuhl, & Goodson, 1989). The effects of TNF on peritoneal wound healing have not been examined.

Summary

TNF is a pleiotropic hormone that may affect wound healing at many steps. It is a moderate enhancer of fibroblast proliferation and protease secretion. It is also procoagulatory and angiogenic but does not accelerate wound healing. Alternatively, TNF may enhance tissue destruction and remodeling through inhibiting collagen and proteoglycan synthesis and enhancing respiratory burst and other inflammatory activities of leukocytes.

Transforming Growth Factor-β

Transforming growth factors (TGFs) were initially identified as proteins that induce a phenotypic transformation of cultured cells (deLarco & Todaro, 1978). Two types of TGFs have been identified. TGF-α shares a receptor with EGF and regulates many of the biologic activities of EGF (Marquardt & Todaro, 1982; Marquardt et al., 1983, 1984; Derynck, Roberts, Winkler, Chen, & Goeddel, 1984). However, TGF-α synergistically interacts with TGF-β in the induction of a neoplastic phenotype (Anzano, Roberts, & Sporn, 1986). TGF-β is another type of TGF and does not compete with EGF for binding to its receptor (Cheifetz et al., 1987). TGF-β is a homodimeric protein of 25 kd and 112 amino acids (Derynck et al., 1985). Originally, TGF-β was isolated from platelets, kidney, and placenta (Assoian, Komoriya, Meyers, Miller, & Sporn, 1983; Frolik, Dart, Meyers, Smith, & Sporn, 1983; Roberts, Anzano, Meyers, & Sporn, 1983). Since that time, several isoforms of TGF-β, e.g., TGF-β1, TGF-β1.2, and TGF-β2, have been identified, but it is not yet known if they have distinct biologic effects (Seyedin, Thomas, Thompson, Rosen, & Piez, 1985; Roberts & Sporn 1989a).

TGF-β is secreted in a biologically inactive or latent form (Roberts & Sporn, 1988b). Latent TGF-β is unable to bind to its receptor and must be cleaved prior to receptor binding (Wakefield, Smith, Masui, Harris, & Sporn, 1987). Although the mechanism by which TGF-β is activated in vivo is unknown, it may occur as a result of interaction with cell-associated proteases (Keski-Oja, Lyones, & Moses, 1987). The latent complex may be activated by acidification (acidic environments are found in the vicinity of healing wounds) or by cleavage by proteases such as plasmin or cathepsin D. Due to the constitutive expression of the TGF-β receptor, the mechanism by which TGF-β is activated in vivo is of importance in understanding the regulation of the TGF-β activity (Wakefield et al., 1987).

Biological Activity

TGF-β was initially found to induce anchorage-dependent, nonneoplastic cells to lose contact inhibition and undergo anchorage-independent growth, i.e., transformation. The effect of TGF-β on cell growth is complex (Figure 3.11). TGF-β is bifunctional; that is, it can inhibit as well as stimulate cell growth (Tucker, Shipley, Moses, & Holley, 1985, Roberts & Stern, 1988a). TGF-β may act through increasing the number of EGF receptors (Assoian, Frolik, Roberts, Miller, & Sporn, 1984). TGF-β is consistently inhibitory to the proliferation of epithelial cells, but its effects on the proliferation of mesenchymal cells are more complex (Tucker et al., 1985; Massague, 1985; Roberts et al., 1985; Assoian & Sporn, 1986). TGF-β is both inhibitory and stimulatory to fibroblast and osteoblast proliferation (Moses et al., 1985; Centrella, McCarthy, & Canalis, 1987; Robey et al., 1987).

Like many growth factors, TGF-β seems to have a role in the modulation of inflammatory response. Inflammatory cell recruitment, i.e., platelets followed by neutrophils, macrophages, lymphocytes, and fibroblasts, can be induced by subcutaneous injection of TGF-β (Roberts et al., 1986). In vivo administration of TGF-β also induces angiogenesis and causes the formation of granulation tissue (Roberts et al., 1986).

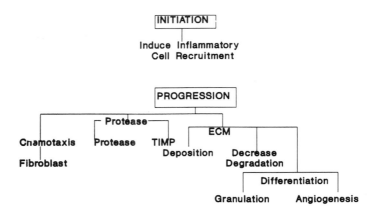

FIGURE 3.11. The activities involved in wound healing that are modulated by transforming growth factor-β. TIMP, tissue inhibitor of metalloproteinase.

TGF-β Effects on Endothelial Cells

TGF-β, unlike many other growth factors, inhibits the growth of endothelial cells when added to monolayers but enhances growth and capillary tube formation when added to three-dimensional collagen gels (Heimark, Twardzik, & Schwartz, 1986; Takehara, LeRoy, & Grotendorst, 1987; Madri, Pratt, & Tucker, 1988; Mignatti, Tsuboi, Robbins, & Rifkin, 1989). This inhibition of proliferation may be due to a decrease in EGF receptors and EGF-induced expression of competence genes (Takehara et al., 1987). TGF-β also inhibits chemotaxis of endothelial cells, and IL-1–induced neutrophil adhesion to endothelial cells (Gamble & Vadas, 1988; Mignatti et al., 1989).

Modulation of Monocyte/Macrophage Function by TGF-β

TGF-β stimulates monocyte chemotaxis and recruitment to the site of release (Wahl et al., 1987). Monocytes undergo chemotaxis in response to very low concentrations of TGF-β. Upon exposure to higher levels of TGF-β, a few monocyte functions are modulated. Upon exposure to picomolar concentration of TGF-β, monocytes show increased gene expression for inflammatory mediators including IL-1, PDGF, FGF and TNF (Wahl et al., 1987; Wiseman, Polverini, Kamp, & Leibovich, 1987; Chantry, Turner, & Feldman, 1988). TGF-β also induces its own production by monocytes (Assoian et al., 1987; Wahl, McCartney-Francis, & Mergenhagen, 1989). Upon differentiation of monocytes into macrophages, the macrophages are less susceptible to modulation by TGF-β. This may be due to the fact that macrophages down regulate their receptors for TGF-β (Wahl et al., 1987).

Other Cell Types

TGF-β also affects the differentiation of a variety of cell types. TGF-β is a strong inhibitor of adipogenic and myogenic differentiation under conditions in which it does not alter the proliferation of preadipocytes or myoblasts (Ignotz & Massague 1986; Massague, Cheifetz, Endo, & Nadal-Ginard, 1986). Many cells also respond to TGF-β not only through alterations in growth and differentiation, but also with an increase in the production and accumulation of the extracellular matrix proteins, fibronectin and collagen, by fibroblasts from a variety of origins (Ignotz & Massague, 1986; Roberts AB et al., 1986). TGF-β is also chemotactic for fibroblasts. TGF-β increases the levels of types I, III, and IV collagens and fibronectin mRNA through stimulation of the promoter for these genes (Ignotz, Endo, & Massague, 1987).

Effects on Tissue Repair

In addition to the modulation of extracellular matrix proteins, TGF-β modulates protease production and thus inhibits proteolytic degradation of matrix proteins (Keski-Oja, Blasi, Leof, & Moses, 1988). TGF-β was shown to modulate the secretion of plasminogen activator (PA) and plasminogen activator inhibitor (PAI-1) (Laiho, Sakesela, Andreasen, & Keski-Oja, 1986; Keski-Oja et al., 1988). TGF-β also induces the synthesis and secretion of a tissue inhibitor of metalloproteinase. TGF-β decreases the secretion of PA, a thiolprotease and a metalloprotease, by fibroblasts (Chiang & Nilsen-Hamilton, 1986; Laiho et al., 1986; Matrisian, Leroy, Ruhlmann, Gesnel, & Breathnach, 1986). Since TGF-β was shown to regulate both extracellular matrix formation and extracellular proteolytic activity, a study was conducted that compared the effects of TGF-β on PAI-1 mRNA synthesis with its effects on the synthesis of fibronectin and procollagen mRNAs. PAI-1 mRNA synthesis was elevated rapidly following exposure to TGF-β and this elevation was not altered by protein synthesis inhibition. Fibronectin, β-actin, and procollagen mRNA synthesis was also induced by TGF-β but this enhancement was abrogated by inhibition of protein synthesis (Keski-Oja et al., 1988). Studies indicate that the regulation of fibronectin and procollagen mRNAs by TGF-β occurs through posttranslational modifications (Raghow, Postlethwaite, Keski-Oja, Moses, & Kang, 1987).

TGF-β is an immunosuppressive peptide hormone inhibitory to the proliferation of cells of the T- and B-cell lineage (Kehrl et al., 1986a, 1986b; Wahl et al., 1988a, 1988b). TGF-β antagonizes IL-1–dependent T-cell proliferation, but does not block the transduction of the signal of IL-1 binding to produce IL-2 and IL-2 receptor by T cells (Like & Massague, 1986; Wahl et al., 1988a). TGF-β must therefore interfere with a postreceptor-binding event of IL-1 on T cells that does not affect IL-2 or

IL-2 receptor production (Like & Massague 1986). Although TGF-β stimulates the production of IL-1 by monocytes, it also inhibits the ability of IL-1 to cause T-lymphocyte proliferation and may be the mediator of the immune suppression observed in chronic inflammatory lesions (Wahl et al., 1988b).

Mechanism of Action

Several laboratories reported that receptors for TGF-β are universally and constitutively expressed (Figure 3.3). However, unlike other growth factor receptors, such as EGF and PDGF, no tyrosine kinase activity has been associated with the mitogenic effects of TGF-β (Tucker et al., 1985; Moses et al., 1985; Anzano et al., 1986; Baird & Durkin, 1986; Fanger, Wakefield, & Sporn, 1986; Libby, Martinez, & Weber, 1986c; Like & Massague, 1986). Although the mitogenic effect of these factors is antagonized by TGF-β, the very early steps following signal transduction by these growth factors, such as increases in phospholipid turnover, protein kinase C activation, the activity of the Na^+/H^+ antiport, or ornithine decarboxylase activity, are not blocked by TGF-β. Therefore, TGF-β may interfere with a distal step in DNA synthesis that has not been identified.

TGF-β stimulates extracellular matrix formation through interaction with the promoter for collagen and fibronectin. Recently, it was shown that TGF-β activates the nuclear factor-I binding site on the alpha$_2$ (I) collagen gene. This binding site is present in the promoter of many genes and may explain the common point of action of many of the pleiotropic effects of TGF-β.

Wound Healing

Sporn et al. (1983) showed that addition of TGF-β to wound chambers in rats increased the amounts of collagen, DNA, and protein in the chambers. Addition of TGF-β with or without PDGF significantly reversed the deficit of wound healing induced by Adriamycin (Lawrence, Norton, Sporn, Gorschboth, & Grotendorst, 1988). Other studies showed that a single direct application of TGF-β accelerated the healing of incisional wounds in rats as measured by wound strength and collagen deposition (Mustoe et al., 1987).

Upon injection of TGF-β into a subcutaneous polyvinyl sponge in the rat, the collagen content of the sponge was increased. In an incisional model, TGF-β increased the tensile and breaking strength (McGee, et al., 1989). Histological analysis of treated wounds showed an in vivo chemotactic response of macrophages and the synthesis of procollagen type I (Pierce, Mustoe, & Deuel, 1988a; Pierce et al., 1989a).

Longitudinal dermal wounds on the dorsum of guinea pigs were treated with TGF-β2 in a sponge composed of collagen and heparin as a vehicle.

Eight days after wounding, there was increased connective tissue and wound strength in the wounds of treated animals (Ksander et al., 1990). In partial-thickness wounds on swine, application of TGF-β produced new connective tissue and increased collagen content, maturity, and angiogenesis. In addition, TGF-β increased the number of inflammatory cells in the wound (Lynch, 1991).

Peritoneum

The effect of TGF-β on the proliferation and protein synthetic capability of rabbit TRCs harvested from various postsurgical days was tested. TGF-β suppressed TRC proliferation but increased the production of the extracellular matrix (Table 3.1); that is, incubation of TRCs with TGF-β enhances the incorporation of radiolabeled proline, but inhibits the incorporation of thymidine (Figure 3.12). In this context, TGF-β may function as a modulator of TRC differentiation in that it may induce these mesothelial cells to enter a secretory stage rather than proliferate.

Recent studies implicated TGF-β in the formation of peritoneal adhesions. In one study, it was shown, through immunohistochemical staining, that there was increased production of TGF-β, especially in inflam-

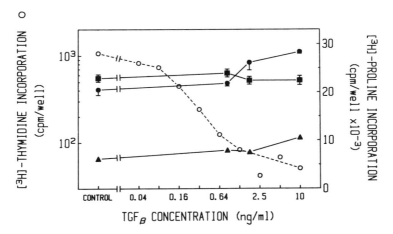

FIGURE 3.12. Effect of TGF-β on protein synthesis by tissue repair cells (TRCs) recovered from the peritoneal cavity of rabbits on postsurgical day 10. Protein synthetic activity was determined using incorporation of acid-precipitable tritiated proline. Data represent means ± SEM (cpm/well). (O), [^{3}H]Thymidine incorporation into TRC; (■), [^{3}H]proline incorporation into TRC; (●), [^{3}H]proline incorporation into trichloroacetic acid precipitable supernatant; (△), [^{3}H]proline incorporation into trypsin-labile protein from cultured cells. (From Fukasawa et al., 1989. Reproduced by permission of Academic Press.)

matory cells and fibroblasts, after injury to rat uterine tissue (Chegini, Simms, Williams, Rossi, & Masterson, 1991). In addition, as with IL-1 above, administration of TGF-β to rats after peritoneal trauma increased the formation of adhesions, but did not induce adhesion formation in nonsurgical rats (Williams, Rossi, Chegini, & Shultz, 1992).

Summary

TGF-β is a mediator of many cellular functions central to tissue repair. TGF-β can enhance fibroblast proliferation, fibroblast and macrophage chemotaxis, and synthesis and accumulation of extracellular matrix, and decrease the proteolytic activity of wound environments through enhancement of protease inhibitor synthesis and inhibition of protease production.

Other Factors

Insulin

Diabetic patients frequently have poorly healing wounds. In animals in which diabetes was induced, wound tensile strength and hydroxyproline levels were diminished (Prakash, Pandit, & Sharma, 1974; Goodson & Hunt, 1977). In both of these models, healing was improved if insulin was administered early in the repair process.

Eye-Derived Growth Factor

A factor that stimulates the growth of keratinocytes, termed eye-derived growth factor, was isolated. This factor stimulates re-epithelialization and neovascularization when regeneration of epidermis occurs (Fourtanier et al., 1986).

Nerve Growth Factor

Removal of submandibular glands in mice decreased the rate of wound contraction. In these mice, application of high molecular weight nerve growth factor (NGF) increased wound contraction (Li, Koroby, Schattenkerk, Malt, & Young, 1980). In contrast, no effect of high molecular weight NGF was observed in full-thickness wounds in the hamster (Leitzel, Cano, Marks, & Lipton, 1982).

Growth Hormone

One study reported that recombinant human grown hormone in rats augmented the tear strength in wounds of full-thickness dorsal skin incisions at postoperative days 6 and 12 (Pessa, Bland, Sitren, Miller, & Copeland, 1985).

Wound Healing and Growth Factor Interactions

Several studies show that growth factors interact to promote wound healing. In animal studies, highly purified preparations of PDGF or TGF-β did not affect wound healing, but when placed in combination with one another and other factors (such as EGF or IGF-I) they were more effective at the promotion of wound healing (Franklin & Lynch, 1979; Greaves, 1980; Thonton, Hess, Cassingham, & Bartlett, 1981; Niall et al., 1982; Arturson, 1984; Buckley et al., 1985; Brown et al., 1986; Hennessey, Black, & Andrassy, 1989; Lynch, Colvin, & Antoniades, 1989). In a recent study using a swine model in which several growth factors were examined alone or in combination, combining PDGF with IGF-1 significantly increased the thickness of new epidermis, the number and depth of epithelial extensions, and the hydroxyproline content of the wound. In addition, TGF-β in combination with PDGF synergistically increased new connective tissue (Lynch, 1991).

Studies conducted using crude preparations of serum, platelets, and keratinocytes on wound healing of patients with nonhealing wounds showed some improvement in healing (Carter et al., 1988). When a crude preparation of platelets was placed in petroleum-impregnated gauze in a nonrandomized study of patients with chronic nonhealing wounds, 97% of the wounds improved (Knighton et al., 1988). Another study treated 32 patients for 8 weeks with a crude preparation of autologous platelets (Knighton et al., 1986, 1990). Re-epithelization occurred in this study in 100% of treated patients compared to 15% of the controls. Upon crossover of the nonhealing controls to the treatment group, 100% of these patients' wounds re-epithelialized. Most recently, treatment of patients with homologous platelet-derived wound healing factor showed improvement in the healing of diabetic neurotrophic ulcers in many patients (Steed et al., 1991).

Peritoneum and Growth Factor Interactions

Several studies by Fukasawa et al. (discussed in Chapter 4), demonstrated that conditioned medium from postsurgical macrophages accelerates the proliferation and alters the morphology of TRC harvested from various postsurgical days compared to condition media of macrophages from nonsurgical rabbits. The proliferative response of TRC harvested 10 days after abrasion of the peritoneal side wall and cultured for 8 days in response to growth factors and an extract of conditioned medium from

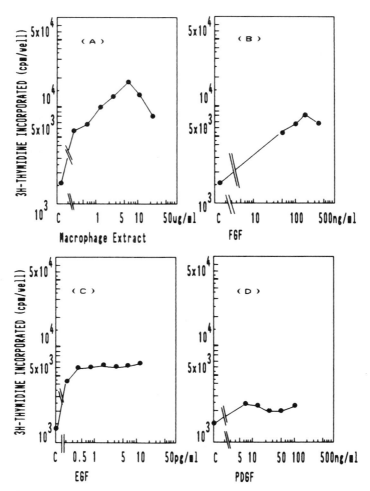

FIGURE 3.13. Effect of growth factors and an extract of macrophage-spent medium on [³H]thymidine incorporation into TRCs. TRCs recovered from the peritoneal cavity of rabbits on postsurgical day 10 were treated with various concentrations of the extract of macrophage-spent medium (A), FGF (B), EGF (C), and PDGF (D). Each data point represents the mean ± SEM (cpm/well). C, media control. (From Fukasawa et al., 1990. Reproduced by permission of Academic Press.)

cultures of postsurgical macrophages was studied (Fukasawa, Campeau, Yanigihara, Rodgers, & diZerega, 1990). Again these studies show significant proliferation of TRCs in response to EGF and FGF but not to PDGF (Figure 3.13). TGF-β was a potent inhibitor of TRC proliferation with an ED_{50} of approximately 0.1 ng/ml (Figure 3.12). However, maximal stimulation on a per weight basis of TRC proliferation was achieved by the extract of macrophage-conditioned medium (Figures 3.5 and 3.13).

Macrophages are potent secretory cells and this conditioned medium contains many soluble mediators of tissue repair. In fact, this study would suggest that macrophages secrete growth factors in an appropriate ratio to promote peritoneal re-epithelialization (Fukasawa et al. 1990).

Wound Fluid

Many studies have been conducted to determine the constituents of wound fluid or the extracellular environment in which wound healing occurs. In this fluid, the presence of angiogenic factors, TGF-β, interleukins, IGF-1, and TNF was demonstrated (Hunt, 1991).

IL-1 and TNF were shown to be present in peritoneal wound fluid at early time points after a laparotomy and intraperitoneal trauma (Kuraoka, personal communication). Studies by Abe, Rodgers, Ellefson, & diZerega (1991) showed that IL-1 and TNF are spontaneously secreted into culture medium by postsurgical macrophages harvested from the peritoneal cavity (see Chapter 6). In these same studies, TNF was shown to be present in peritoneal lavage fluid and secreted by postsurgical peritoneal macrophages without further stimuli.

Conclusion

This chapter reviewed the actions and mechanisms of actions of many growth factors that may regulate peritoneal healing (Table 3.1). Several of these growth factors were shown in animal models to accelerate healing of skin wounds. However, most of these data indicate that the greatest benefit may be derived through combinations of growth factors.

References

Abe H, Rodgers KE, Ellefson D, diZerega GS. (1991). Kinetics of interleukin-1 and tumor necrosis factor secretion by rabbit macrophages recovered from the peritoneal cavity after surgery. *J Invest Surg.* 4:141–151.

Abraham RT, Ho SN, Barna TJ, McKean DJ. (1987). Transmembrane signaling during interleukin-1–dependent T cell activation. Interactions of signal 1- and 2-type mediators with the phosphoinositide-dependent signal transduction mechanism. *J Biol Chem.* 262:2719–2728.

Adashi EY, Resnick CE, Bergeman CS, Gospodarowicz D. (1987). Fibroblast growth factor as a regulator of ovarian granulosa cell differentiation: a novel non-mitogenic role. *J Biol Chem.* 262:1–13.

Aggarwal BB, Eessalu TE, Hass PE. (1985). Characterization of receptors for human tumor necrosis factor and their regulation by γ-interferon. *Nature.* 318:665–667.

Akahoshi T, Oppenheim JJ, Matsushima K. (1988). Interleukin-1 stimulates its own receptor expression on human fibroblasts through the endogenous production of prostaglandins. *J Clin Invest.* 82:1219–1224.

Alexander RB, Nelson WG, Coffey DS. (1987). Synergistic enhancement by tumor necrosis factor of in vitro cytotoxicity from chemotherapeutic drug targeted at DNA topoisomerase II. *Cancer Res.* 47:2403–2406.

Anzano MA, Roberts AB, Sporn MB. (1986). Anchorage-independent growth of primary rat embryo cells in induced by platelet-derived growth factor and inhibited by type-beta transforming growth factor. *J Cell Physiol.* 126:312–318.

Arend WP, D'Angelo S, Massoni RJ, Joslin FG. (1985a). Interleukin-1 production by human monocytes: effects of different stimuli. In: Kluger MJ, Oppenheim JJ, Powanda MX, eds. *The Physiologic, Metabolic and Immunologic Actions of Interleukin.* New York: Alan Liss; 399–426.

Arend WP, Joslin FG, Massoni RJ. (1985b). Effects of immune complexes on production by human monocytes of interleukin 1 or an interleukin 1 inhibitor. *J Immunol.* 134:3868–3875.

Arend WP, Gordon DF, Wood WM, Janson RW, Joslin FG, Jameel S. (1989). IL-1β production in cultured human monocytes is regulated at multiple levels. *J Immunol.* 143:118–126.

Arenzana-Seisdedos F, Virelizier J-L. (1983). Interferons as macrophage activating factors. II. Enhanced secretion of interleukin-1 by lipopolysaccharide-stimulated human monocytes. *Eur J Immunol.* 13:437–440.

Armelin HA, Armelin MCS, Kelly K, Stewart T, Leder P, Cochran BH, Stiles CD. (1984). Functional role of c myc in mitogenic response to platelet derived growth factor precedes activation of c myc. *Nature.* 310:655–660.

Arturson G. (1984). Epidermal growth factor in the healing of corneal wounds, epidermal wounds and partial thickness scalds. *Scand J Plast Reconstr Surg.* 18:33–37.

Assoian RK, Komoriya K, Meyers CA, Miller DM, Sporn MB. (1983). Transforming growth factor-β in human platelets. Identification of a major storage site, purification and characterization. *J Biol Chem.* 258:7155–7160.

Assoian RK, Frolik CA, Roberts AB, Miller DM, Sporn MB. (1984). Transforming growth factor beta controls receptor levels for epidermal growth factor in NRK fibroblasts. *Cell.* 36:35–41.

Assoian RK, Sporn MB. (1986). Type beta transforming growth factor in human platelets: release during platelet degranulation and action on vascular smooth muscle cells. *J Cell Biol.* 142:1217–1223.

Assoian RK, Fleurdelys BE, Stevenson HC, Miller PJ, Madtes DK, Raines EW, Ross R, Sporn MB. (1987). Expression and secretion of type beta transforming growth factor by activated human macrophages. *Proc Natl Acad Sci USA.* 84:1681–1687.

Auron PE, Webb AC, Rosenwasser LJ, Mucci SF, Rich A, Wolff SM, Dinarello CA. (1984). Nucleotide sequence of human monocyte interleukin-1 precursor cDNA. *Proc Natl Acad Sci USA.* 81:7907–7911.

Auron PE, Warner SJ, Webb AC, Cannon JG, Bernheim HA, McAdam KJP, Rosenwasser LJ, LoPreste G, Mucci SF, Dinarello CA. (1987). Studies on the molecular nature of interleukin-1. *J Immunol.* 138:1447–1456.

Bachelet M, Masliah J, Vargaftig BB, Bereziat G, Colard O. (1986). Changes induced by PAF-acether in diacyl and ether phospholipids from guinea-pig alveolar macrophages. *Biochim Biophys Acta.* 878:177–183.

Bagby GC, Dinarello CA, Wallace P, Wagner C, Hefeneider S, McCall E. (1986). Interleukin-1 stimulates granulocyte macrophage colony stimulating activity release by vascular endothelial cells. *J Clin Invest.* 78:1316–1323.

Baglioni C, McCandless S, Tavernier J, Fiers W. (1985). Binding of human tumor necrosis factor to high affinity receptors on HELA and lymphoblastoid cells sensitive to growth inhibition. *J Biol Chem.* 260:13395–13397.

Baird A, Durkin T. (1986). Inhibition of endothelial cell proliferation by type-beta transforming growth factor: interactions with acidic and basic fibroblast growth factors. *Biochem Biophys Res Commun.* 138:476–482.

Baird A, Esch F, Mormede P, Ueno N, Ling N, Bohlen P, Ying SY, Wehrenberg WB, Guillemin R. (1986). Molecular characterization of fibroblast growth factor: distribution and biological activities in various tissues. *Recent Prog Horm Res.* 42:143–205.

Bakouche O, Ichinose Y, Heicappell R, Fidler IJ, Lachman LB. (1988). Plasma membrane associated tumor necrosis factor: a non-integral membrane protein possibly bound to its own recepter. *J Immunol.* 142:1142–1147.

Balavoine JF, de Rochemonteix B, Williamson K, Sekinger P, Cruchaud A, Dayer J-M. (1986). Prostaglandin E2 and collagenase production by fibroblasts and synovial cells is regulated by urine-derived human interleukin-1 and inhibitor(s). *J Clin Invest.* 78:1120–1124.

Barak V, Treves AJ, Yanai P, Halperin M, Wasserman D, Birin S, Brown S. (1986). Interleukin-1 inhibitory activity secreted by a human myelomonocytic cell line (C20). *Eur J Immunol.* 16:1449–1452.

Barrett TB, Gajdusek CM, Schwartz SM, McDougall JK, Benditt EP. (1984). Expression of the sis gene by endothelial cells in culture and in vivo. *Proc Natl Acad Sci USA.* 81:6772–6774.

Beck G, Habicht GS, Benach JL, Miller F. (1986). Interleukin-1: a common endogenous mediator of inflammation and the local Shwartzman reaction. *J Immunol.* 136:3025–3031.

Berk BC, Alexander RW, Brock TA, Gimbrone MA, Webb CR. (1986). Vasoconstriction: a new activity for platelet-derived growth factor. *Science.* 232:87–90.

Berman MA, Sandberg CI, Calabia BS, Andrews BS, Friou GJ. (1987). Interleukin-1 inhibitor masks high interleukin-1 production in acquired immune deficiency syndrome (AIDS). *Clin Immunol Immunopathol.* 42:133–140.

Bernheim HA, Dinarello CA. (1985). Effects of purified human interleukin-1 on the release of prostaglandin E2 from fibroblasts. *Br J Rheumatol.* 24:122–127.

Bernton EW, Beach JE, Holaday JW, Smallbridge RC, Fein HG. (1987). Release of multiple hormones by a direct action of interleukin-1 on pituitary cells. *Science.* 238:519–521.

Bertolini DR, Nedwin GE, Bringman TS, Smith DD, Mundy GR. (1986). Stimulation of bone marrow resorption and inhibition of bone marrow formation in vitro by human tumor necrosis factors. *Nature.* 319:516–519.

Beutler B, Greenwald D, Hulmes JD, Chang M, Pan YC, Mathison J, Ulevitck R, Cerami A. (1985a). Identity of tumor necrosis factor and the macrophage secreted factor cachectin. *Nature.* 316:552–554.

Beutler B, Mahoney J, LeTrang N, Pekala P, Cerami A. (1985b). Purification of cachectin, a lipoprotein lipase-suppressing hormone secreted by endotoxin-induced RAW 264.7 cells. *J Exp Med.* 161:984–995.

Beutler B, Cerami A. (1986). Cachectin and tumor necrosis factor as two sides of the same biological coin. *Nature.* 320:584–588.

Beutler B, Tkacenko V, Milsark I, Krockin N, Cerami A. (1986). Effect of gamma interferon on cachectin expression by mononuclear phagocytes. Reversal of lpsd (endotoxin resistance) phenotype. *J Exp Med.* 164:1791–1796.

Bevilacqua MP, Pober JS, Majeau GR, Contran RA, Gimbrone MA. (1984). Interleukin-1 (IL-1) induces biosynthesis and cell surface expression of procoagulant activity in human vascular endothelial cells. *J Exp Med.* 160:618–623.

Bevilacqua MP, Pober JS, Wheeler ME, Cotran RS, Gimbrone MA. (1985). Interleukin-1 acts on cultured human vascular endothelium to increase the adhesion of polymorphonuclear leukocytes, monocytes and related leukocyte lines. *J Clin Invest.* 76:2003–2007.

Bevilacqua MP, Schleef RR, Gimbrone MA, Loskutoff DJ. (1986a). Regulation of the fibrinolytic system of cultures of human endothelium by interleukin-1. *J Clin Invest.* 78:587–591.

Bevilacqua MP, Pober JS, Majeau GR, Fiers W, Cotran RS, Gimbrone MA. (1986b). Recombinant tumor necrosis factor induces procoagulant activity in cultured human vascular endothelium: characterization and comparison with the actions of interleukin-1. *Proc Natl Acad Sci USA.* 83:4533–4537.

Bird TA, Saklatvala J. (1987). Studies on the fate of receptor-bound 125I-interleukin 1β in porcine synovial fibroblasts. *J Immunol.* 139:92–97.

Black RA, Kronheim SR, Cantrell M, Deeley MC, March CJ, Prickett KS, Wignall J, Conlon PJ, Cosman D, Hopp TP, Mochizuki DY. (1988). Generation of biologically active interleukin-1β by proteolytic cleavage of the inactive precursor. *J Biol Chem.* 263:9437–9442.

Bohlen P, Esch F, Baird A, Gospodarowicz D. (1985). Acidic fibroblast growth factor from bovine brain. Amino terminal sequence and comparison to basic fibroblast growth factor. *EMBO J.* 4:1951–1956.

Bonin PD, Singh JP. (1988). Modulation of interleukin-1 receptor expression and interleukin-1 response in fibroblasts by platelet-derived growth factor. *J Biol Chem.* 263:11052–11055.

Bonney RJ, Humes JL. (1984). Physiological and pharmalogical regulation of prostaglandin and leukotriene production by macrophages. *J Leukocyte Biol.* 35:1–10.

Boraschi D, Tagliabue A. (1984). Multiple modulation of macrophage functions by lymphokines: different effects of interferon and macrophage activating factor. In: Pick E, ed. *Lyymphokines.* San Diego: Academic Press; 9:71–99.

Bowen-Pope DF, Ross R. (1985). Methods for studying the platelet-derived growth factor receptors. Methods. *Enzymology.* 109:69–100.

Bron C, MacDonald HR. (1987). Identification of a plasma membrane receptor for interleukin-1 on mouse thymoma cells *FEBS Lett.* 219:365–368.

Bronson RE, Bentilami CN, Siebert EP. (1987). Modulation of fibroblast growth and glycosaminoglycan synthesis by interleukin-1. *Coll Relat Res.* 7:323–332.

Broudy VC, Kaushansky K, Harlan JM, Adamson JW. (1987). Interleukin-1 stimulates endothelial cells to produce granulocyte-macrophage colony-stimulating factor and granulocyte colony stimulating factor. *J Immunol.* 139:464–468.

Brown GL, Curtsinger, LJ III, Brightwell JR, Ackerman DM, Polk HE, Schultz GS. (1985). Human epidermal growth factor accelerates epithelialization of partial-thickness burns (abstract). Presented at the Association for Academic Surgery 19th Annual Meeting, p. 67.

Brown GL, Curtsinger L III, Brightwell JR, Ackerman DM, Tobin GR, Polk HC Jr, George-Nascimento C, Valenzuela P, Schultz GS. (1986). Enhancement of epidermal regeneration by biosynthetic epidermal growth factor. *J Exp Med.* 163:1319–1324.

Brown GL, Curtsinger LJ III, White M, Mitchell RO, Pietsch J, Nordquest R, von Fraunhofer A, Schultz GS. (1988). Acceleration of tensile strength of incisions treated with EGF and TGF-β. *Ann Surg.* 208:788–794.

Brown GL, Nanney LB, Griffen J, Cramer AB, Yancey JM, Curtsinger LJ III, Holtzin L, Schultz GS, Jurkiewicz MJ, Lynch JB. (1989). Enhancement of wound healing by topical treatment with epidermal growth factor. *N Engl J Med.* 321:76–79.

Brown K. (1986). Uromodulin, an immunosuppressive protein derived from pregnancy urine, is an inhibitor of interleukin-1. *Proc Natl Acad Sci USA.* 83:9119–9123.

Broxmeyer HE, Williams DE, Lu L, Cooper S, Anderson SL, Beyer GS, Hoffman R, Rubin BY. (1986). The suppressive influences of human tumor necrosis factor on bone marrow hematopoietic progenitor cells from normal donors and patients with leukemia: synergism of tumor necrosis factor and interferon-gamma. *J Immunol.* 136:4487–4495.

Bucher NLR. (1978). Hormonal factors and liver growth. *Adv Enzyme Regul.* 16:205–215.

Buckley A, Davidson JM, Kamerath CD, Wolt TB, Woodward SC. (1985). Sustained release of epidermal growth factor accelerates wound repair. *Proc Natl Acad Sci USA.* 82:7340–7344.

Bunning RA, Crawford A, Richardson HJ, Openakker G, Van Damme J, Russell RG. (1987). Interleukin-1 preferentially stimulates the production of tissue type plasminogen activator by human articular chondrocytes. *Biochim Biophys Acta.* 924:473–482.

Burchett SK, Weaver WM, Westall JA, Larsen A, Kronheim S, Wilson CB. (1988). Regulation of tumor necrosis factor/cachectin and IL-1 secretion in human mononuclear phagocytes. *J Immunol.* 140:3473–3481.

Canalis R. (1986). Interleukin-1 has independent effects on DNA and collagen synthesis in cultures of rat calvariae. *Endocrinology.* 118:74–81.

Caput D, Beutler B, Hartog K, Thayer R, Brown-Shimer S, Cerami A. (1986). Identification of a common nucleotide sequence in the 3′ untranslated region of mRNA molecules specifying inflammatory mediators. *Proc Natl Acad Sci USA.* 83:1670–1674.

Carpenter G, Cohen S. (1976a). ^{125}I-labeled human epidermal growth factor (hEGF): binding, internalization and degradation in human fibroblasts. *J Cell Biol.* 71:159–171.

Carpenter G, Cohen S. (1976b). Human epidermal growth factor and the proliferation of human fibroblasts. *J Cell Physiol.* 88:227–237.

Carpenter G, Cohen S. (1979). Epidermal growth factor. *Annu Rev Biochem.* 48:193–216.

Carpenter G, King L, Cohen S. (1979). Epidermal growth factor–receptor-protein kinase interactions. *J Biol Chem.* 255:4834–4842.

Carpenter G. (1985). Epidermal growth factor: biology and receptor metabolism. *J Cell Sci Suppl.* 3:1–9.

Carswell EA, Old LJ, Kassel RL, Green S, Fiore N, Williamson B. (1975). An endotoxin-induced serum factor that causes necrosis of tumors. *Proc Natl Acad Sci USA.* 72:3666–3670.

Carter DM, Balin AK, Gottliet AB, Eisenger M, Lin A, Pratt L, Sherbany A, Caldwell D. (1988). Clinical experience with crude preparation of growth factors in healing of chronic wounds in human subjects. In: Barbul A, Pines E, Caldwell M, Hunt TK, eds. *Growth Factors and Other Aspects of Wound Healing: Biological and Clinical Research.* New York: Alan Liss; 266:303–317.

Catterton WZ, Escobedo MB, Sexson WR, Gray ME, Sundell HW, Stahlman MT. (1979). The effects of epidermal growth factor on lung maturation in fetal rabbit. *Pediatr Res.* 13:104–108.

Cavender DE, Haskard DO, Joseph B, Ziff M. (1986). Interleukin-1 increases the binding of human B and T lymphocytes to endothelial cell monolayers. *J Immunol.* 136:203–207.

Centrella M, McCarthy TL, Canalis E. (1987). Transforming growth factor beta is a bifunctional regulator of replication and collagen synthesis in osteoblast-enriched cell cultures from fetal rat bone. *J Biol Chem.* 262:2869–2874.

Chantry D, Turner M, Feldman M. (1988). Regulation of interleukin-1 and tumor necrosis factor mRNA and protein by transforming growth factor beta. *Lymphokine Res.* 7:283–306.

Chapman HA, Stone OL. (1985). Characterization of macrophage derived plasminogen activator inhibitor (similarities with placental urokinase inhibitor). *Biochem J.* 230:109–116.

Chegini N, Simms JS, Williams RS, Rossi AMK, Masterson BJ. (1991). Identification of transforming growth factors alpha and beta (TGF-α and TGF-β) in postoperative adhesion formation. 38th Annual Meeting for Society of Gynecological Investigation, San Antonio, TX, pp. 331.

Cheifetz S, Weatherbee JA, Tsang MLS, Anderson JIC, Mole JE, Lucas R, Massague J. (1987). The transforming growth factor–beta system, a complex pattern of cross-reactive legends and receptors. *Cell.* 48:409–415.

Chen WS, Lazar CS, Poenie M, Tsien RY, Gill G, Rosenfeld MG. (1987). Requirement for intrinsic protein tyrosine kinase in the immediate and late actions of the EGF receptor. *Nature.* 328:820–823.

Chiang C-P, Nilsen-Hamilton M. (1986). Opposite and selective effects of epidermal growth factor and human platelet transforming growth factor–beta on the production of secreted proteins by murine 3T3 cells and human fibroblasts. *J Biol Chem.* 261:10478–10481.

Chinkers M, McKanna JA, Cohen S. (1979). Rapid induction of morphological changes in human carcinoma cells A-431 by epidermal growth factor. *J Cell Biol.* 83:260–265.

Chuo P, Francis L, Atkins F. (1977). The release of an endogenous pyrogen from guinea pig leukocytes in vitro. A new model for investigating the role of lymphocytes in fevers induced by antigens in hosts with delayed hypersensitivity. *J Exp Med.* 145:1288–1298.

Chvapil M, Gaines JA, Gilman T. (1988). Lanolin and epidermal growth factor in healing of partial thickness pig wounds. *J Burn Care Rehabil.* 9:279–284.

Cohen S. (1962). Isolation of a mouse submaxillary gland protein accelerating incisor eruption and eyelid opening in the newborn animal. *J Biol Chem.* 237:1562–1568.

Cohen S, Elliott GA. (1963). The stimulation of epidermal keratinization by a protein isolated from the submaxillary gland of the mouse. *J Invest Dermatol.* 40:1–5.

Cohen S. (1965). The stimulation of epidermal proliferation by a specific protein (EGF). *Dev Biol.* 12:394–407.

Cohen S, Taylor JM. (1974). Epidermal growth factor: chemical and biological characterization. *Recent Prog Horm Res.* 30:533–550.

Coley WB. (1893). The treatment of malignant tumors by repeated inoculations of erysipelas with a report of ten original cases. *Am J Med Sci.* 105:487–511.

Collins MKL, Sinnett-Smith JW, Rozengurt E. (1983). Platelet derived growth factor treatment decreases the affinity of the epidermal growth factor receptors of swiss 3T3 cells. *J Biol Chem.* 258:11689–11693.

Collins T, Lapierre LA, Riers W, Strominger JL, Pober JS. (1986). Recombinant human tumor necrosis factor increases mRNA levels and surface expression of HLA-A,B antigens in vascular endothelial cells and dermal fibroblasts in vitro. *Proc Natl Acad Sci USA.* 83:446–450.

Conlon PJ, Grabstein KH, Alpert A, Prickett KS, Hopp TP, Gillis S. (1987). Localization of human mononuclear cell interleukin-1. *J Immunol.* 139:98–102.

Cooper ML, Hansbrough JF, Foreman TJ, Sakabu SA, Laxer JA. (1991). The effects of epidermal growth factor and basic fibroblast growth factor on epithelialization of meshed skin graft interstices. In: Caldwell MD, Hunt TK, Pines E, Skovee G, eds. *Clinical and Experimental Approaches to Dermal and Epidermal Repair Normal and Chronic Wounds.* New York: Wiley-Liss; 365:429–442.

Czarnetzki G. (1983). Increased monocyte chemotaxis towards leukotriene B_4 and platelet activating factor in patients with inflammatory dermatoses. *Clin Exp Immunol.* 54:486–492.

Davidson J, Bulkley A, Woodward S, Nichols W, McGee G, Demerriou A. (1988). Mechanisms of accelerated wound repair using epidermal growth factor and basic fibroblast growth factor. In: Barbul A, Pines E, Caldwell M, Hunt TK, eds. *Growth Factors and Other Aspects of Wound Healing: Biological and Clinical Research.* New York: Alan R. Liss; 266:63–75.

Davis L, Lipsky PE. (1986). Signals involved in T cell activation. II. Distinct roles of intact accessory cells, phorbol esters, and interleukin-1 in activation and cell cycle progression of resting T lymphocytes. *J Immunol.* 136:3588–3596.

Dayer J-M, Beutler B, Cerami A. (1985). Cachectin/tumor necrosis factor stimulates collagenase and prostaglandin-E_2 production by human synovial cells and dermal fibroblasts. *J Exp Med.* 162:2163–2168.

Decker SJ, Harris P. (1989). Effects of platelet-derived growth factor on phosphorylation of the epidermal growth factor receptor in human skin fibroblasts. *J Biol Chem.* 264:9204–9209.

Degliantoni G, Murphy M, Kobayashi M, Francis MK, Perussia B, Trinchieri G. (1985). Natural killer (NK) cell–derived hematopoietic colony-inhibiting activity and NK cytotoxic factor: relationship with tumor necrosis factor and synergism with immune interferon. *J Exp Med.* 162:1512–1530.

Dejana E, Brevario F, Erroi A, Bussolino F, Mussoni L, Gramse M, Pintucci G, Casali B, Dinarello CA, Van Damme J, Mantovani A. (1987). Modulation of endothelial cell function by different molecular species of interleukin-1. *Blood.* 69:695–699.

Dejana E, Bertocchi F, Bortolami MC, Regonesi A, Tonta A, Breviario F, Giavazzi R. (1988). Interleukin-1 promotes tumor cell adhesion to cultured human endothelial cells. *J Clin Invest.* 82:1466–1470.

DeLarco JE, Todaro GJ. (1978). Growth factors from murine sarcoma virus transformed cells. *Proc Natl Acad Sci USA.* 75:4001–4005.

Demczuk S, Baumberger C, Mach B, Dayer J-M. (1987). Expression of human IL-1α and β messenger RNAs and IL-1 activity in human peripheral blood mononuclear cells. *J Mol Cell Immunol.* 3:255–265.

Demopoulos CA, Pinckard RN, Hanahan DJ. (1979). Platelet-activating factor. Evidence for 1-O-alkyla-2acetyl-sn-glyceryl-α-1-phosphorylcholine as the active component (a new class of lipid chemical mediators). *J Biol Chem.* 254:9355–9358.

Derynck R, Roberts AB, Winkler ME, Chen EY, Goeddel DV. (1984). Human transforming growth factor-α: precursor structure and expression in *E. coli. Cell.* 38:287–297.

Derynck R, Jarrett JA, Chen EY, Eaton DH, Bell JR, Assoian RK, Roberts AB, Sporn MB, Goeddel DV. (1985). Human transforming factor beta cDNA sequence and expression in tumor cell lines. *Nature.* 316:701–705.

Deuel TF, Huang JS. (1983). Platelet-derived growth factor: purification, properties, and biological activities. *Prog Hematol.* 13:201–221.

Deuel TF. (1987). Polypeptide growth factors: roles in normal and abnormal cell growth. *Annu Rev Cell Biol.* 3:443–492.

DiCorleto PE, Bowen-Pope DF. (1983). Cultured endothelial cells produce a platelet-derived growth factor–like protein. *Proc Natl Acad Sci USA.* 80:1919–1923.

Dinarello CA, Renfer L, Wolff SM. (1977). Human leukocytic pyrogen: purification and development of a radioimmunoassay. *Proc Natl Acad Sci USA.* 74:4624–4627.

Dinarello CA. (1985). The physiologic, metabolic, and immunologic actions of interleukin-1. In: Kluger MJ, Oppenheim JJ, Powanda MC, eds. *Biology of Interleukin-1.* New York: Alan R. Liss; 1–19.

Dinarello CA, Cannon JG, Mier JW, Bernheim HA, LoPreste G, Lynn DL, Love RN, Webb AC, Auron PE, Reuben RC, Rich A, Wolff SM, Putney SD. (1986a). Multiple biological activities of human recombinant interleukin-1. *J Clin Invest.* 77:1734–1739.

Dinarello CA, Cannon JG, Wolff SM. (1986b). Tumor necrosis factor (cachectin) is an endogenous pyrogen and induces production of interleukin-1. *J Exp Med.* 163:1443–1450.

Doolittle RF, Hunkapiller MW, Hood LE, Devare SG, Robbins K, Aaronson SA, Antoniades HN. (1983). Simian sarcoma virus one gene, v-sis, is derived from the gene (or genes) encoding a platelet-derived growth factor. *Science.* 221:275–277.

Dower SK, Kronheim SR, March CJ, Conlon PJ, Hopp TP, Gillis S, Urdal DL. (1985). Detection and characterization of high affinity receptors for human interleukin-1. *J Exp Med.* 162:501–515.

Dower SK, Urdal DL. (1987). The interleukin-1 receptor. *Immunol Today.* 8:46–51.

Duff GW, Forre O, Waalen K, Dickens SE, Kvamesh L, Nuki G. (1985). Interleukin-1 activity produced by human rheumatoid and normal dendritic cells. *Br J Rheumatol.* 24:94–98.

Durum SK, Higuchi C, Ron Y. (1984). High affinity interleukin-1 receptors. *Immunobiology.* 168:213–231.

Eisinger M, Sadan S, Soehnchen R, Silver IA. (1988). Wound healing by epidermal-derived factors: experimental and preliminary clinical studies. In: Dicken SF, Kvarmes L, Nuko G, eds. *Growth Factors and Other Aspects of Wound Healing: Biological and Clinical Research.* New York: Alan R. Liss; 266:291–302.

Ek B, Westermark B, Wasteson A, Heldin C-H. (1982). Stimulation of tyrosine-specific phosphorylation by platelet-derived growth factor. *Nature.* 295:419–420.

Elias JA, Gustilo K, Baeder W, Freundlich B. (1987). Synergistic stimulation of fibroblast prostaglandin production by recombinant interleukin-1 and tumor necrosis factor. *J Immunol.* 138:3812–3816.

Elias L, Moore PB, Rose SM. (1988). Tumor necrosis factor induced DNA fragmentation of HL-60 cells. *Biochem Biophys Res Commun.* 157:963–969.

Emeis JJ, Kooestra J. (1986). Interleukin-1 and lipopolysaccharide induce an inhibitor of tissue-type plasminogen activator in vivo and in cultured endothelial cells. *J Exp Med.* 163:1260–1266.

Engrav LH, Richey KJ, Kao CC, Murray MJ. (1989). Topical growth factors and wound contraction in the rat: Part II. Platelet-derived growth factor and wound contraction in normal and steroid-impaired rats. *Ann Plast Surg.* 23:245–248.

Esch F, Baird A, Ling N, Ueno N, Hill F, Deneroy L, Klepper R, Gospodarowicz D, Bohlen P, Guillemin R. (1985). Primary structure of bovine pituitary basic fibroblast growth factor (FGF) and comparison with the amino terminal sequence of bovine brain acidic FGF. *Proc Natl Acad Sci USA.* 85:6507–6511.

Estes JE, Pledger WJ, Gillespie GY. (1984). Macrophage derived growth factor for fibroblasts and interleukin-1 are distinct entities. *J Leukoc Biol.* 35:115–129.

Fanger BO, Wakefield LM, Sporn MB. (1986). Structure and properties of the cellular receptor for transforming growth factor type beta. *Biochemistry.* 25:3083–3091.

Farr AG, Dorf ME, Unanue ER. (1977). Secretion of mediators following T lymphocyte–macrophage interaction is regulated by the major histocompatability complex. *Proc Natl Acad Sci USA.* 74:3542–3546.

Fenton MJ, Clark BD, Collins KL, Webb AC, Rich A, PE Auron. (1987). Transcriptional regulation of the human prointerleukin 1β gene. *J Immunol.* 138:3972–3979.

Fontana A, Kristinsen F, Pub R, Gemsa D, Weber E. (1982). Production of prostaglandin E and an interleukin-1 by cultured astrocytes and C_6 glioma cells. *J Immunol.* 129:2413–2419.

Fourtanier AY, Courty J, Muller E, Courtois Y, Prunieras M, Berritault D. (1986). Eye-derived growth factor isolated from bovine retina and used for epidermal wound healing in vivo. *J Invest Dermatol.* 87:76–80.

Franklin JD, Lynch JB. (1979). Effects of topical applications of epidermal growth factor on wound healing. *Plast Reconstr Surg.* 64:766–770.

Franklin TJ, Gregory H, Morris WP. (1986). Acceleration of wound healing by recombinant human urogastrone (epidermal growth factor). *J Lab Clin Med.* 108:103–108.

Fransen L, Van Der Heyden J, Ruysschaert R, Fiers W. (1986). Recombinant tumor necrosis factor: its effect and its synergism with interferon-γ on a variety of normal and transformed human cell lines. *Eur J Cancer Clin Oncol.* 22:419–426.

Frolik CA, Dart LL, Meyers CA, Smith DM, Sporn MB. (1983). Purification and initial characterization of a type β transforming growth factor from human placenta. *Proc Natl Acad Sci USA.* 80:3676–3680.

Fukasawa M, Yanagihara DL, Rodgers KE, diZerega GS. (1989). The mitogenic activity of peritoneal tissue repair cells: control by growth factor. *J Surg Res.* 47:45–51.

Fukasawa M, Campeau JD, Yanigihara DL, Rodgers KE, diZerega GS. (1990). Regulation of proliferation of peritoneal tissue repair cells by peritoneal macrophages. *J Surg Res.* 49:81–87.

Fulbrigge RC, Chaplin DD, Kiely J-M, Unanue ER. (1987). Regulation of interleukin-1 gene expression by adherence and lipopolysaccharide. *J Immunol.* 138:3799–3802.

Furutani Y, Notake M, Yamayoshi M, Yamagishi J, Nomura H, Ohue M, Fukui T, Yamada M, Nakamura S. (1985). Cloning and characterization of cDNAs for human and rabbit interleukin-1 precursor. *Nucleic Acids Res.* 13:5869–5882.

Gahring L, Baltz M, Pepys MB, Daynes R. (1984). Effect of ultraviolet radiation on production of epidermal cell thymocyte activating factor/interleukin-1 in vivo and in vitro. *Proc Natl Acad Sci USA.* 81:1198–1202.

Gajusek C, Carbon S, Ross R, Nawroth P, Stern D. (1986). Activation of coagulation releases endothelial cell mitogens. *J Cell Biol.* 103:419–428.

Gamble JR, Harlan JM, Klebanoff SJ, Vadas MA. (1985). Stimulation of the adherence of neutrophils to umbilical vein endothelium by human recombinant tumor necrosis factor. *Proc Natl Acad Sci USA.* 82:8667–8771.

Gamble JR, Vadas MA. (1988). Endothelial adhesiveness for blood neutrophils is inhibited by transforming growth factor beta. *Science.* 242:97–99.

Gery I, Waksman BH. (1972). Potentiation of the T-lymphocyte response to mitogens. II. The cellular source of potentiating mediator(s). *J Exp Med.* 136:143–155.

Ghezzi P, Saccardo B, Villa P, Rossi V, Bianchi M, Dinarello CA. (1986). Role of interleukin-1 in the depression of liver drug metabolism by endotoxin. *Infect Immun.* 54:837–840.

Gilman SC, Rosenberg JS, Feldman JD. (1984). Immune complexes in endocarditis. *J Immunol.* 133:217–221.

Giri I, Lepe-Zuniya JL. (1983). Lymphocyte activating factors. In: Pick EJ, ed. *Lymphokines.* San Diego: Academic Press: 9:109–126.

Giri JG, Lomedico PT, Mizel SB. (1985). Studies on the synthesis and secretion of interleukin-1. I. A 33,000 molecular weight precursor for interleukin-1. *J Immunol.* 134:343–349.

Goodson WH III, Hunt TK. (1977). Studies of wound healing in experimental diabetes mellutes. *J Surg Res.* 22:221–227.

Gorden P, Carpentier JL, Cohen S, Orci L. (1978). Epidermal growth factor: morphological demonstration of binding, internalization and lysosomal association in human fibroblasts. *Proc Natl Acad Sci USA.* 75:5025–5029.

Gospodarowicz D. (1974). Localization of a fibroblast growth factor and its effect alone and with hydrocortisone on 3T3 cell growth. *Nature.* 249:123–127.

Gospodarowicz D, Moran JS. (1974). Effect of fibroblast growth factor, insulin, dexamethasone and serum on the morphology of BALB/c 3T3 cells. *Proc Natl Acad Sci USA.* 71:4648–4652.

Gospodarowicz D, Moran JS. (1975). Mitogenic effect of fibroblast factor on early passage of human and murine fibroblasts. *J Cell Biol.* 66:451–456.

Gospodarowicz D, Weseman F, Moran J. (1975). Presence in the brain of a mitogenic agent distinct from fibroblast growth factor that promotes the proliferation of myoblasts in low density in culture. *Nature.* 256:216–219.

Gospodarowicz D, Bialecki H. (1978). The effects of the epidermal and fibroblast growth factor and the replicative lifespan of bovine granulosa cells in culture. *Endocrinology.* 103:854–865.

Gospodarowicz D, Brown KS, Birdwell CR, Zetter B. (1978a). Control of proliferation of human vascular endothelial cells of human origin: I. Characterization of the response of human umbilical vein endothelial cells to fibroblast growth factor, epidermal growth factor, and thrombin. *J Cell Biol.* 77:774–788.

Gospodarowicz D, Greenburg G, Bialecki H, Zetter B. (1978b). Factors involved in the modulation of cell proliferation in vivo and in vitro: the role of fibroblast and epidermal growth factors in the proliferative response of mammalian cells. *In Vitro.* 14:85–118.

Gospodarowicz D, Mescher AL, Moran JS. (1978c). Cellular specificity of fibroblast growth factor and epidermal growth factor. In: *Symposia of the Society for Developmental Biology.* New York: Academic Press; 35:33–61.

Gospodarowicz D, Vlodavsky I, Greenburg G, Alvarado J, Johnson LK, Moran J. (1979a). Cellular shape is determined by the extracellular matrix and is responsible for the control of cellular growth and function. Cold Spring Harbor Conference on Cell Proliferation 9:561–592.

Gospodarowicz D, Tauber J-P. (1980). Growth factors and extracellular matrix. *Endocrinol Rev.* 1:201–267.

Gospodarowicz D, Mescher AL. (1981). Fibroblast growth factor and vertebrate regeneration. *Adv Neurol (Neurofibromatosis).* 29:149–171.

Gospodarowicz D, Vlodavsky I, Savion N. (1981). The role of fibroblast growth factor and the extracellular matrix in the control of proliferation and differentiation of corneal endothelial cells. *Vision Res.* 21:87–103.

Gospodarowicz D. (1983a). Growth factors and their action in vivo and in vitro. *J Pathol.* 141:201–233.

Gospodarowicz D. (1983b). The control of mammalian cell proliferation by growth factors, basement lamina and lipoproteins. *J Invest Dermatol.* 81:405–503.

Gospodarowicz D. (1984). Fibroblast growth factor. In: Li CH, ed. *Hormonal Proteins and Peptides.* New York: Academic Press; 12:205–230.

Gospodarowicz D, Cheng J, Lui G-M, Bohlen P. (1984). Isolation by heparin-sepharose affinity chromatography of brain fibroblast growth factor: identity with pituitary fibroblast growth factor. *Proc Natl Acad Sci USA.* 81:6963–6967.

Gospodarowicz D. (1985). Biological activity in vivo and in vitro of pituitary and brain fibroblast growth factor. In: Ford RJ, Maizel AL, ed. *Mediators in Cell Growth and Differentiation.* New York: Raven Press; 109–134.

Gospodarowicz D, Massaglia S, Cheng J, Lui G-M, Bohlen P. (1985). Isolation of bovine pituitary fibroblast growth factor purified by fast protein liquid chromatography (FPLC). Partial chemical and biological characterization. *J Cell Physiol.* 122:323–332.

Gospodarowicz D. (1986). Purification of brain and pituitary FGF. In: Barnes D, Sirbasku D, eds. *Methods in Enzymology.* New York: Academic Press; 147:106–119.

Gospodarowicz D, Cheng J. (1986). Heparin protects basic and acidic FGF from inactivation. *J Cell Physiol.* 128:475–484.

Gospodarowicz D, Neufeld G, Schweigerer L. (1986). Fibroblast growth factor. *Mol Cell Endocrinol.* 46:187–204.

Goto K, Nakamura S, Goto F, Myoshinagu M. (1984). Generation of an interleukin 1–like lymphocyte stimulating factor at inflammatory sites: correlation with the infiltration of polymorphonuclear leukocytes. *Br J Exp Pathol.* 65:521–532.

Goustin AS, Betsholtz C, Pfeiffer-Ohlsson S, Persson H, Ryndert J. (1985). Coexpression of the sis and myc proto-oncogenes in developing human placenta suggests autocrine control of trophoblast growth. *Cell.* 41:301–312.

Granstein RD, Margolis R, Mizel SB, Sauder DN. (1985). In vivo inflammatory activity of epidermal cell–derived thymocyte activating factor and recombinant interleukin-1 in the mouse. *J Clin Invest.* 77:1020–1027.

Gray PW, Aggarwal BB, Benton CV, Bringman TS, Henzel WJ, Jarrett JA, Leung DW, Moffat B, Ng P, Svedersky LP. (1984). Cloning and expression of cDNA for human lymphotoxin, a lymphokine with tumor necrosis activity. *Nature.* 312:721–724.

Greaves MW. (1980). Lack of effect of typically applied epidermal growth factor (EGF) on epidermal growth in man in vivo. *Clin Exp Dermatol.* 5:101–103.

Green H, Kehinde O, Thomas J. (1979). Growth of cultured human epidermal cells into multiple epithelia suitable for grafting. *Proc Natl Acad Sci USA.* 76:5665–5668.

Greenburg G, Vlodavsky I, Foidart JM, Gospodarowicz D. (1980). Conditioned medium from endothelial cell cultures can restore the normal phenotypic expression of vascular endothelium maintained in vitro in the absence of fibroblast growth factor. *J Cell Physiol.* 103:333–347.

Gregory H. (1975). Isolation and structure of urogastrone and its relationship to epidermal growth factor. *Nature.* 257:325–327.

Grotendorst GR, Chang T, Seppa HEJ, Kleinman HK, Martin GR. (1982). Platelet-derived growth factor is a chemoattractant for vascular smooth muscle cells. *J Cell Physiol.* 113:261–266.

Grotendorst GR, Martin GR, Penceu D, Sodek J, Harvey AK. (1985). Stimulation of granulation tissue by platelet-derived growth factor in normal and diabetic rats. *J Clin Invest.* 76:2323–2329.

Guy MW. (1975). Serum and tissue fluid lipids in rabbits experimentally infected with *Trypanosoma brucei. Trans R Soc Trop Med Hyg.* 69:429–435.

Habernicht AJR, Dresel HA, Goerig M, Weber JA, Stoehr M, Glomset JA, Ross R, Schettles G. (1986). Low-density lipoprotein receptor-dependent prostaglandin synthesis in Swiss 3T3 cells stimulated by platelet-derived growth factor. *Proc Natl Acad Sci USA.* 83:1344–1348.

Hackett RJ, Davis LS, Lipsky PE. (1988). Comparative effects of tumor necrosis factor-α and IL-2β on mitogen-induced T cell activation. *J Immunol.* 140:2639–2644.

Haigler HT, McKanna JA, Cohen S. (1979a). Direct visualization of the binding and internalization of epidermal growth factor in human carcinoma cells A-431. *J Cell Biol.* 81:382–395.

Haigler HT, McKanna JA, Cohen S. (1979b). Rapid stimulation of pinocytosis in human carcinoma A431 by epidermal growth factor. *J Cell Biol.* 83:82–90.

Haigler HT, Carpenter G. (1980). Production and partial characterization of antibody blocking epidermal growth factor: receptor interactions. *Biochim Biophys Acta.* 598:314–325.

Hamilton RT, Nilsen-Hamilton M, Adams G. (1985). Superinduction by cycloheximide of mitogen induced secreted protein produced by Balb/c 3T3 cells. *J Cell Physiol.* 123:201–208.

Hanazawa S, Hanaizumi C, Amano S, Hirose K, Ohmori Y, Kumegawa M, Yamaura K, Kitano S. (1988). Inductive effect of recombinant interleukin-1α and β on differentiation of macrophage-like tumor cell line P388D1. *J Cell Physiol.* 136:543–546.

Hartung H-P. (1983). Acetyl glyceryl ether phosphorylcholine (platelet-activating factor) mediates heightened metabolic activity in macrophages. *FEBS Lett.* 160:209–212.

Hartung H-P, Parnham MJ, Winkelmann J, Engleberger W, Hadding U. (1983). Platelet-activating factor (PAF) induces the oxidative burst in macrophages. *Int J Immunopharmacol.* 5:115–121.

Haskill S, Johnson C, Eierman D, Becker S, Warren K. (1988). Adherence induces selective mRNA expression of monocyte mediators and proto-oncogenes. *J Immunol.* 140:1690–1694.

Hazuda DJ, Lee JC, Young PR. (1988). The kinetics of interleukin-1 secretion from activated monocytes. Differences between interleukin-1α and interleukin-1β. *J Biol Chem.* 263:8473–8479.

Heimark RL, Twardzik DR, Schwartz SM. (1986). Inhibition of endothelial regeneration by type-beta transforming growth factor from platelets. *Science.* 233:1078–1080.

Heldin CH, Westermark B. (1984). Growth factors: mechanism of action and relation to oncogenes. *Cell.* 37:9–20.

Hennessey PJ, Black J, Andrassy RJ. (1989). Growth factors and diabetic wound healing: epidermal growth factor and insulin. *Current Surg.* 46:285–286.

Herman J, Dinarello CA, Kew MC, Rabson AR. (1985). The role of interleukin-1 in tumor NK cell interaction: correction of defective NK cell activity in cancer patients by treating target cells with IL-1. *J Immunol.* 135:2882–2886.

Herschlag A, Herness IGO, Wimberly HC, Bleven ML, Diamond MP, Polan ML. (1991). The effect of interleukin-1 on adhesion formation in the rat. *Am J Obstet Gynecol.* 165:771–774.

Hesse DG, Tracey KJ, Fong Y, Manoque KR, Palladino MA, Cerami A, Shires GT, Lowrey SF. (1988). Cytokine appearance in human endotoxemia and primate bacteremia. *Surg Gynecol Obstet.* 166:147–153.

Hirano T, Yasukawa K, Harada H, Taga T, Watanabe Y, Matsuda T, Kashiwamura S, Nakajima K, Koyama K, Iwasmatsu A, Tsunasawa S, Sakiyama F, Matsui H, Takahara Y, Taniguchi T, Kishimoto T. (1986). Complementary DNA for a novel human interleukin (BSF-2) that induces B lymphocytes to produce immunoglobulin. *Nature.* 324:73–76.

Hollenberg MD, Gregory H. (1976). Human urogastrone and mouse epidermal growth factor share a common receptor site in cultured human fibroblasts. *Life Sci.* 20:267–274.

Honegger AM, Szapary D, Schmidt A, Lyall R, Van Obberghen E, Dull TJ, Ullrich A, Schlessinger J. (1987a). A mutant epidermal growth factor receptor with defective protein tyrosine kinase is unable to stimulate protooncogene expression and DNA synthesis. *Mol Cell Biol.* 7:4568–4571.

Honegger AM, Dull TJ, Felder S, Van Obberghen E, Bellot F, Szapary D, Schmidt A, Ullrich A, Schlessinger J. (1987b). Point mutation at the ATP binding site of EGF receptor abolishes protein-tyrosine kinase activity and alters cellular routing. *Cell.* 51:199–209.

Hunt TK. (1991). Wound fluid: the growth environment. In: Caldwell MD, Hunt TK, Pines E, Skover G, eds. *Clinical and Experimental Approaches to Dermal and Epidermal Repair Normal and Chronic Wounds.* New York: Wiley-Liss; 365:223–230.

Hunter T, Cooper JA. (1985). Protein-tyrosine kinases. *Annu Rev Biochem.* 54:879–930.

Ignotz R, Massague J. (1986). Transforming growth factor beta stimulates the expression of fibronectin and collagen and their incorporation into the extracellular matrix. *J Biol Chem.* 261:4337–4345.

Ignotz RA, Endo T, Massague J. (1987). Regulation of fibronectin and type I collagen mRNA levels by transforming growth factor-beta. *J Biol Chem.* 262:6443–6446.

Imamura K, Spriggs D, Kufe D. (1987). Expression of tumor necrosis factor receptors on human monocytes and internalization of receptor bound ligand. *J Immunol.* 139:2989–2992.

Iribe H, Koga T, Kotani S, Kusumoto S, Shiba T. (1983). Stimulating effect of MDP and its adjuvant active analogues on guinea pig fibroblasts for the production of thymocyte activating factor. *J Exp Med.* 157:2190–2195.

Jacob CO, McDevitt HO. (1988). Tumor necrosis factor alpha in murine autoimmune 'lupus' nephritis. *Nature.* 331:356–358.

Jelink DF, Lipsky PE. (1987). Enhancement of human B cell proliferation and differentiation by tumor necrosis factor-**a** and interleukin-1. *J Immunol.* 139:2970–2976.

Jijon AJ, Gallup DG. (1989). Assessment of epidermal growth factor in the healing process of clean full thickness skin wounds. *Am J Obstet Gynecol.* 161:1658–1662.

Jiminez de Asua L, O'Farrell MK, Clinigan D, Rudland PS. (1977). Temporal sequence of hormonal interactions during the prereplicative phase of quiescent cultured 3T3 fibroblasts. *Proc Natl Acad Sci USA.* 74:3845–3849.

Johnson LK, Baxter JD, Vlodavsky I, Gospodarowicz D. (1980). EGF and expression of specific genes: effect on cultured rat pituitary cells are dissociable from the mitogenic response. *Proc Natl Acad Sci USA.* 77:394–398.

Johnson SE, Baglioni C. (1988). Tumor necrosis factor receptors and cytocidal activity are down-regulated by activators of protein kinase C. *J Biol Chem.* 263:5686–5692.

Kaibuchi K, Tsuda T, Kikuchi A, Tanimoto T, Yamashita T, Takai Y. (1986). Possible involvement of protein kinase C and calcium ions in growth factor induced expression of c myc oncogene in Swiss 3T3 cells. *J Biol Chem.* 261:1187–1192.

Kamata N, Chida K, Kimaru KR, Horikoshi M, Enomoto S, Kuroki T. (1986). Growth inhibitory effects of epidermal growth factor and overexpression of its receptors on human squamous cell carcinomas. *Cancer Res.* 46:1648–1653.

Kato Y, Gospodarowicz D. (1985). Sulfated proteoglycan synthesis by rabbit costal chondrocytes grown in the presence and absence of fibroblast growth factor. *J Cell Biol.* 100:477–485.

Kaye J, Gillis S, Mizel SB, Shevach EM, Malek TA, Dinarello CA, Lachman LB, Janeway C. (1984). Growth of a cloned helper T cell line induced by a monoclonal antibody specific for the antigen receptor: interleukin-1 is required for the expression of receptors of interleukin-2. *J Immunol.* 133:1339–1345.

Kehrl JH, Roberts AB, Luakefield LM, Jakowlew SB, Sporn MB, Fauci AS. (1986a). Transforming growth factor beta is an important immunomodulatory protein for human B lymphocytes. *J Immunol.* 137:3855–3860.

Kehrl JH, Wakefield LM, Roberts AB, Jakowlew SB, Alvarez-Mon MA, Derynck R, Sporn MB, Fauci AS. (1986b). Production of transforming growth factor beta by human T lymphocytes and its potential role in the regulation of T cell growth. *J Exp Med.* 163:1037–1050.

Kemp A, Mellow L, Sabbadini E. (1986). Inhibition of interleukin-1 activity by a factor in sub-mandibular glands of rats. *J Immunol.* 137:2245–2251.

Keski-Oja J, Lyones RM, Moses HL. (1987). Inactive secreted form(s) of transforming growth factor-beta: activation by proteolysis. *J Cell Biochem Suppl.* 11A:60.

Keski-Oja J, Blasi F, Leof EB, Moses HL. (1988). Regulation of the synthesis and activity of urokinase plasminogen activator in A549 human lung carcinoma cells by transforming growth factor beta. *J Cell Biol.* 106:451–459.

Kilian PA, Kafka KL, Stern AS, Woehle D, Benjamin LR, DeChiarg TM, Gubler U, Farrar JJ, Mizel SB, Lomedico PT. (1986). Interleukin-1α and interleukin-1β bind to the same receptor on T cells. *J Immunol.* 136:4509–4515.

Knighton DR, Ciresi KF, Fiegel VD, Austin LL, Butler EL. (1986). Classification and treatment of chronic nonhealing wounds. Successful treatment with autologous platelet-derived wound healing factors. *Ann Surg.* 204:322–330.

Knighton DR, Dowcette M, Fiegel VD, Ciresi K, Butler E, Austin L. (1988). The use of platelet derived wound healing formula in human clinical trials. In: Barbul A, Pines E, Caldwell M, Hunt TK, eds. *Growth Factors and Other Aspects of Wound Healing: Biological and Clinical Research.* New York: Alan R. Liss; 266:319–329.

Knighton DR, Ciresi K, Fiegel VD, Schumerk S, Bulter E, Kind A, Cerra F. (1990). Stimulation of repair in chronic, nonhealing, cutaneous ulcers using platelet-derived wound healing formula. *Surg Gynecol Obstet.* 170:56–60.

Koch KS, Leffert HL. (1979). Increased sodium ion influx is necessary to initiate rat hepatocyte proliferation. *Cell.* 18:153–163.

Kohler N, Lipton A. (1974). Platelets as a source of fibroblast growth promoting activity. *Exp Cell Res.* 87:297–301.

Krane SM, Dayer J-M, Simon LS, Bryne S. (1985). Mononuclear cell-conditioned medium containing mononuclear cell factor (MCF), homologous with interleukin-1, stimulates collagen and fibronectin synthesis by adherent rheumatoid synovial cells : effects of prostaglandin E2 and indomethacin. *Coll Relat Res.* 5:99–117.

Kreuger JM, Walter J, Dinarello CA, Wolff SM, Chedid L. (1984). Sleep-promoting effects of endogenous pyrogen (interleukin-1). *Am J Physiol.* 246:R994–R999.

Kriegler M, Perez C, DeFay K, Albert I, Lu SD. (1988). A novel form of TNF/cachectin is a cell surface cytotoxic transmembrane protein: ramifications for the complex physiology of TNF. *Cell.* 53:45–53.

Kroggel R, Martin M, Pingoud V, Dayer J-M, Resch K. (1988). Two-chain structure of interleukin-1 receptor. *FEBS Lett.* 229:59–62.

Ksander GA, Ogawa Y, Chu GH, McMullin H, Rosenblatt JS, McPherson JM. (1990). Exogenous transforming growth factor–Beta$_2$ enhances connective tissue formation and wound strength in guinea pig dermal wounds healing by secondary intent. *Ann Surg.* 211:288–294.

Kull FC, Jacobs S, Cuatrecasas P. (1985). Cellular receptor for ^{125}I-labeled tumor necrosis factor: specific binding, affinity labeling and relationship to sensitivity. *Proc Natl Acad Sci USA.* 82:5756–5760.

Kunkumian GK, Lafyatis R, Rennmers EF, Case JP, Kim SJ, Wilder RL. (1989). Platelet-derived growth factor and IL-1 interactions in rheumatoid arthritis. Regulation of synoviocyte proliferation, prostaglandin production and collagenase transcription. *J Immunol.* 143:833–837.

Kuraoka S, Campeau JD, Rodgers KE, Nakamura RM, diZerega GS. (1992). Effects of interleukin-1 (IL-1) on postsurgical macrophage secretion of protease and protease inhibitor activities. *J Surg Res.* 52:71–78.

Laato M, Ninikoshi J, Gerdin B, Lebel L. (1985). Stimulation of wound healing by epidermal growth factor: a dose-dependent effect. *Ann Surg.* 203:379–381.

Laiho M, Sakesela O, Andreasen PA, Keski-Oja J. (1986). Enhanced production of extracellular deposition of the endothelial type plasminogen activator inhibitor in cultured human lung fibroblasts by transforming growth factor beta. *J Cell Biol.* 103:2403–2410.

Lawrence WT, Norton JA, Sporn B, Gorschboth C, Grotendorst GR. (1988). The reversal of an Adriamycin-induced healing impairment with chemoattractants and growth factors. *Ann Surg.* 203:142–147.

Lee MD, Zentella A, Pekala PH, Cerami A. (1987). Effect of endotoxin-induced monokines on glucose metabolism in the muscle cell line L6. *Proc Natl Acad Sci USA.* 84:2590–2594.

Leffert HL, Koch KS. (1982). Hepatocyte growth regulation by hormones in chemically defined medium: a two-signal hypothesis. Cold Spring Harbor Symposium on Cell Proliferation 9:597–619.

Leibovich SJ, Polverini PJ, Shepard HM, Wiseman DM, Shwely V, Nuseir N. (1987). Macrophage induced angiogenesis is mediated by tumor necrosis factor α. *Nature.* 329:630–632.

Leitzel K, Cano C, Marks J, Lipton A. (1982). Failure of nerve growth factor to enhance wound healing in the hamster. *J Neurosci Res.* 8:413–417.

Leizer T, Clarris BJ, Ash PE, Van Damme J, Saklatvah J, Hamilton JA. (1987). Interleukin-1 beta and interleukin-1 alpha stimulate the plasminogen activator activity and prostaglandin E$_2$ levels of human synovial cells. *Arthritis Rheum.* 30:562–566.

Leizer T, Hamilton JA. (1989). Plasminogen activator and prostaglandin E$_2$ levels in human synovial fibroblasts. Differential stimulation by synovial activator and other cytokines. *J Immunol.* 143:971–978.

Lemmon SK, Rielly MC, Thomas KA, Hoover GA, Maciag T, Bradshaw R.

(1982). Bovine fibroblast growth factor: comparison of brain and pituitary preparations. *J Cell Biol.* 95:162–169.

Li AKC, Koroby MJ, Schattenkerk ME, Malt RA, Young M. (1980). Nerve growth factor: acceleration of the rate of wound healing in mice. *Proc Natl Acad Sci USA.* 77:4379–4381.

Libby P, Ordovas JM, Auger KR, Robbins AH, Birinyi LK, Dinarello CA. (1986a). Endotoxin and tumor necrosis factor induce interleukin-1 gene expression in adult human vascular endothelial cells. *Am J Pathol.* 123:16–24.

Libby P, Ordovas JM, Auger KR, Robbins AH, Birinyi LK, Dinarello CA. (1986b). Inducible interleukin-1 gene expression in vascular smooth muscle cells. *J Clin Invest.* 78:1432–1438.

Libby J, Martinez R, Weber MJ. (1986c). Tyrosine phosphorylase in cells treated with transforming growth factor-beta. *J Cell Physiol.* 129:159–166.

Libby P, Warner SJC, Salomon RN, Birinyi LK. (1988). Production of platelet-derived growth factor-like mitogen by smooth-muscle cells from human atheroma. *N Engl J Med.* 318:1493–1498.

Like B, Massague J. (1986). The antiproliferative effect of type beta transforming growth factor occurs at a level distal from receptors for growth-activating factors. *J Biol Chem.* 261:13426–13429.

Limjuco G, Galuska S, Chin J, Cameron P, Boger J, Schmidt JA. (1986). Antibodies of predetermined specificity to the major charged species of interleukin 1. *Proc Natl Acad Sci USA.* 83:3972–3976.

Lobb R, Sasse J, Sullivan R, Shing Y, D'Amore P, Jacobs J, Klagsbrun M. (1986). Purification and characterization of heparin binding endothelial cell growth factor. *J Biol Chem.* 261:1924–1928.

Lomedico PT, Gubler U, Hellman CP, Dukovich M, Giri JG, Pan YE, Collier K, Semionow R, Chua AO, Mizel SB. (1984). Cloning and expression of murine interleukin-1 in *Escherichia coli. Nature.* 312:458–462.

Lovett DH, Ryan JL, Sterzel RB. (1983). A thymocyte activating factor derived from glomerular mesangial cells. *J Immunol.* 130:1796–1801.

Lowenthal JW, MacDonald HR. (1986). Binding and internalizing of interleukin-1 by T cells. Direct evidence for high- and low-affinity classes of interleukin-1 receptor. *J Exp Med.* 164:1060–1074.

Lowenthal JW, Cerrottini J-C, MacDonald HR. (1986). Interleukin-1–dependent induction of both interleukin-2 secretion and interleukin-2 receptor expression by thymoma cells. *J Immunol.* 137:1226–1231.

Luger TA, Stadler BM, Katz SI, Oppenheim JJ. (1981). Epidermal cell (keratinocyte)-derived thymocyte-activating factor (ETAF). *J Immunol.* 127:1493–1498.

Luger TA, Charon JA, Colot M, Micksche M, Oppenheim JJ. (1983). Chemotactic properties of partially purified human epidermal cell-derived thymocyte activating factor (ETAF) for polymorphonuclear and mononuclear cells. *J Immunol.* 131:816–820.

Lynch SE, Nixon JC, Colvin RB, Antoniades HN. (1987). Role of platelet-derived growth factors in wound healing: synergistic effects with other growth factors. *Proc Natl Acad Sci USA.* 84:7696–7700.

Lynch SE, Colvin RB, Antoniades HN. (1989). Growth factors in wound healing: single and synergistic effects on partial thickness porcine skin wounds. *J Clin Invest.* 84:640–646.

Lynch SE. (1991). Interactions of growth factors in tissue repair. In: Caldwell MD, Hunt TK, Pines E, Skover G, eds. *Clinical and Experimental Approaches to Dermal and Epidermal Repair Normal and Chronic Wounds*. New York: Wiley-Liss; 365:341–358.

Macaig R, Cerundolo J, Isley S, Kelley PR, Forand R. (1979). An endothelial cell growth factor from bovine hypothalamus: identification and partial characterization. *Proc Natl Acad Sci USA*. 76:5674–5679.

Madri JA, Pratt BM, Tucker AM. (1988). Phenotypic modulation of endothelial cells by transforming growth factor beta depends upon the composition and organization of the extracellular matrix. *J Cell Biol*. 106:1375–1384.

March CJ, Mosley B, Larsen A, Ceretti DP, Braedt G, Price V, Gillis S, Henney CS, Kronheim SR, Grabstein K, Conlon PJ, Hopp TP, Cosman D. (1985). Cloning, sequence and expression of two distinct human interleukin-1 complementary DNAs. *Nature*. 315:641–647.

Marquardt H, Todaro GJ. (1982). Human tranforming growth factor. Production by a melanoma cell line; purification and initial characterization. *J Biol Chem*. 257:5220–5225.

Marquardt H, Hunkapiller HW, Hood LE, Tiuardzik DR, deLarco JE, Stephenson JR, Todaro GJ. (1983). Transforming growth factors produced by retrovirus transformed rodent fibroblasts and human melanoma cells: amino acid sequence homology with epidermal growth factor. *Proc Natl Acad Sci USA*. 80:4684–4688.

Marquardt H, Hunkapiller HW, Hood LE, Todaro GJ. (1984). Rat transforming growth factor 1: structure and relation to epidermal growth factor. *Science*. 223:1079–1082.

Martinet Y, Bitterman PB, Mornex J-F, Grotendorst GR, Martin GR, Crystal RG. (1986). Activated human monocytes express the c-sis proto-oncogene and release a mediator showing PDGF-like activity. *Nature*. 319:158–160.

Massague J. (1985). Transforming growth factor-beta modulates the high affinity receptors for epidermal growth factor and transforming growth factor beta. *J Cell Biol*. 100:1508–1514.

Massague J, Cheifetz S, Endo T, Nadal-Ginard B. (1986). Type-beta transforming growth factor is an inhibitor of myogenic differentiation. *Proc Natl Acad Sci USA*. 83:8206–8210.

Matrisian LM, Leroy P, Ruhlmann C, Gesnel M-C, Breathnach R. (1986). Isolation of the oncogene and epidermal growth factor-induced transferin gene: complex control in rat fibroblasts. *Mol Cell Biol*. 6:1679–1686.

Matsushima K, Kimball ES, Durum SK, Oppenheim JJ. (1985a). Purification of human interleukin-1 from a human monocyte culture supernatants and identity of thymocyte comitogenic factor, fibroblast proliferation factor, acute phase protein inducing factor and endogenous pyrogen. *Cell Immunol*. 92:290–301.

Matsushima K, Bano M, Kidwell WR, Oppenheim JJ. (1985b). Interleukin-1 increase collagen type IV production by murine mammary epithelial cells. *J Immunol*. 134:904–909.

Matsushima K, Propopio A, Abe H, Scala G, Ortaldo JR, Oppenheim JJ. (1985c). Production of interleukin-1 activity by normal peripheral blood B lymphocytes. *J Immunol*. 135:1132–1136.

Matsushima K, Taguchi M, Kovaks EJ, Young HA, Oppenheim JJ. (1986a). Intracellular localization of human monocyte associated interleukin-1 activity and release of biologically active IL-1 from monocytes by trypsin and plasmin. *J Immunol.* 136:2883–2891.

Matsushima K, Akahoshi T, Yamada M, Furutani Y, Oppenheim JJ. (1986b). Properties of specific interleukin-1 receptor on human Epstein-Barr virus-transformed B lymphocytes: identity of the receptor for IL-1α and IL-1β. *J Immunol.* 136:4496–4501.

Maury CP, Teppo AM. (1987). Raised serum levels of cachectin/tumor necrosis factor alpha in renal allograft rejection. *J Exp Med.* 166:1132–1137.

McAdam KPWJ, Dinarello CA. (1980). Induction of serum amyloid A synthesis by human leukocytic pyrogen. In: Agawal MK, ed. *Bacterial Endotoxins and Host Response.* Amsterdam: Elsevier North Holland; 167–178.

McBride WH, Mason K, Withers HR, Davis C. (1989). Effect of interleukin-1, inflammation, and surgery on the incidence of adhesion formation after abdominal irradiation in mice. *Cancer Res.* 49:169–173.

McCroskery PA, Arai A, Amento EP, Krane SM. (1985). Stimulation of procollagenase synthesis in human rheumatoid synovial fibroblasts by mononuclear cell factor/interleukin-1. *FEBS Lett.* 191:7–12.

McGee GS, Davidson JM, Buckley A, Sommer A, Woodward SC, Aquino AM, Barbour R, Demetriou AA. (1988). Recombinant basic fibroblast growth factor accelerates wound healing. *J Surg Res.* 45:145–153.

McGee GS, Broadley KN, Buckley A, Aquino A, Woodward SC, Demetriou AA, Davidson JM. (1989). Recombinant transforming growth factor beta accelerates incisional wound healing. *Curr Surg.* March:103–106.

McGowan JA, Strain AJ, Bucher NLR. (1981). DNA synthesis in primary cultures of adult rat hepatocytes in a defined medium: effect of epidermal growth factor, insulin, glucagon, and cyclic AMP. *J Cell Physiol.* 108:353–364.

McManus LM, Hanahan DJ, Demopoulos CA, Pinckard RN. (1980). Pathobiology of the intravenous infusion of acetyl glyceryl ether phosphorylcholine (AGPEC), and synthetic platelet-activating factor (PAF), in the rabbit. *J Immunol.* 124:2919–2924.

McManus LM, Fitzpatrick FA, Hanahan DJ, Pinckard RN. (1983). Thromboxane B$_2$ release following acetyl glyceryl ether phosphorylcholine (AGEPC) infusion in the rabbit. *Immunopharmacology.* 5:197–207.

Medcalf RL, Hamilton JA. (1986). Human synovial fibroblasts produce urokinase-type plasminogen activator. *Arthritis Rheum.* 29:1397–1401.

Mescher AL, Gospodarowicz D, Moran JS. (1979). Mitogenic effect of a growth factor derived from myelin on denervated regenerates of newt forelimbs. *J Exp Zool.* 207:497–503.

Mestan J, Digel W, Mittnacht S, Hillen H, Blohm D, Moeller A, Jacoben H, Kirchner H. (1986). Antiviral effects of recombinant tumor necrosis factor in vitro. *Nature.* 323:816–819.

Michel JB, Quertermous T. (1989). Modulation of mRNA levels for urinary- and tissue-type plasminogen activator and plasminogen activator inhibitors 1 and 2 in human fibroblasts by interleukin-1. *J Immunol.* 143:890–895.

Mignatti P, Tsuboi R, Robbins E, Rifkin DB. (1989). In vitro angiogenesis on the human amniotic membrane: requirement for basic fibroblast growth factor-induced proteinases. *J Cell Biol.* 108:671–682.

Mira Y, Lopez R, Joseph-Silverstein J, Rifkin DB, Ossowski L. (1986). Identification of a pituitary factor responsible for enhancement of plasminogen activator activity in breast tumor cells. *Proc Natl Acad Sci USA.* 83:7780–7788.

Mizel SB, Mizel D. (1981). Purification to apparent homogeneity of murine interleukin-1. *J Immunol.* 126:834–842.

Mondschein JS, Schomberg DW. (1981). Growth factors modulate gonadotropin receptor induction in granulosa cell cultures. *Science.* 211:1179–1180.

Montesano R, Vassalli JD, Baird A, Guillemin R, Orci L. (1986). Basic fibroblast growth factor induces angiogenesis in vitro. *Proc Natl Acad Sci USA.* 83:7297–7301.

Morrison RS, Sharma A, De Veillis J, Bradshaw RA. (1986). Basic fibroblast growth factor supports the survival of cerebral cortical neurons in primary culture. *Proc Natl Acad Sci USA.* 83:7537–7541.

Moscatelli D, Presta M, Rifkin DB. (1986). Purification of a factor from human placenta that stimulates capillary endothelial cell protease production, DNA synthesis, and cell migration. *Proc Natl Acad Sci USA.* 83:2091–2095.

Moses HL, Tucker RF, Leof EB, Coffey RJ, Halper J, Shipley GD. (1985). Type beta transforming growth factor in a growth stimulator and a growth inhibitor. *Cancer Cells* (Cold Spring Harbor). 3:65–71.

Muchmore AV, Decker JM. (1985). Uromodulin a unique 85-kilodalton immunosuppressive glycoprotein from urine of pregnant women. *Science.* 229:479–481.

Muchmore AV, Decker JM. (1986). An immunosuppressive 85-kilodalton glycoprotein isolated from human pregnancy urine is a high affinity ligand for recombinant interleukin-1a. *J Biol Chem.* 261:13404–13407.

Mueller R, Bravo R, Burkshardt J, Curran T. (1984). Induction of c fos gene and protein by growth factors precedes activation of c myc. *Nature.* 312:716–720.

Munker R, Gasson J, Ogawa M, Koeffler HP. (1986). Recombinant human TNF induces production of granulocyte-monocyte colony-stimulating factor. *Nature.* 323:79–82.

Muraguchi A, Kehrl JH, Butler JL, Fauci AS. (1984). Regulation of human B-cell activation, proliferation and differentiation by soluble factors. *J Clin Immunol.* 4:337–347.

Murphy PA, Chesney J, Wood WB. (1974). Further purification of rabbit leukocyte pyrogen. *J Lab Clin Med.* 83:310–322.

Murphy PA, Simon PL, Willoughby WF. (1980). Endogenous pyrogens made by rabbit peritoneal exudate cells are identical with lymphocyte activating factors made by rabbits alveolar macrophages. *J Immunol.* 124:2498–2501.

Mustoe TA, Pierce GF, Thomason A, Gramates P, Sporn MB, Deuel TF. (1987). Accelerated healing of incisional wounds in rats induced by transforming growth factor-β. *Science.* 237:1333–1336.

Nachman RL, Hajjar KA, Silverstein RL, Dinarello CA. (1986). Interleukin-1 induces endothelial cell synthesis of plasminogen activator inhibitor. *J Exp Med.* 163:1545–1547.

Nathan CF. (1987). Neutrophil activation on biological surfaces: massive secretion of hydrogen peroxide in response to products of macrophages and lymphocytes. *J Clin Invest.* 80:1550–1560.

Nauts HC. (1980). *The Beneficial Effects of Bacterial Infections on Host Resistance to Cancer: End Results in 449 Cases.* 2nd ed. New York: Cancer Research Institute (Cancer Research Institute Monograph); vol 8.

Nawroth PP, Stern DM. (1986). Modulation of endothelial cell hemostatic properties by tumor necrosis factor. *J Exp Med.* 163:740–745.

Nawroth PP, Handley DA, Esmon CT, Stern DM. (1986a). Interleukin-1 induces endothelial cell procoagulant while suppressing cell surface anti-coagulant activity. *Proc Natl Acad Sci USA.* 83:3460–3464.

Nawroth PP, Bank I, Handley D, Cassimeris J, Chess L, Stern D. (1986b). Tumor necrosis factor/cachectin interacts with endothelial cell receptors to induce release of interleukin-1. *J Exp Med.* 163:1363–1375.

Neufeld G, Gospodarowicz D. (1985). The identification and partial characterization of the fibroblast growth factor receptor of baby hamster kidney cells. *J Biol Chem.* 260:13860–13868.

Neufeld G, Gospodarowicz D. (1986). Basic and acidic fibroblast growth factor interact with the same cell surface receptor. *J Biol Chem.* 261:5631–5637.

Newton RC. (1985). Effect of interferon on the induction of human monocyte secretion of interleukin-1 activity. *Immunology.* 56:441–449.

Niall M, Ryan GB, O'Brien BM. (1982). The effect of epidermal growth factor on wound healing in mice. *J Surg Res.* 33:164–169.

Nieuwkoop PD. (1969). The formation of mesoderm in Urodelean amphibians. I. Induction by the ectoderm. *Wilhelm Roux' Arch Entw Mech Org.* 162:341–373.

Nilsen-Hamilton M, Shapiro JM, Massoglia SL, Hamilton RT. (1980). Selective stimulation by mitogens of incorporation of S-methionine into a family of proteins released into the medium by 3T3 cells. *Cell.* 20:19–28.

Nilsen-Hamilton M, Hamilton RT, Allen WR, Massoglia S. (1981). Stimulation of the release of two glycoproteins from mouse 3T3 cells by growth factors and by agents that increase intralysosomal pH. *Biochem Biophys Res Commun.* 101:411–417.

O'Malley WE, Achinstein B, Shear MJ. (1962). Action of bacterial polysaccharide on tumors. II. Damage of sarcoma 37 by serum of mice treated with *Serratia marcescens* polysaccharide and induce tolerance. *J Nat Cancer Inst.* 29:1169–1175.

Oliff A, Defeo-Jones D, Boyer M, Martinez D, Kiefer D, Vuocolo G, Wolfe A, Socher SH. (1987). Tumors secreting human TNF/cachectin induce cachexia in mice. *Cell.* 50:555–563.

Olwin BB, Hauschka SD. (1986). Identification of the fibroblast growth factor receptor of Swiss 3T3 cells and mouse skeletal myoblasts. *Biochemistry.* 25:3487–3492.

Panaretto BA, Leish Z, Moore GP, Robertson DMJ. (1984). Inhibition of DNA synthesis in dermal tissue of merino sheep treated with depilatory doses of mouse epidermal growth factor. *J Endocr.* 100:25–31.

Parfett CLJ, Hamilton RT, Howell BW, Edwards DR, Nilsen-Hamilton M, Denhardt DT. (1985). Characterization of a cDNA clone encoding murine mitogen regulated protein: regulation of mRNA levels in mortal and immortal cell lines. *Mol Cell Biol.* 5:3289–3292.

Pennica D, Nedwin GE, Hayflick JS, Seeburg PH, Derynck R, Palladino MA, Kohr WJ, Aggarwall BB, Goeddel DV. (1984). Human tumor necrosis factor: precursor, structure, expression and homology to lymphotoxin. *Nature.* 312:724–729.

Pennica D, Hayflick JS, Bringham TS, Palladino MA, Goeddal DV. (1985). Cloning and expression in *E. coli* of the cDNA for murine tumor necrosis factor. *Proc Natl Acad Sci USA.* 82:6060–6064.

Perlmutter D, Goldberger G, Dinarello CA, Mizel SB, Colten HR. (1986a). Regulation of class II major histocompatability complex gene products by interleukin-1. *Science.* 232:850–852.

Perlmutter D, Dinarello CA, Punsal P, Colten HR. (1986b). Cachectin/tumor necrosis factor regulates hepatic acute phase gene expression. *J Clin Invest.* 78:1349–1354.

Pessa ME, Bland KI, Sitren HS, Miller GJ, Copeland EM III. (1985). Improved wound healing in tumor-bearing rats treated with perioperative synthetic human growth hormone. *Surg Forum.* 36:6–8.

Pierce GF, Mustoe TA, Deuel TF. (1988a). Transforming growth factor β induces increased directed cellular migration and tissue repair in rats. In: Barbul A, Pines E, Caldwell M, Hunt TK, eds. *Growth Factors and Other Aspects of Wound Healing: Biological and Clinical Research.* New York: Alan R. Liss; 266:93–102.

Pierce GF, Mustoe TA, Senior RM, Reed J, Griffin GL, Thomason A, Deuel TF. (1988b). In vivo incisional wound healing augmented by platelet-derived growth factor and recombinant c-sis gene homodimeric proteins. *J Exp Med.* 167:974–987.

Pierce GF, Mustoe TA, Lingelbach J, Masakowski VR, Griffin GL, Senior RM, Deuel TF. (1989a). Platelet-derived growth factor and transforming growth factor-β enhance tissue repair activities by unique mechanisms. *J Cell Biol.* 109:429–440.

Pierce GF, Mustoe TA, Lingelbach J, Masakowski V, Gramates P, Deuel TF. (1989b). Transforming growth factor β reverses the glucocorticoid-induced wound healing deficit in rats and is regulated by platelet-derived growth factor in macrophages. *Proc Natl Acad Sci USA.* USA 86:2229–2233.

Pierce GF, Yanagihara D, Thomason A, Fox GM. (1990). PDGF, TGF-β and basic FGF differentially induce extracellular matrix, neovessel formation and re-epithelialization in lapine excisional wounds. *FASEB J.* 4(3):A624.

Piguet PF, Grau GE, Allet B, Vassalli P. (1987). Tumor necrosis factor/cachectin is an effector of skin and gut lesions of the acute phase of graft-vs-host disease. *J Exp Med.* 166:1280–1289.

Pinckard RN, McManus LM, Demopoulos CA, Halonen M, Clark PO, Shaw JO, Kniker WT, Hanahan DJ. (1980). Molecular pathobiology of acetyl glyceryl ether phosphorylcholine (AGEPC): Evidence for the structural identity with platelet-activating factor (PAF). *J Reticuloendothel Soc.* 28:95s–103s.

Pincus SH, Whitcomb EA, Dinarello CA. (1986). Interaction of interleukin-1 and TPA in modulation of eosinophil function. *J Immunol.* 137:3509–3514.

Pober JS, Gimbrone MA, Lapierre LA, Mendrick DL, Fiers W, Rothlein R, Springer TA. (1986a). Overlapping patterns of activation of human endothelial cells by interleukin-1, tumor necrosis factor and immune interferon. *J Immunol.* 137:1893–1896.

Pober JS, Bevilacqua MP, Mendrick DL, Lapierre PA, Fiers W, Gimbrone MA. (1986b). Two distinct monokines, interleukin-1 and tumor necrosis factor, each independently induce biosynthesis and transient expression of the same antigen on the surface of cultured human vascular endothelial cells. *J Immunol.* 136:1680–1683.

Pober JS. (1987). Effects of tumor necrosis factor and related cytokines on vascular endothelial cells. In: Bock G, Marsh J, eds. *Tumor Necrosis Factor and Related Cytokines.* Ciba Foundation Symposium 131. Chichester: John Wiley; 88–108.

Pohlman TH, Stanness KA, Beatty PG, Ochs HE, Harlan JM. (1986). An endothelial cell surface factor(s) induced in vitro by lipopolysaccharide, interleukin-1, and tumor necrosis factor-α increases neutrophil adherence by a CDw18-dependent mechanism. *J Immunol.* 136:4548–4553.

Postlethwaite AE, Lachman LB, Mainardi CL, Kang AH. (1983). Interleukin-1 stimulation of collagenase production by cultured fibroblasts. *J Exp Med.* 157:801–806.

Prakash A, Pandit PN, Sharma LK. (1974). Studies in wound healing in experimental diabetes. *Int Surg.* 59(1):25–36.

Raghow R, Postlethwaite AK, Keski-Oja J, Moses HL, Kang AH. (1987). Transforming growth factor-beta increases steady state levels of type I procollagen and fibronectin mRNAs post transcriptionally in cultured human dermal fibroblasts. *J Clin Invest.* 79:1285–1288.

Ramadori G, Sipes JD, Dinarello CA, Mizel SB, Colter HR. (1985). Pretranslational modulation of acute phase hepatic protein synthesis by murine recombinant interleukin-1 and purified human IL-1. *J Exp Med.* 162:930–942.

Richman RA, Claus TH, Pilkis SJ, Friedman DL. (1976). Hormonal stimulation of DNA synthesis in primary cultures of adult rat hepatocytes. *Proc Natl Acad Sci USA.* 60:1620–1624.

Risau W. (1986). Developing brain produces an angiogenesis factor. *Proc Natl Acad Sci USA.* 83:3855–3859.

Roberts AB, Anzano MA, Meyers CA, Sporn MB. (1983). Purification and properties of a type-β transforming growth factor from bovine kidney. *Biochemistry.* 22:5692–5698.

Roberts AB, Anzano MA, Wakefield LM, Roche NS, Stern DF, Sporn MB. (1985). Type beta transforming growth factor: a bifunctional regulator of cellular growth. *Proc Natl Acad Sci USA.* 82:119–123.

Roberts AB, Sporn MB, Assoian RK, Smith JM, Roche NS, Wakefield PM, Heine UI, Liotta LA, Falanga V, Kehrl JH, Fauci AS. (1986). Transforming growth factor type-beta; rapid induction of fibrosis and angiogenesis in vivo and stimulation of collagen formation in vitro. *Proc Natl Acad Sci USA.* 83:4167–4171.

Roberts AB, Sporn MB. (1988a). Transforming growth factor beta: new chemical forms and new biological roles. *Biofactors.* 1:89–93.

Roberts, AB, Sporn MB. (1988b). Transforming growth factor beta. *Adv Cancer Res.* 51:107–145.

Roberts NJ, Prill AH, Mann TN. (1986). Interleukin-1 and interleukin-1 inhibitor production by human macrophages exposed to influenza virus or respiratory syncytial virus. *J Exp Med.* 163:511–519.

Robey PG, Young MF, Flanders KC, Roche NS, Kondaiah P, Reddi AH, Termine JD, Sporn MB, Roberts AB. (1987). Osteoblasts synthesize and respond to TGF-beta in vitro. *J Cell Biol.* 105:457–463.

Rodgers BC, Scott DM, Mundin J, Sissons JGP. (1985). Monocyte-derived inhibitor of interleukin-1 induced by human cytomegalovirus. *J Virol.* 55:527–532.

Rodgers KE, diZerega GS. Modulation of peritoneal re-epithelialization by postsurgical macrophages. *J Surg Res.* (in press).

Roger PP, Dumont JE. (1982). Epidermal growth factor controls the proliferation and the expression of differentiation in canine thyroid cells in primary culture. *FEBS Lett.* 144:209–212.

Rosenwasser LJ, Dinarello CA, Rosenthal A. (1979). Adherent cell function in murine T-lymphocyte recognition by human leukocytic pyrogen. *J Exp Med.* 150:709–714.

Rosoff PM, Savage N, Dinarello CA. (1988). Interleukin-1 stimulates diacylglycerol production by T lymphocytes by a novel mechanism. *Cell.* 54:73–81.

Ross R, Glomset JA, Kariya B, Harker L. (1974). A platelet-derived serum factor that stimulates the proliferation of arterial smooth muscle cells in vitro. *Proc Natl Acad Sci USA.* 71:1207–1210.

Ross R. (1986). The pathogenesis of atherosclerosis: an update. *N Engl J Med.* 314:488–500.

Ross R, Raines EW, Bowen-Pope DF. (1986). The biology of platelet-derived growth factor. *Cell.* 46:155–169.

Rossi V, Breviario F, Ghezzi P, Dejana E, Mantovani A. (1985). Interleukin-1 induces prostacyclin in vascular cells. *Science.* 229:1174–1176.

Rouzer CA, Cerami A. (1980). Hypertriglyceridemia associated with *Trypanosoma brucei* infection in rabbits: role of defective triglyceride removal. *Mol Biochem Parasitol.* 2:31–38.

Rozengurt E, Heppel LA. (1975). Serum rapidly stimulates ouabain-sensitive ^{86}Rb+ influx in quiescent 3T3 cells. *Proc Natl Acad Sci USA.* 72:4492–4495.

Ruggiero V, Tavernier J, Fiers W, Baglioni C. (1986). Induction of the synthesis of tumor necrosis factor receptors by interferon-gamma. *J Immunol.* 136:2445–2450.

Ruggiero V, Latham K, Baglioni C. (1987). Cytostatic and cytotoxic activity of tumor necrosis factor on human cancer cells. *J Immunol.* 138:2711–2717.

Saklatvala J, Sarsfield SJ, Townsend Y. (1985). Pig interleukin-1: purification of two immunologically different leukocyte proteins that cause cartilage resorption, lymphocyte activation and fever. *J Exp Med.* 162:1208–1222.

Saklatvala J. (1986). Tumor necrosis factor α stimulates resorption and inhibits synthesis of proteoglycan in cartilage. *Nature.* 322:547–549.

Sapolsky R, Rivier C, Yamamoto G, Plotsky P, Vale W. (1987). Interleukin-1 stimulates the secretion of hypothalamic corticotropin-releasing factor. *Science.* 238:522–524.

Sauder DN, Dinarello CA, Morhenn VB. (1984a). Langerhans cell production of interleukin-1. *J Invest Dermatol.* 82:605–607.

Sauder DN, Mounessa NL, Katz SI, Dinarello CA, Gallin JI. (1984b). Chemotactic cytokines. The role of leukocytic pyrogen and epidermal cell thymocyte activating factor in neutrophil chemotaxis. *J Immunol.* 132:828–832.

Sayers TJ, Wiltrout TA, Bull CA, Denn AC, Pilaro AM, Lokesh B. (1988). Effects of cytokines on polymorphonuclear neutrophil infiltration in the mouse. Prostaglandin- and leukotriene-independent induction of infiltration by IL-1 and tumor necrosis factor. *J Immunol.* 141:1670–1677.

Schlessinger J, Schechter Y, Willingham MC, Pastan I. (1978). Direct visualization of binding, aggregation and internalization of insulin and epidermal growth factor on living fibroblast cells. *Proc Natl Acad Sci USA.* 75:2659–2663.

Schlessinger J, Geiger B. (1981). Epidermal growth factor induces redistribution of actin and actinin in human epidermal carcinoma cells. *Exp Cell Res.* 134:273–279.

Schlessinger J. (1987). Allosteric regulation of the epidermal growth factor receptor kinase. *J Cell Biol.* 103:2067–2072.

Schmidt JA, Mizel SB, Cohen D, Green I. (1982). Interleukin-1, a potential regulator of fibroblast proliferation. *J Immunol.* 128:2177–2182.

Schnyder J, Payne T, Dinarello CA. (1987). Human monocyte or recombinant interleukin-1s are specific for the secretion of a metalloproteinase from chondrocytes. *J Immunol.* 138:496–503.

Schonbrunn A, Krashoff M, Westerdorf JM, Tashyan AH. (1980). EGF and TRH act similarly on a clonal pituitary cell strain. *J Cell Biol.* 85:786–797.

Schwartz T, Urbanska A, Gschnait F, Luger TA. (1987). UV-irradiated epidermal cells produce a specific inhibitor of interleukin-1 activity. *J Immunol.* 138:1457–1463.

Seckinger P, Lowenthal JW, Williamson K, Dayer J-M, MacDonald HR. (1987). An urine inhibitor of interleukin-1 activity that blocks ligand binding. *J Immunol.* 139:1546–1549.

Seifert RA, Hart CE, Phillips PE, Forstran JW, Ross R, Murray MJ, Bowen-Pope DF. (1989). Two different subunits associate to create isoform-specific PDGF receptors. *J Biol Chem.* 264:8771–8778.

Seyedin SM, Thomas TC, Thompson AY, Rosen DM, Piez KA. (1985). Purification and characterization of two cartilage-inducing factors from bovine demineralized bone. *Proc Natl Acad Sci USA.* 82:2267–2271.

Shalaby MR, Aggarwal BB, Rinderknecht E, Svedersky LP, Finkle BS, Palladino MA. (1985). Activation of human polymorphonuclear neutrophil functions by interferon-γ and tumor necrosis factors. *J Immunol.* 135:2069–2073.

Shaw JO, Pinckard RN, Ferrigni KS, McManus LM, Hanahan DJ. (1981). Activation of human neutrophils with 1-O-hexadecyl/octadecyl-2-acetyl-sn-glyceryl-3-phosphorylcholine (platelet-activating factor). *J Immunol.* 127:1250–1255.

Shear MJ. (1944). Chemical treatment of tumors. IX. Reactions of mice with primary subcutaneous tumors to injection of a hemorrhage-producing bacterial polysaccharide. *J Nat Cancer Inst.* 4:461–476.

Shechter Y, Hernaez L, Cuatrecasas P. (1978). Epidermal growth factor: biological activity requires persistent occupation of high-affinity cell surface receptors. *Proc Natl Acad Sci USA.* 75:5788–5791.

Shimokado K, Raines EW, Madres DK, Barrett TB, Benditt EP, Ross R. (1985). A significant part of macrophage-derived growth factor consists of at least two forms of PDGF. *Cell.* 43:277–286.

Shirai T, Yamaguchi H, Ito H, Todd CW, Wallace RB. (1985). Cloning and expression in *Escherichia coli* of the gene for human tumor necrosis factor. *Nature.* 313:803–806.

Simonian MH, Hornsby PJ, Ill CR, O'Hare MJ, Gill GN. (1979). Characterization of cultured bovine adrenal cortical and derived clonal lines: regulation of steroidogenesis and culture life span. *Endocrinology.* 105:99–108.

Sims JE, March CJ, Cosman D, Widmar MB, MacDonald HR, McMahan CJ, Grubin CE, Wignall JM, Jackson JL, Call SM. (1988). cDNA expression cloning of the IL-1 receptor a member of the immunoglobulin super family. *Science.* 241:585–589.

Slack JMW, Darlington BF, Heath HK, Godsave SF. (1987). Heparin binding growth factors as agents of mesoderm induction in early xenopus embryo. *Nature.* 326:197–200.

Smith JC, Dale L, Slack JMW. (1985). Cell lineage and region-specific markers in the analysis of inductive interactions. *J Embryol Exp Morphol.* 89(suppl): 317–331.

Smith RJ, Bowman BJ, Iden SS. (1984). Stimulation of the human neutrophil superoxide anion-generating system with 1-O-hexadecyl/octadecyl-2-acetyl-sn-glyceryl-3-phosphorylcholine. *Biochem Pharmacol.* 33:973–978.

Smith RJ, Bowman BJ, Speziale SC. (1986). Interleukin-1 stimulates granule exocytosis from human neutrophils. *Int J Immunopharmacol.* 8:33–40.

Solis-Herruzo JA, Brenner DA, Chojkier M. (1988). Tumor necrosis factor-d inhibits collagen gene transcription and collagen synthesis in cultured human fibroblast. *J Biol Chem.* 263:5841–5845.

Sporn MS, Roberts PB, Shull JH, Smith JM, Ward JM, Sodek J. (1983). Polypeptide transforming growth factors isolated from bovine sources and used for wound healing in vivo. *Science.* 219:1329–1331.

Sprugel KH, Greenhalgh DG, Murray MJ, Ross R. (1991). Platelet-derived growth factor and impaired wound healing. In: Caldwell MD, Hunt TK, Pines E, Skover G. eds. *Clinical and Experimental Approaches to Dermal and Epidermal Repair Normal and Chronic Wounds.* New York: Wiley-Liss; 365:325–340.

Steed D, Goslen B, Hambley R, Abell E, Hebda P, Webster M. (1991). Clinical trials with purified platelet releasate. In: Caldwell MD, Hunt TK, Pines E, Skover G, eds. *Clinical and Experimental Approaches to Dermal and Epidermal Repair Normal and Chronic Wounds.* New York: Wiley-Liss; 365:103–114.

Steenfos HH, Hunt TK, Scheuenstuhl H, Goodson WH. (1989). Selective effects of tumor necrosis factor-alpha on wound healing in rats. *Surgery.* 106:171–176.

Stephenson ML, Golding MB, Burkhead JR, Krane SM, Rhamsdorf HJ, Angel P. (1987). Stimulation of procollagenase synthesis parallels increases in cellular procollagenase mRNA in human articular chondrocytes exposed to recombinant interleukin-1 or phorbol ester. *Biochem Biophys Res Commun.* 144:583–590.

Stiles CD, Capne GT, Scher CD, Antoniades HM, Van Wyk JJ, Pledger WJ. (1979). Dual control of cell growth by somatomedins and "competence factors." *Proc Natl Acad Sci USA.* 76:1279–1283.

Stiles CD. (1983). The molecular biology of platelet-derived growth factor. *Cell.* 33:653–655.

Subramanian N, Bray MA. (1987). Interleukin-1 releases histamine from human basophils and mast cells in vitro. *J Immunol.* 138:271–275.

Sugarman BJ, Aggarwal BB, Hass PE, Figari IS, Palladino MA, Shepard HM. (1985). Recombinant tumor necrosis factor alpha: Effects on proliferation of normal and transformed cells in vitro. *Science.* 230:943–945.

Sun TT, Green H. (1977). Cultured epithelial cells of cornea, conjunctiva and skin: absence of marked intrinsic divergence of their differentiated states. *Nature.* 269:489–492.

Sundell HW, Senenius RS, Barthe P, Friedman Z, Kanarek KS, Escobedo MB, Orth DN, Stahlman MT. (1975). The effect of EGF on fetal lamb lung maturation. *Pediatr Res.* 9:371.

Sundell HW, Gray ME, Serenius RS, Scobedo MBE, Stahlman MT. (1980). Maturation in fetal lamb. *Am J Pathol.* 10:707–726.

Takehara K, LeRoy EC, Grotendorst GR. (1987). TGF-beta inhibition of endothelial cell proliferation: alteration of EGF binding and EGF-induced growth-regulatory (competence) give expression. *Cell.* 49:415–422.

Takeda K, Iwamoto S, Sugimoto H, Takuma T, Kawatani N, Noda M, Masaki A, Morise H, Arimura H, Konro K. (1986). Identity of differentiation inducing factor and tumor necrosis factor. *Nature.* 323:338–340.

Thornton JW, Hess CA, Cassingham V, Bartlett RH. (1981). Epidermal growth factor in the healing of second degree burns. A controlled animal study. *Burns* 8:156–160.

Tiku K, Tiku ML, Liu S, Skosey JL. (1986). Normal human neutrophils are a source of specific interleukin-1 inhibitor. *J Immunol.* 136:3686–3692.

Togari A, Dickens G, Huzuya H, Guroff G. (1985). The effect of fibroblast growth factor on PC-12 cells. *J Neurosci.* 5:307–316.

Torti FM, Dieckmann B, Beutler B, Cerami A, Ringold GM. (1987). A macrophage factor inhibits adipocyte gene expression: an in vitro model of cachexia. *Science.* 229:867–869.

Tracey KJ, Beutler B, Lowry SF, Merryweather J, Wolfe S, Milsark IW, Hariri RJ, Fahey TJ, Zentella A, Albert JD. (1986). Shock and tissue injury induced by recombinant human cachectin. *Science.* 234:470–474.

Tracey KJ, Lowry SF, Fahey TJ III, Albert JD, Fong Y, Hesse D, Bieutler B, Manoque KR, Calvano S, Wei H. (1987). Cachectin/tumor necrosis factor induces lethal shock and stress hormone responses in the dog. *Surg Gynecol Obstet.* 164:415–422.

Tracey KJ, Wei H, Manogue KR, Fong Y, Hesse DG, Nguyen HT, Kuo GC, Beutler B, Cotran RS, Cerami A. (1988). Cachectin/tumor necrosis factor induces cachexia, anemia and inflammation. *J Exp Med.* 167:1211–1227.

Trinchieri G, Kobayashi M, Rosen M, Louden R, Murphy M, Perussia B. (1986). Tumor necrosis factor and lymphotoxin induce differentiation of human myeloid cell lines in synergy with immune interferon. *J Exp Med.* 164:1206–1225.

Tseng S, Savion N, Stern R, Gospodarowicz D. (1982). Fibroblast growth factor modulates synthesis of collagen in cultured vascular endothelial cells. *Eur J Biochem* 122:355–360.

Tsuda T, Kaibuchi K, Kawahara Y, Fukuzaki H, Takai Y. (1985). Induction of protein kinase C and calcium ion mobilization by fibroblast growth factor in Swiss 3T3 cells. *FEBS Lett.* 191:205–210.

Tsujimoto M, Kip YK, Vilcek J. (1985). Tumor necrosis factor: specific binding and internalization in sensitive and resistant cells. *Proc Natl Acad Sci USA.* 82:7626–7630.

Tucker RF, Shipley GD, Moses HL, Holley RW. (1985). Growth inhibitor from BSC-1 cells closely related to platelet type beta transforming growth factor. *Science.* 226:705–707.

Ullrich A, Coussens L, Haylick JS, Dull TJ, Gray A, Tam AW, Lee J, Yarden Y, Liberman TA, Schlessinger J, Downward J, Bye J, Whittle N, Waterfield MD, Seeburg PH. (1984). Human epidermal growth factor receptor cDNA sequence and aberrant expression of the amplified gene in A431 epidermoid carcinoma cells. *Nature.* 309:418–425.

Urdal DL, Call SM, Jackson JL, Dower SK. (1988). Affinity purification and chemical analysis of the interleukin-1 receptor. *J Biol Chem.* 263:2870–2875.

Ushiro H, Cohen S. (1980). Identification of phosphotyrosine as a product of epidermal growth factor-activated protein kinase in A-431 cell membrane. *J Biol Chem.* 255:8363–8365.

Van Damme J, De Ley M, Opdenakker G, Biliau A, De Somer P. (1985). Homogeneous interferon-inducing 22K factor is related to endogenous pyrogen and interleukin-1. *Nature.* 314:266–268.

Van Damme J, Billiau A. (1987). Interferon beta-2 and plasmacytoma growth factor are identical to B-cell stimulating factor 2. *J Exp Med.* 163:145–168.

Vilcek J, Palombell VJ, Henryksen-DeStefano D, Swenson C, Feinman R, Hirai M, Tsujimoto M. (1986). Fibroblast growth enhancing activity of tumor necrosis factor and its relationship to other polypeptide growth factors. *J Exp Med.* 163:632–642.

Vlodavsky I, Gospodarowicz D. (1979). Structural and functional alterations in the surface of vascular endothelial cells associated with the formation of a confluent cell monolayer and with the withdrawal of fibroblast growth factor. *J Supramol Struct.* 12:73–114.

Vlodavsky I, Johnson LK, Greenburg G, Gospodarowicz D. (1979). Vascular endothelial cells maintained in the absence of fibroblast growth factor undergo structural and functional alterations that are incompatible with their in vivo differentiated properties. *J Cell Biol.* 83:468–486.

Vuk-Pavlovic S, Svingen P, Vroman B, Kovach JS. (1987). Inhibition of colony formation and DNA degradation by tumor necrosis factor-alpha in human epithelial tumors. Proc Am Assoc *Cancer Res.* 28:400–405.

Vuk-Pavlovic S, Kovach JS. (1989). Recycling of tumor necrosis factor-α receptor in MCF-7 cells. *FASEB J.* 3:2633–2640.

Wagner JA, D'Amore P. (1986). Neurite outgrowth induced by an endothelial cell mitogen isolated from retina. *J Cell Biol.* 103:1363–1367.

Wahl SM, Hunt DA, Wakefield LM, McCartney-Frances N, Wahl LM, Roberts AB, Sporn MB. (1987). Transforming growth factor beta (TGF-beta) induces monocyte chemotaxis and growth factor production. *Proc Natl Acad Sci USA.* 84:5788–5792.

Wahl SM, Hunt DA, Wong HL, Dougherty S, McCartney-Francis N, Wahle LM. (1988a). Transforming growth factor-β is a potent immunosuppressive agent that inhibits IL-1 dependent lymphocyte proliferation. *J Immunol.* 140:3026–3032.

Wahl SM, Hunt DA, Bansal G, McCartney-Francis N, Ellingsworth L, Allan JB. (1988b). Bacterial cell wall induced immunosuppression. Role of TGF-β. *J Exp Med.* 168:1403–1417.

Wahl SM, McCartney-Francis N, Mergenhagen SE. (1989). Inflammatory and immunomodulatory roles of TGF-β. *Immunol Today.* 10:258–261.

Wakefield LM, Smith MDM, Masui T, Harris CC, Sporn MB. (1987). Distribution and modulation of the cellular receptor for transforming growth factor-beta. *J Cell Biol.* 105:965–975.

Walicke P, Cowan M, Ueno N, Baird B, Guillemin R. (1986). Fibroblast growth factor promotes survival of dissociated hippocampal neurons and enhances neurite extension. *Proc Natl Acad Sci USA.* 83:3012–3016.

Walsh LJ, Lander PE, Seymour GJ, Powell RN. (1987). Isolation and purification of 1LS, an interleukin-1 inhibitor produced by human gingival epithelial cells. *Clin Exp Immunol.* 68:366–374.

Warren RS, Donner DB, Starnes HF, Brennan MF. (1987). Modulation of endogenous hormone action by recombinant human tumor necrosis factor. *Proc Natl Acad Sci USA.* 84:8619–8622.

Waterfield MD, Scrace GT, Whittle N, Stroobant P, Johnsson A, Bornert JM,

Staub A. (1985). Platelet-derived growth factor is structurally related to the putative transforming protein P 28 sis of simian sarcoma virus. *Nature.* 304:35–39.

Westermark B, Heldin C-H, Ek B, Westermark K. (1983). Biochemistry and biology of platelet-derived growth factor. In: Guroff G, ed. *Growth and Maturation Factors.* Philadelphia: Wiley; 73–92.

Westermark K, Karlsson FA, Westermark B. (1983). Epidermal growth factor modulates thyroid growth and function in culture. *Endocrinology.* 112:1680–1686.

Williams RS, Rossi AM, Chegini N, Shultz G. (1992). Effect of transforming growth factor beta on postoperative adhesion formation and intact peritoneum. *J Surg Res* 52(1):65–70.

Williamson BD, Carswell EA, Rubin BY, Prendergast YS, Old LJ. (1983). Human tumor necrosis factor produced by human B-cell lines: synergistic cytotoxic interaction with human interferon. *Proc Natl Acad Sci USA.* 80:5397–5401.

Wiseman DM, Polverini PJ, Kamp DW, Leibovich SJ. (1987). Transforming growth factor beta (TGF-β) is a chemoattractant for monocytes and induces their expression of angiogenic activity. *J Cell Biol.* 105:163a.

Wood DD, Bayne EK, Goldring MB, Gowen M, Hamerman D, Humes JL, Ihrie EJ, Lipsky PE, Staruch MJ. (1985). The four biochemically distinct species of human interleukin-1 exhibit similar biologic activities. *J Immunol.* 134:895–903.

Wrann M, Fox CF, Ross R. (1980). Modulation of epidermal growth factor receptors on 3T3 cells by platelet derived growth factor. *Science.* 210:1363–1365.

Yarden Y, Ullrich A. (1988). Molecular analysis of signal transduction by growth factors. *Biochemistry.* 27:3113–3119.

Yasaka T, Boxer LA, Baehner RL. (1982). Monocyte aggregation and superoxide anion release in response to formyl-methionyl-leucyl-phenylalanine (FMLP) and platelet-activating factor (PAF). *J Immunol.* 128:1939–1944.

Zucali JR, Dinarello CA, Oblon DJ, Gross MA, Anderson I, Werner RS. (1986). Interleukin-1 stimulates fibroblasts to produce granulocyte-macrophage colony stimulating activity and prostaglandin-E$_2$. *J Clin Invest.* 77:1857–1863.

Zucali JR, Elfenbein GJ, Barth KC, Dinarello CA. (1987). Effects of human interleukin-1 and human tumor necrosis factor on human T lymphocyte colony formation. *J Clin Invest.* 80:772–777.

Zullo JN, Cochran BH, Huang A, Stiles CD. (1985). Platelet-derived growth factor and double-stranded ribonucleic acids stimulate expression of the same genes in 3T3 cells. *Cell.* 43:793–800.

4

Fibroblasts and Tissue Repair Cells

FIBROBLASTS ARE SPECIALIZED CELLS THAT DEVELOP FROM EMBRYONIC mesenchyme. They provide an important source of the cellular response to peritoneal injury. As fibroblasts migrate they send out lamellipodia, which adhere to surfaces and allow the fibroblast to move to the new attachment site by contraction of the filaments (Abercrombie, Heaysman, & Pegrum, 1971, 1972; Harris & Dunn, 1972). Fibroblasts synthesize matrix components and direct organization of the resulting connective tissue matrix (e.g., collagens, fibronectin, proteoglycans, and other proteins). The matrix is constantly being turned over and remodeled by fibroblasts and the degradative enzymes they secrete (e.g., collagenases, proteoglycanases, glycosaminodases, and other proteases).

Matrix

Three components (collagens, fibronectin, and elastin) of the connective tissue matrix provide chemotactic signals for fibroblasts (Postlethwaite, Seyer, & Kang, 1978; Postlethwaite, Keski-Oja, & Kang, 1981; Senior, Griffin, & Mecham, 1982; Postlethwaite, 1983; Senior et al., 1984). Activation of serum complement by the classical or alternative pathways generates an 80,000 molecular weight C5-derived fragment that is chemotactic for fibroblasts (Postlethwaite, Snyderman, & Kang, 1979). Some of the degradation peptides from these components are also chemotactic for fibroblasts. Therefore, complement fragments provide chemotactic signals for fibroblasts from sites of virtually all types of inflammatory reactions in the peritoneum.

Several matrix components possess important biological properties in addition to their structural properties: response to inflammation and tissue repair processes. Matrix components are degraded at sites of tissue injury, and such degradation products may provide important signals to inflammatory cells. Solubilized collagens and collagenous peptides generated by the action of collagenase and proteinases may provide chemotactic signals for peripheral blood monocytes (Postlethwaite, 1983; Postlethwaite & Kang, 1988) and neighboring connective tissue fibroblasts to migrate into the area of tissue inflammation and injury in vivo.

Fibronectin is a potent chemoattractant for fibroblasts in vitro (Postlethwaite & Kang, 1980; Seppae, Seppae, & Yamada, 1980; Postlethwaite et al., 1981). Other properties of fibronectin promote attachment, spreading, and proliferation of fibroblasts. Fibronectin also promotes attachment and spreading of platelets on collagen fibers and cell attachment to fibrin clots (Kleinman, McGoodwin, & Klebe, 1976; Kleinman, Klebe, & Martin, 1981). Some intermediate fragments from fibronectin degradation retain biologic activity, such as binding and chemotaxis (Ginsberg, Pierschbacher, Ruoslahti, Marguerie, & Plow, 1985). These matrices bind fibroblasts and other cell types regulate cellular functions. For example, fibronectin binds to collagen and to proteoglycans (heparin, heparan sulfate, and hyaluronic acid) as well as fibroblasts and other cells, thereby facilitating matrix organization (Klebe, 1974; Kleinman et al., 1976; Yamada, Kennedy, Kimata, & Pratt, 1980; Laterra & Culp, 1982; Oldberg & Ruoslahti, 1982). Studies of wound healing in laboratory animals show that hyaluronic acid is produced in the early phases of the repair process and probably serves to promote the migration of inflammatory cells and fibroblasts by interfering with cell-cell and cell-substrate interactions (Dunphy & Udupa, 1955).

Matrix Degradation

Extracellular collagenases are metalloproteases requiring both Ca^{2+} and Zn^{2+}, which manifest optimal activity at neutral pH (Woolley, 1984). Net collagenolytic activity is regulated by proteolytic activation of procollagenase and inhibitors that complex with the collagenases which include α_2-macroglobulin and β_1-anticollagenase (Woolley, 1984; Welgus, Campbell, Bar-Shavit, Senior & Teitelbaum, 1985). The degradation of collagen in normal and inflamed tissues likely depends on the balance between collagenase and its inhibitors. Unlike mammalian collagenases, elastases lack specificity and are general and potent proteases. Neutrophil elastases are serine proteases and are inhibited by α_1-antiprotease (Gosline & Rosenbloom, 1984).

Proliferation

Fibroblasts require two signals for DNA synthesis to be affected. Scher, Shepard, Antoniades, and Stiles (1979) called these "competence" and "progression" signals. The "competence factors" do not stimulate DNA synthesis but render cells in the G_0 or G_1 phase "competent" to do so.

"Progression factors" stimulate DNA synthesis in competent cells (Scher et al., 1979). Growth factors can be classified into one of these two groups by a "complementation" test, in which fibroblasts are rendered quiescent by reducing serum concentration in medium so that the fibroblasts are growth-arrested (Stiles et al., 1979). The growth factor being tested is then added before and after known progression factors to determine under which conditions fibroblast DNA synthesis is stimulated. Some of the known fibroblast growth factors have been classified as being either competence or progression factors (Figure 4.1).

Tissue Repair Cells

Mesothelial and other epithelial cells collected from the site of peritoneal injury at various times after trauma will be referred to in this chapter as tissue repair cells (TRCs). To study the re-epithelialization of peritoneal injury and the changing character of these cells, a standardized excision of rabbit parietal peritoneum was used to initiate peritoneal repair (Fukasawa, Bryant, Nakamura, & diZerega, 1987; Fukasawa, Bryant, & diZerega, 1988; Fukasawa, Yanagihara, Rodgers, & diZerega, 1989a; Fukasawa, Campeau, Yanagihara, Rodgers, & diZerega, 1989b). At 4 days after peritoneal injury, the surface of the healing peritoneum contains proliferating mesothelial cells that actively secrete connective tissue matrix (Raftery, 1973a, 1973b). The cells on the surface of the parietal defect are harvested and grown in culture for 4 to 8 days to allow for the generation of a confluent layer of adherent cells. This layer is essentially devoid of leukocytes. The activity of TRCs, as measured by protein and collagen synthesis, increases after surgery, reaching peak levels on postsurgical days 5 to 7 (Fukasawa, et al., 1989b). These TRCs respond to a

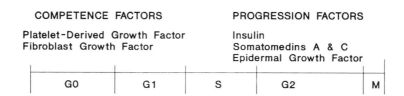

FIGURE 4.1. The growth of connective tissue cells is regulated by polypeptide growth factors that act through specific cell surface receptors. Two classes of these factors have been described: "competence" and "progression" factors. Competence factors act during the G0–G1 phase of the cell cycle preparing the cell to enter the S-phase. However, the cells cannot enter the S-phase unless progression factors are present. Factors from both classes must be present in order for cell replication to occur. (From Grotendorst, Pencer, Martin, & Sodek, 1984. Reproduced by permission of Greenwood Publishing Group, Inc., Westport, CT.)

variety of stimuli including monokines in a manner distinctly different from that of established fibroblast cell lines (Fukasawa et al., 1989a; Rodgers & diZerega, 1992).

Postsurgical Differentiation

At day 5 after peritoneal surgery in rabbits, TRCs incorporate greater amounts of thymidine compared to day 2 TRCs (Figure 4.2; Fukasawa et al., 1989a). Thereafter, mitogenic activity decreases during extended postsurgical times. Day 2 TRCs might not be fully capable of mitogenesis, whereas day 5 TRCs are more active in vivo. At postsurgical day 7 and day 10 TRCs differentiate, allowing for production of extracellular matrix. TRCs are morphologically transformed and activated to proliferate when cocultured with postsurgical macrophages (Orita, Campeau, Nakamura, & diZerega, 1986). The mitogenic activity of TRCs cocultured with postsurgical macrophages or spent media from postsurgical macrophages is greater than that measured when they are cultured with nonsurgical macrophages (Figure 4.3).

How do postsurgical macrophages modulate the proliferation of TRCs during peritoneal healing? The effect of postsurgical macrophages on TRC proliferation changes as a function of postsurgical time. Postsurgical mac-

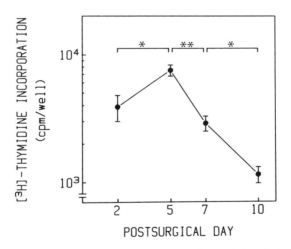

FIGURE 4.2. The proliferative capacity of TRCs is modulated during the postsurgical interval. TRCs were recovered from abraded peritoneum at various days after surgery and incubated for 4 days. TRCs were then plated into 96-well plates. After 48 hours of incubation, TRCs were pulsed with 1 μCi [³H]thymidine for 24 hours. At day 5 after surgery, the peak of TRC mitogenesis was observed. Data represent means ± SEM. *p <.05; **p <.01. (From Fukasawa et al., 1989a. Reproduced by permission of Academic Press.)

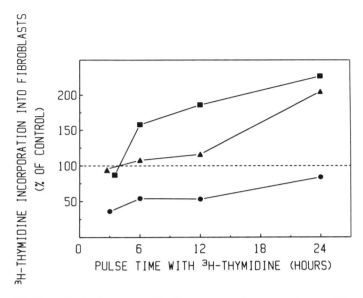

FIGURE 4.3. The effect of spent media from macrophages on the proliferation of TRCs is shown. TRCs were preincubated with resident (●), postsurgical day 4 (■) and postsurgical day 7 macrophage-spent media (▲), and fresh medium as control for 48 hours. TRCs were then pulsed with [³H]thymidine and fresh medium for 3 to 24 hours. Each data point expresses percentage of control incorporation. These data show that the mitogenic activity of TRC cocultured with spent media from postsurgical macrophages is greater than TRC cultured with spent media from resident macrophages. Each point represents the mean of three experiments. (From Fukasawa et al., 1988. Reproduced by permission of Academic Press.)

rophages alter the composition of their secretory products as a function of time (Fukasawa et al., 1988; Abe, Rodgers, Ellefson & diZerega, 1989; Abe, Rodgers, Ellefson & diZerega, 1991). Initially macrophages may stimulate the proliferation of TRCs; later macrophages modulate differentiation of TRCs to produce extracellular matrix (Bryant, Fukasawa, Orita, Rodgers, & diZerega, 1988; Rodgers & diZerega, 1992).

Response to Growth Factors

Purified growth factors can modulate TRC proliferation. Macrophage-derived growth factor(s) are produced by many types of monocyte-macrophage cell populations (further discussed in Chapter 3). Following stimulation in vivo or in vitro, macrophages produce "factors" that stimulate the proliferation and expression of differentiated functions of a variety of cell types (Schmidt, Mizel, Cohen, & Green, 1982; Estes, Pledger, &

Gillespie, 1984; Aggarwal et al., 1985; Dinarello et al., 1986; Bronson, Bertiolami, & Siebert, 1987). Interleukin-1 (IL-1), which is produced by stimulated macrophages, has the potential to enhance the proliferation and differentiation of fibroblasts (Mizel, Dayer, Krane, & Mergenhagen, 1981; Schmidt et al., 1982; Postlethwaite, Lachman, Mainardi, & Kang, 1983; Postlethwaite, Lachman, & Kang, 1984; Matsushima, Bono, Kidwell, & Oppenheim, 1985). Jimenez de Asua, Clingan, & Rudland (1975) and Jimenez de Asua, Otto, Lingren, & Hammerstom (1983) reported that prostaglandin $F_2\alpha$ ($PGF_2\alpha$) also stimulates the proliferation of fibroblasts. Inhibition of fibroblast mitogenic activity by prostaglandin E_2 (PGE_2) was reported by other investigators (Ko, Page, & Narayanan, 1977; Korn, Halushka, & LeRoy, 1980; Bitterman, Rennard, Hunninghake, & Crystal, 1982; Gleiber & Schiffmann, 1984; Wahl & Wahl, 1985). Thus, macrophage secretory products have the potential to modulate the proliferation of fibroblasts (and TRCs) by both stimulation (macrophage-derived growth factor [MDGF], IL-1, $PGF_2\alpha$, etc.) and inhibition (PGE_2, fibroblast growth inhibitor, transforming growth factor β [TGF-β], interferon-γ [IFN-γ]). However, which product(s) secreted by postsurgical macrophages is the dominant regulator(s) of proliferation during the tissue repair process is dependent upon the amount of secretagogue produced by postsurgical macrophages as well as the responsiveness (i.e., differentiation) of TRC to these factors.

Response to Macrophages

To determine the role of macrophages or peritoneal exudate cells in the repair of injured peritoneum, the influence of peritoneal macrophages on mesothelial re-epithelialization at an injured site was studied using a postsurgical rabbit model. The secretory products of macrophages recovered from peritoneal exudate at various time after surgery initially suppress (during the initial 48 hours of culture) and later enhance (following 48 to 54 hours of incubation) the incorporation of thymidine into fibroblasts (Figure 4.4; Fukasawa et al., 1988). This suppression by postsurgical macrophages is significantly less than that observed with resident (nonsurgical) macrophages (Fukasawa et al., 1987; 1988). Therefore, modulation of TRC proliferation by macrophages appears to be a complex process involving elements of both suppression and stimulation. There may be a lag time during which TRCs are either refractory to proliferative signals from postsurgical macrophages or are controlled by inhibitors of proliferation. Alternatively, TRC may not be initially responsive to macrophage-derived growth factor(s), but the inhibitory signal(s), which is presumably also macrophage-derived, initially predominates. Since the inhibition of TRC proliferation is reduced at later times in culture, the inhibitory signals (1) may be short-lived (as prostaglandins are thought to be), (2) may be overcome (or inactivated) by fibroproliferative factor(s),

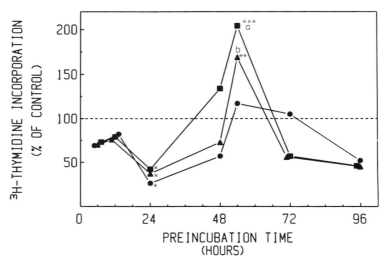

FIGURE 4.4. The effect of macrophage secretory products on TRC proliferation is shown. TRCs were preincubated with resident (●), postsurgical day 4 (■), post-surgical day 7 macrophage-spent media (▲), and fresh medium as control. Each data point represents the percentage of control incorporation. These data show that spent media from postsurgical macrophages modulate TRC proliferation in a complex manner. *p <.05, **p <.01, ***p <.001 compared to control. [a]p <.001, [b]p <.05 compared to group treated with spent media from resident macrophages. (From Fukasawa et al., 1988. Reproduced by permission of Academic Press.)

or (3) changes in TRC responsiveness to inhibitory factors may occur during culture.

Cell Morphology

Microscopic examination of TRCs cultured with spent macrophage media indicates that an alteration in the morphology of TRCs from a flat-oval shape to a more spindly appearance occurs together with the macrophage-induced inhibition of TRC proliferation (Figure 4.5) (Orita et al., 1986). Interestingly, this morphological change seems to be associated with the inhibition of proliferation; the time required for a reduction in thymidine incorporation was the same as that required for morphological changes. Alteration in the morphology of TRCs cultured with macrophage-spent media indicates a complex change in cell metabolism to maximize the potential for migration. In this regard, postsurgical day 4 TRCs are more responsive to postsurgical macrophages than day 8 TRCs (Figure 4.6). This dissociation between basal proliferative activity and responsiveness to stimuli ("transformation") might be related to a time

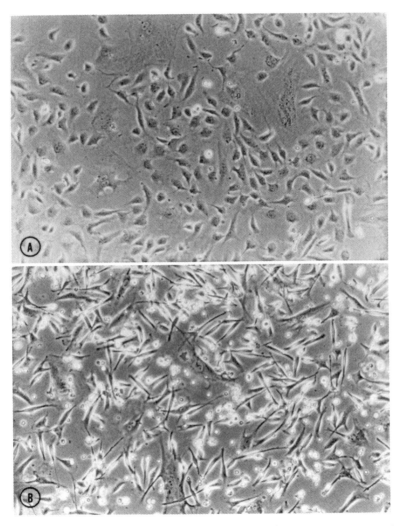

FIGURE 4.5. Microscopic examination of TRCs cultured with spent media from postsurgical macrophages indicates that an alteration in TRC morphology occurs upon cultures with postsurgical macrophages. Appearance of fibroblasts before and 24 hours after the addition of postoperative day 7 macrophages is shown. A: Day 4 fibroblasts before the addition of macrophages. (×200). B: Day 4 fibroblasts 24 hours after the addition of macrophages, (×200). (From Orita et al., 1986. Reproduced by permission of C.V. Mosby.)

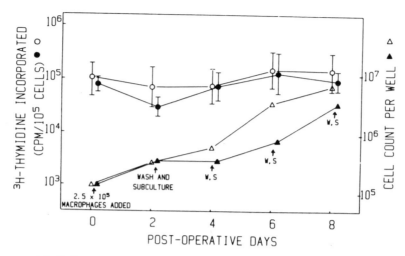

FIGURE 4.6. Cell growth and tritiated thymidine incorporation of peritoneal TRC derived from injured peritoneal wall on postoperative days 4 and 8 after 5 days incubation with macrophages from different postoperative days in vitro. These data show that postsurgical day 4 TRCs are more responsive to postsurgical macrophages than day 8 TRCs. Each data point represents the geometric mean and 95% range of three experiments. △, Number of day 4 fibroblasts; ▲, number of day 8 fibroblasts; ○, tritiated thymidine incorporation of day 4 fibroblasts; ●, tritiated thymidine incorporation by day 8 fibroblasts. (From Orita et al., 1986. Reproduced by permission of C.V. Mosby.)

constraint for the cell to return to the original nonmigratory state prior to division. This time constraint may be related to the TRCs' ability to proliferate or not proliferate at the site of injury (Bryant et al., 1988).

Cell-to-Cell Response

Macrophages are critical in the final resolution of tissue debris and completion of healing, a process that ends in the formation of the connective tissue matrix and mesothelial syncytium (Ryan, Grobety, & Majno, 1973; Bryant, Fukasawa, Orita, Rodgers, & diZerega, 1988). In nonsurgical systems, macrophages provide the primary stimulus for proliferation of fibroblasts (Martin, Gimbrone, Unanue, & Cotran, 1981; Tsukamoto, Helsen, & Wahl, 1981; Postlethwaite & Kang, 1983; Gosline & Rosenbloom, 1984). Factors secreted by activated macrophages in nonsurgical systems can stimulate fibroblast proliferation (further discussed in Chapter 3; macrophage-derived fibroblast growth factor [FGF], IL-1, and tumor necrosis factor [TNF]). As a direct or indirect response to these factors, fibroblasts proliferate and secrete connective tissue proteins including fibronectin, proteoglycans, collagen, and proteases such as collagenase and elastase. Proper coordination of these fibroblast-mediated functions leads to the repair and remodeling of tissue. In addition, the rate and extent to which these factors regulate wound healing may be amenable to modulation by extrinsic intervention.

Fibroproliferative activity in TRCs is increased on postsurgical days 4 and 7 and decreases to resident levels on day 28 (Fukasawa et al., 1988). TRC proliferation is generally suppressed in situ when compared to TRC cultured in medium supplemented with only fetal bovine serum (Fukasawa et al., 1987; 1988). Candidates for mediators of this suppression of proliferation include prostaglandins (Samuelson, Branstrom, Greek, Hamberg, & Hammerstrom, 1971; Opitz, Niethammer, Lemk, Flad, & Huget, 1975), interferons (Gresser, Brouty-Boye, Thomas, & MacLerira-Cuehlo, 1970), arginase (Kung, Brooks, Jakway, Leonard, & Talmadge, 1977), and complement cleavage products (Harris & Dunn, 1972; Prydze, Allison, & Schlorlemner, 1977). The manifestation of these complex signals appears to be a function of (1) the period of time after surgery, and (2) the length of preincubation of the macrophage-spent media with the TRCs.

Growth Factors

A large number of factors contribute to the growth of fibroblasts (Cohen & Carpenter, 1975; Leibovich & Ross, 1976; Ross & Bowen-Pope, 1984; Baird, Mormede, & Bohlen, 1985; Baird et al., 1986; Ignotz & Massaque, 1986). At the injured site, TRCs are involved with other cell types (i.e., lymphocytes, PMN, platelets) that may modulate the in situ proliferative and functional activities of TRCs (Simpson & Ross, 1972; Leibovich & Ross, 1975). Platelet-derived growth factor (PDGF), isolated from platelets, stimulates the proliferation of normal skin and established fibroblast cell lines. PDGF also functions as a chemoattractant for fibroblasts (Seppae, Grotendorst, Seppae, Schiffmann, & Martin, 1982). Ross and his colleagues reported the production of a PDGF-like factor by macrophages (Shimakado et al., 1985). Many factors occur in several compartments involved in tissue repair: serum, wound fluid, platelets, macrophages, and TRC. FGF, readily produced by macrophages (Baird et al., 1985), stimulates the proliferation of fibroblasts and endothelial cells (Korn et al., 1980; Baird et al, 1986). Epidermal growth factor (EGF), initially isolated from the submaxillary gland, is present in serum (Cohen, 1962). Insulin like growth factor-I (IGF-I)/somatomedin-C was isolated from fibroblasts (Clemmons, Underwood, & Van Wyk, 1981; Conover, Hintz, & Rosenfeld, 1985). Transforming growth factor-β (TGF-β) is found in platelets, wound fluid, and macrophages (Assoian, Komoriya, Meyers, Miller, & Sporn, 1983; Assoian et al., 1987; Cromack et al., 1987). Thus, these factors directly modulate the growth of TRCs during postsurgical healing.

EGF and FGF stimulate the incorporation of thymidine into TRCs (Fukasawa et al., 1989a). Interestingly, TRC responsiveness to EGF increases during the postsurgical period with postsurgical day 10 TRC demonstrating the greatest response to EGF (Figure 4.7). PDGF also stimulates the incorporation of thymidine into TRC, but the stimulation is only 30% of control values for postsurgical day 10 TRC (Figure 4.8; Fukasawa et al., 1989a). PDGF stimulates the proliferation of fibroblasts, especially under conditions of confluent culture. The effect of PDGF on proliferation is thought to induce the entry of G_0-arrested cells into the proliferative phase of the cell cycle (Pledger, Stiles, Antoniades, & Scher, 1978). TRCs may be undergoing a mitotic cycle and, therefore, do not manifest as great a response to the addition of PDGF as established fibroblasts. EGF and FGF, which affect the proliferation of TRC, may function as competence factors involved in the transition of cells from the G_0 to S phase (Abercrombie et al., 1972; Pledger et al., 1978).

Interleukin-1 (IL-1) is synthesized and released from monocytes in response to stimulants including lymphokines and phagocytosis of particles. IL-1α and IL-1β exert a variety of effects on fibroblasts in vitro.

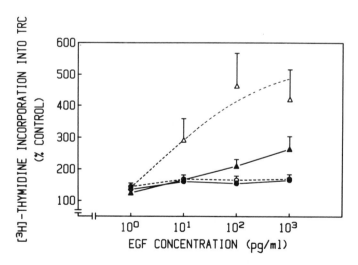

FIGURE 4.7. Dose response to EGF of TRCs recovered from different postsurgical days. [³H]thymidine incorporation was determined. TRC responsiveness to EGF increases during the postsurgical period with postsurgical day 10 TRC demonstrating the greatest response. Data represent percentage of media control culture (means ± SEM). ●, Postsurgical day 2 TRC; ○, postsurgical day 5 TRC; ▲, postsurgical day 7 TRC; △, postsurgical day 10 TRC. (From Fukasawa et al., 1989a. Reproduced by permission of Academic Press).

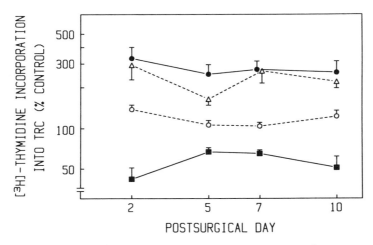

FIGURE 4.8. Response of postsurgical day 10 TRC to growth factors measured by [³H]thymidine incorporation. TRCs were cultured for 8 days prior to the assay. PDGF slightly increases the proliferation of day 10 TRC, FGF and EGF stimulate the proliferation of postsurgical TRC. On the other hand, TGF-β suppresses the proliferative response of postsurgical TRC. Data represent percentage of control culture media (means ± SEM). O, PDGF; ●, 1 ng/ml EGF; △, 100 ng FGF; ■, 0.1 ng TGF-β. (From Fukasawa et al., 1989a. Reproduced by permission of Academic Press.)

Proliferation and production of prostaglandin E_2, collagen, collagenase, and hyaluronic acid are all stimulated by IL-1α and IL-1β (Schmidt et al., 1982; Postlethwaite et al., 1983; Estes et al., 1984; Postlethwaite, Keski-Oja, Moses, & Kang, 1987). Although IL-1 does not stimulate proliferation of TRC, IL-1 stimulates protein synthesis by TRC (Fukasawa et al., 1989a). IL-1 may function as an initiation factor similar to the role played by PDGF or may be more important for the production of extracellular matrix.

IL-2 stimulates the healing of skin wounds (Barbul, Knud-Hansen, Wasserkrug, & Efron, 1986); however, IL-2 does not affect proliferation of fibroblasts or TRCs (Fukasawa et al., 1989a). IL-2 may indirectly affect the growth of TRCs in vivo through stimulation of other cellular elements. For example, macrophages have cell-surface receptors for IL-2 and IL-2 that can stimulate the respiratory burst of macrophages in the absence of other stimuli.

IGF-I does not affect the incorporation of tritiated thymidine into TRC (Fukasawa et al., 1989a). IGF-I/somatomedin-C stimulates the proliferation of fibroblasts by effecting the transition from the S-G_2 phase to the M phase (Pledger et al., 1978). Since IGF-I effects the M phase, and since this factor may be produced by fibroblasts, the growth factors involved in the G_1-S phase of the cell cycle may be more important for the enhancement of TRC proliferation (Kleinman et al., 1976, 1981).

TGF-β stimulates the anchorage-independent proliferation of fibroblasts but not anchorage-dependent growth (Assoian et al., 1983; Roberts et al., 1985; Assoian 1986). TGF-β inhibits the incorporation of thymidine into TRC (Figure 4.9; Fukasawa et al., 1989a; Fukasawa, Campeau, Yanagihara, Rodgers, & diZerega, 1990), and stimulates the production of extracellular matrix (collagen and fibronectin) by fibroblasts (Sporn et al., 1983; Mensing & Czarnetozki, 1984; Assoian, 1986; Ignotz & Massague, 1986; Thalacker & Nilsen-Hamilton, 1987; Varga & Jimenez, 1987; Wahl, McCartney-Francis, & Mergenhagen, 1989). Incubation of TRC with TGF-β enhances the incorporation of radiolabeled proline (to measure protein synthesis); in contrast TGF-β inhibits the proliferation of TRC (Fukasawa et al., 1989a). In this context, TGF-β may function as a mod-

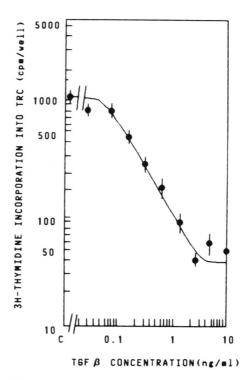

TGF β CONCENTRATION(ng/ml)

FIGURE 4.9. Postsurgical day 10 TRCs previously cultured for 8 days were exposed to various concentrations of TGF-β for 48 hours and then pulsed with 0.2 μCi tritiated thymidine. These data show that TGF-β inhibits the incorporation of thymidine into TRC in a concentration-dependent manner. Incorporation of radiolabel was determined after 24-hour incubation. Each data point represents the mean ± SEM (cpm/well). C, media control (TGF-β free; Fukasawa et al., 1990).

ulator of TRC differentiation in that it may induce these mesothelial cells to enter a functional (secretory) stage rather than to proliferate. Cromack et al. (1987) reported that increase in TGF-β levels in wound fluid occurs late after surgery, not during the early phase of tissue repair.

Although not a monokine in the true sense of the word, macrophage-derived fibronectin is also chemotactic for fibroblasts (Akiyama & Yamada, 1983). The major fibroblast chemoattractants produced by macrophages are PGE_2 (which inhibits fibroblast proliferation) and leukotriene B_4 (which stimulates fibroblast chemotaxis) (Korn et al., 1980; Wyler & Rosenwasser, 1982; Mensing & Czarnetozki, 1984).

Platelets as a Source of Growth Factors

Platelets are a source of two potent fibroblast chemoattractants, PDGF and TGF-beta (Seppae et al., 1980). The aggregation of platelets at sites of inflammation may release PDGF and TGF-β, thereby providing powerful chemotactic signals for fibroblasts. Senior, Huang, Griffin, & Deuel (1985) were able to show that treatment of PDGF with neutrophil elastase and reduction and alkylation yielded some peptides that stimulated fibroblast chemotaxis, whereas others stimulated mitogenesis of fibroblasts. TGF-β is produced by a variety of inflammatory, normal, and neoplastic cells and is thus an almost ubiquitous chemoattractant for fibroblasts (Postlethwaite et al., 1987). It is very potent in its chemotactic effect, inducing migration in the 10- to 50-pg/ml concentration range. The fibrotic response to certain tumors could be related to TGF-β production by such tumors. Transforming growth factor-β (TGF-β) exerts a variety of effects on fibroblasts. It stimulates chemotaxis as well as collagen and fibronectin production, and is a growth factor for fibroblasts (Moses, Nissley, Rechler, Short, & Podskalny, 1979; Ignotz & Massaque, 1986; Kehrl et al., 1986; Postlethwaite et al., 1987).

Effect of Culture Time

Proliferative and functional activities of TRC collected directly from injured peritoneum were determined in vitro to study activation and differentiation of TRCs in vivo. Although TRCs rapidly proliferate after recovery from injured peritoneum, this activity gradually decreases during culture. In addition, collagen production (as measured by ^{3}H-proline incorporation) by TRCs also decreases during culture (Fukasawa et al., 1989b). Since sulfate is found mainly in glycosaminoglycans, ^{35}S-sulfate was used to monitor the production of glycosaminoglycans by TRCs. Interestingly, ^{35}S-sulfate incorporation into TRCs gradually increases during culture (Table 4.1; Fukasawa et al., 1989b). TGF-β stimulates production of extracellular matrix by fibroblasts but does not stimulate the proliferation of fibroblasts (Assoian et al., 1983, Roberts et al., 1985;

TABLE 4.1. Incorporation of radiolabel into tissue repair cells.

Peritoneal exudate cell	[14C]Proline[c] (cpm/well)	[14C]Glucosamine[c] (cpm/well)	Cell number × 10^5 cells
48-hr incubation			
Medium control	100	100	0.68 ± 0.04**,b,*,a
Resident	90 ± 4	67 ± 15	2.1 ± 0.2**,b
Day 4	123 ± 5*,a	146 ± 15**,a	1.8 ± 0.2**,b
Day 7	107 ± 4*,a	123 ± 16**,a	1.3 ± 0.2**,b
Day 10	128 ± 7*,a	114 ± 11**,a	1.5 ± 0.1**,b
96-hr incubation			
Medium control	100	100	1.4 ± 0.1
Resident	353 ± 23*,b	1570 ± 281*,b	10.1 ± 0.6**,b
Day 4	249 ± 39*,b	698 ± 100	7.0 ± 0.8**,b
Day 7	185 ± 26*,b	493 ± 162**,a	5.7 ± 0.6**,b,*,a
Day 10	185 ± 26*,b,*,a	600 ± 138*,a	6.9 ± 0.6**,b

[a]Compared to resident group.
[b]Compared to fresh medium control.
[c]Data expressed as percentage control of results obtained using fresh Medium 199 with 3% fetal calf serum. Data expressed are the x̄ ± SEM of five to seven rabbits per group.
*$p <.05$.
**$p <.002$.
Modified from Fukasawa et al., 1989b.

Assoian, 1986; Ignotz & Massague, 1986). Thus, mitogenic and secretory activities of TRCs are not necessarily concurrent events.

Summary

TRCs are not simply "fibroblasts" and appear to change functional characteristics during postsurgical peritoneal re-epithelialization mediated by macrophage secretory products. TRCs contain different characteristics from established fibroblast cell lines (Orita et al., 1986, Bryant et al., 1988; Fukasawa et al., 1988, 1989a) and reflect a differential responsiveness of surgically elicited cells that may not be present in maintained cell lines.

Macrophages produce soluble mediators that modulate TRC growth during peritoneal repair (Figure 4.10). Interaction between TRCs and regulatory proteins from surgically elicited macrophages is important for peritoneal re-epithelialization. Maximal stimulation of TRC proliferation can be achieved by an extract of macrophage spent media. Macrophages are potent secretory cells and spent medium contains many soluble mediators for peritoneal repair including growth factors, prostaglandins (PGs), and plasminogen activator (Abercrombie et al., 1971; Lemke, Hugert, & Flad, 1975; Leibovich & Ross, 1976; Leibovich, 1978; Martin et

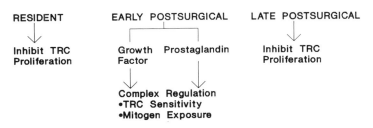

FIGURE 4.10. Peritoneal macrophages (both resident and postsurgical) modulated the proliferation of tissue repair cells (TRCs). Resident and late postsurgical macrophages inhibit TRC proliferation. In contrast, early postsurgical macrophages both up-regulate and down-regulate TRC proliferation depending upon the time of exposure and the sensitivity of the TRCs.

al., 1981; Bitterman et al., 1982; Takemura & Werb, 1984; Bleiberg, Harvey, Smale, & Grotendorst, 1985). PGE$_2$ inhibits the proliferation of fibroblasts, whereas PGF$_2\alpha$ is usually stimulatory (Jimenez et al., 1975, 1983; Mizel et al., 1981). Although resident (nonactivated) macrophages may function as negative modulators of fibroblast proliferation, a facilitation of TRC proliferation and protein secretion may occur after interaction between TRCs and macrophages elicited and subsequently activated by surgical injury. In this way, macrophages may function in many aspects of peritoneal tissue repair after surgery (Calderon, Williams, & Unanue, 1974; Carpenter, 1981; Schmidt et al., 1982).

The net effect result of macrophage growth factor secretion is TRC proliferation in an appropriate ratio during peritoneal re-epithelialization. TGF-β enhances the anchorage-independent proliferation of fibroblasts but does not stimulate anchorage-dependent growth (Roberts et al., 1985; Fukasawa et al., 1989a). However, stimulation of extracellular matrix production may be a more specific activity of TGF-β rather than enhancement of cell proliferation.

From the foregoing observation, the following hypothesis was developed: the mobilization and proliferation of TRCs are responsive to factors secreted by postsurgical macrophages (Figure 4.11). Although resident macrophages may function as negative modulators of TRC proliferation, the postsurgical macrophage secretes substances that induce migration and proliferation of TRCs. The effect of postsurgical macrophages on TRC function may thus be dependent upon (1) the responsiveness of TRCs to these substances and (2) the populations of macrophages present (resident or suppressor versus activated or helper macrophages). This concept is supported by the observation that after surgical trauma in vivo, migration and proliferation of TRCs are accelerated and then stop once tissue repair is complete. In addition, postsurgical macrophages can modulate the proliferation, morphology, and secretory products of post-

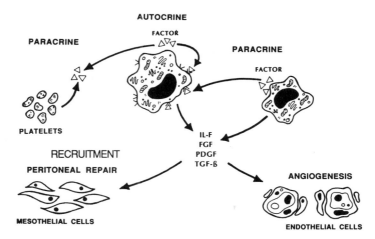

FIGURE 4.11. Early release of factors by cells is probably instrumental in mononuclear cell recruitment and activation. Release of factors by activated macrophages is involved in autoregulation and in attraction, proliferation, and matrix synthesis by mesothelial cells. These effects of factors on mesothelial and also on endothelial cells can be direct or indirect through the stimulation of macrophage-derived polypeptide growth factor synthesis: tumor necrosis factor (TNF), interleukin-1 (IL-1), platelet-derived growth factor (PDGF), and basic fibroblast growth factor (FGF). TGF-β inhibits T-cell proliferation, which may reduce the inflammatory response while promoting healing (adapted from Wahl et al., 1989).

surgical TRCs in vitro. Accordingly, peritoneal wound healing may be controlled by the regulation of macrophage migration and/or TRC proliferation.

References

Abe H, Rodgers KE, Ellefson D, diZerega GS. (1989). Kinetics of interleukin-1 secretion by murine post-surgical peritoneal macrophages. *J Surg Res.* 47:178–182.

Abe H, Rodgers KE, Ellefson D, diZerega GS. (1991). Kinetics of interleukin-1 and tumor necrosis factor secretion by rabbit macrophages recovered from the peritoneal cavity after surgery. *J Invest Surg.* 4:141–151.

Abercrombie M, Heaysman JEM, Pegrum SM. (1971). The locomotion of fibroblasts in culture. IV. Electron microscopy of the leading lamella. *Exp Cell Res.* 67:359–367.

Abercrombie M, Heaysman JEM, Pegrum SM. (1972). Locomotion of fibroblasts in culture. V. Surface marking with concanavalin A. *Exp Cell Res.* 73:536–539.

Aggarwal BB, Kohn WJ, Hass PE, Moffat B, Spencer SA, Henzel WJ, Bringman TS, Nedwin GW, Goeddel DV, Harkins RN. (1985). Human tumor necrosis factor: production, purification and characterization. *J Biol Chem.* 260:2345–2354.

Akiyama SK, Yamada KM. (1985). The interaction of plasma fibronectin with fibroblastic cells in suspension. *J Biol Chem.* 260:4492.

Assoian RK, Komoriya A, Meyers CA, Miller DM, Sporn MB. (1983). Transforming growth factor-β in human platelets. *J Biol Chem.* 258:7155–7160.

Assoian RK. (1986). Biphasic effect of type β transforming growth factor on epidermal growth factor receptors in NRK fibroblasts: functional consequences for epidermal growth factor stimulated mitosis. *J Biol Chem.* 260:9613–9617.

Assoian RK, Fleurdelys BE, Stevenson HC, Miller PJ, Madtes DK, Raines EW, Ross R, Sporn M. (1987). Expression secretion of type β transforming growth factor by activated human macrophage. *Proc Natl Acad Sci USA.* 84:6020–6024.

Baird A, Mormede P, Bohlen P. (1985). Immunoreactive fibroblast growth factor in cells of peritoneal exudate suggest its identity with macrophage derived growth factor. *Biochem Biophys Res Commun.* 126:358–364.

Baird A, Esch F, Mormede P, Veno N, Ling N, Bohlen P, Ying SY, Wehrenberg WB, Guillemin R. (1986). Molecular characteristics of fibroblast growth factors distribution and biological activities in various tissues. *Recent Prog Horm Res.* 42:143–205.

Barbul A, Knud-Hansen J, Wasserkrug HL, Efron G. (1986). Interleukin-2 enhances wound healing in rats. *J Surg Res.* 40:315–319.

Bitterman PB, Rennard SI, Hunninghake GW, Crystal RB. (1982). Human alveolar macrophage growth factor: regulation and partial characterization. *J Clin Invest.* 70:806–822.

Bleiberg I, Harvey AK, Smale G, Grotendorst GR. (1985). Identification of a PDGF-like chemoattractant produced by NIH/3T3 cells after transformation with SV40. *J Cell Biol.* 123:161–166.

Bronson RE, Bertiolami CN, Siebert EP. (1987). Modulation of fibroblast growth and glycosaminoglycan synthesis by interleukin-1. *Coll Relat Res.* 7:323–332.

Bryant SM, Fukasawa M, Orita H, Rodgers KE, diZerega GS. (1988). Mediation of post-surgical wound healing by macrophages. In: Hunt TK, Barbul A, Pines E, eds. *Growth Factors and Other Aspects of Wound Healing: Biological Clinical Research.* New York: Alan R. Liss; 266:273.

Calderon J, Williams RT, Unanue ER. (1974). An inhibitor of cell proliferation related by cultures of macrophages. *Proc Natl Acad Sci USA.* 71:4273.

Carpenter G. (1981). Vanadate, epidermal growth factor and the stimulation of DNA synthesis. *Biochem Biophys Res Commun.* 102:1115–1121.

Clemmons DR, Underwood LE, Van Wyk JJ. (1981). Hormonal control of immunoreactive somatomedin production by cultured human fibroblasts. *J Clin Invest.* 64:10–19.

Cohen S. (1962). Isolation of a mouse submaxillary gland protein accelerating incisor eruption and eyelid opening in the newborn animal. *J Biol Chem.* 237:1555–1568.

Cohen S, Carpenter G. (1975). Human epidermal growth factor: isolation and chemical and biological properties. *Proc Natl Acad Sci USA.* 72:1317–1323.

Conover CA, Hintz R, Rosenfeld RG. (1985). Comparative effects of somatomedin C and insulin on the metabolism and growth of cultured human fibroblasts. *J Cell Physiol.* 122:133–141.

Cromack DT, Sporn MB, Roberts AB, Meuno JJ, Dart LL, Norton TA. (1987). Transforming growth factor β levels in rat wound chambers. *J Surg Res.* 42:622–628.

Dinarello CA, Cannon JG, Mier JW, Berkhein HA, Loprest G, Lynn DL, Love RN, Webb AC, Auron PE, Reuben RC, Rich A, Wolft SM, Putney SD. (1986). Multiple biological activities of human recombinant interleukin 1. *J Clin Invest.* 77:1734–1739.

Dunphy JE, Udupa KN. (1955). Chemical and histochemical sequences in the normal healing of wounds. *N Engl J Med.* 20:847–851.

Estes JE, Pledger WJ, Gillespie GY. (1984). Macrophage-derived growth factor for fibroblasts and interleukin-1 are distinct entities. *J Leukocyte Biol.* 35:115–129.

Fukasawa M, Bryant SM, Nakamura RM, diZerega GS. (1987). Modulation of fibroblast proliferation by postsurgical macrophages. *J Surg Res.* 43:513–520.

Fukasawa M, Bryant SM, diZerega GS. (1988). Incorporation of thymidine into fibroblasts evidence for complex regulation by postsurgical macrophages. *J Surg Res.* 45:460–466.

Fukasawa M, Yanagihara DL, Rodgers KE, diZerega GS. (1989a). The mitogenic activity of peritoneal tissue repair cells: control by growth factors. *J Surg Res.* 47:45–51.

Fukasawa M, Campeau JD, Yanagihara DL, Rodgers KE, diZerega GS. (1989b). Mitogenic and protein synthetic activity of tissue repair cells: control by the postsurgical macrophage. *J Invest Surg.* 2:169–180.

Fukasawa M, Campeau JD, Yanigihara DL, Rodgers KE, diZerega GS. (1990). Regulation of proliferation of peritoneal tissue repair cells by peritoneal mactrophages. *J Surg Res.* 49:81–87.

Ginsberg M, Pierschbacher MD, Ruoslahti E, Marguerie G, Plow EF. (1985). Inhibition of fibronectin binding to platelets by proteolytic fragments and synthetic peptides which support fibroblast adhesion. *J Biol Chem.* 260:3931–3936.

Gleiber WE, Schiffmann E. (1984). Identification of a chemoattractant for fibroblasts produced by human breast carcinoma cell lines. *Cancer Res.* 44:3398–3402.

Gosline JM, Rosenbloom J. (1984). Elastin. In: Piez KA, Reddi AH, eds. *Extracellular Matrix Biochemistry.* New York: Elsevier; 191–227.

Gresser J, Brouty-Boye K, Thomas MG, MacLerira-Cuehlo A. (1970). Interferon and cell division. I. Inhibition of the multiplication of mouse leukemia C12106/ β in vitro by interferon preparations. *Proc Natl Acad Sci USA.* 66:1052–1058.

Grotendorst GR, Pencev D, Martin GR, Sodek J. (1984). Molecular mediators of tissue repair. In: Hunt TK, Heppenstall RB, Pines E, Rovee D, eds. *Soft and Hard Tissue Repair: Biological and Clinical Aspects.* New York: Praeger; 20–41.

Harris A, Dunn G. (1972). Centripetal transport of attached peptides on both surfaces of moving fibroblasts. *Exp Cell Res.* 73:519–523.

Ignotz RA, Massaque J. (1986). Transforming growth factor β stimulates the expression of fibronectin and collagen and their incorporation into the extracellular matrix. *J Biol Chem.* 261:4337–4345.

Jimenez de Asua L, Clingan D, Rudland PS. (1975). Initiation of cell proliferation in cultured mouse fibroblasts by prostaglandin $F_2\alpha$. *Proc Natl Acad Sci USA.* 72:2724–2728.

Jimenez de Asua LL, Otto AM, Lingren J, Hammerstom S. (1983). The stimulation of the initiation of DNA synthesis and cell division in Swiss mouse 3T3 cells by prostaglandin $F_2\alpha$ requires specific functional groups in the molecule. *J Biol Chem.* 258:8774–8777.

Kehrl JH, Wakefield LM, Roberts AB, Jakowlew S, Alvarez-Mon M, Derynck R, Sporn MB, Fauci AS. (1986). Production of transforming growth factor β by human T lymphocytes and its potential role in the regulation of T cell growth. *J Exp Med.* 163:1037–1050.

Klebe RU. (1974). Isolation of a collagen-dependent cell attachment factor. *Nature.* 250:248–251.

Kleinman HK, McGoodwin EB, Klebe RJ. (1976). Localization of the cell attachment region in types I and II collagen. *Biochem Biophys Res Commun.* 72:426–432.

Kleinman HK, Klebe RJ, Martin GR. (1981). Role of collagenous matrices in adhesion and growth of cells. *J Cell Biol.* 88:473–485.

Ko SD, Page RC, Narayanan AS. (1977). Fibroblast heterogeneity and prostaglandin regulation of subpopulation. *Proc Natl Acad Sci USA.* 74:3429–3436.

Korn JH, Halushka PV, LeRoy EC. (1980). Mononuclear cell modulation of connective tissue function: suppression of fibroblast growth by stimulation of endogenous prostaglandin production. *J Clin Invest.* 65:543–554.

Kung JT, Brooks SB, Jakway JB, Leonard LL, Talmadge DW. (1977). Suppression of in vitro cytotoxic response by macrophage due to induced arginase. *J Exp Med.* 146:665–680.

Laterra J, Culp LA. (1982). Differences in hyaluronate binding to plasma and cell surface fibronectin. *J Biol Chem.* 257:719–726.

Leibovich SJ, Ross R. (1975). The role of macrophages in wound repair. A study with hydrocortisone and anti-macrophage serum. *Am J Pathol.* 78:71–100.

Leibovich SJ, Ross R. (1976). A macrophage-dependent factor that stimulates the proliferation of fibroblast in vitro. *Am J Pathol.* 84:501–513.

Leibovich SJ. (1978). Production of macrophage-dependent fibroblast-stimulating activity (M-FSA) by murine macrophages. *Exp Cell Res.* 113:47–56.

Lemke H, Huget R, Flad HD. (1975). Biochemical characterization of a factor released by macrophages. *Cell Immunol.* 18:70–75.

Martin BM, Gimbrone MA Jr, Unanue ER, Cotran RS. (1981). Stimulation of nonlymphoid mesenchymal cell proliferation by a macrophage-derived growth factor. *J Immunol.* 126:1510–1515.

Matsushima K, Bano M, Kidwell WR, Oppenheim JJ. (1985). Interleukin-1 increases collagen type IV production by murine mammary epithelial cells. *J Immunol.* 134:904–909.

Mensing H, Czarnetozki BM. (1984). Leukotriene B_4 induces in vitro fibroblast chemotaxis. *J Invest Dermatol.* 82:9–12.

Mizel SB, Dayer JM, Krane SM, Mergenhagen SE. (1981). Stimulation of rheumatoid synovial cell collagenase and prostaglandin production by partially purified lymphocyte activating factor. *Proc Natl Acad Sci USA.* 78:2474–2477.

Moses AC, Nissley SP, Rechler MM, Short A, Podskalny JM. (1979). The purification and characterization of multiplication stimulating activity (MSA) from media conditioned by a rat liver cell line. In: Geordano G, Van Wyk JJ, Minuto F, eds. *Somatomedins and Growth.* New York: Academic Press; 45–49.

Muller R, Bravo R, Burckhardt J, Curran T. (1984). Induction of C-fos gene and protein by growth factors precedes activation of C-myc. *Nature.* 312:716–720.

Oldberg A, Ruoslahti E. (1982). Interaction between chondroitin sulfate proteoglycan, fibronectin and collagen. *J Biol Chem.* 257:4859–4863.

Opitz HG, Niethammer D, Lemk H, Flad HD, Huget R. (1975). Inhibition of ^{3}H-thymidine incorporation of lymphocytes by a soluble factor from macrophages. *Cell Immunol.* 16:379–388.

Orita H, Campeau JD, Nakamura RM, diZerega GS. (1986). Modulation of fibroblast proliferation by post-surgical macrophages: a time and dose-response study during postsurgical peritoneal re-epithelialization. *Am J Obstet Gynecol.* 155:905–911.

Pledger WJ, Stiles CD, Antoniades HN, Scher CD. (1978). An ordered sequence of events in required before BALB/c-3T3 cells have become committed to DNA synthesis. *Proc Natl Acad Sci USA.* 74:2839–2848.

Postlethwaite AE, Seyer JM, Kang AH. (1978). Chemotactic attraction of human fibroblasts to type I, II and III collagens and collagen-derived peptides. *Proc Natl Acad Sci USA.* 75:871–875.

Postlethwaite AE, Snyderman R, Kang AH. (1979). Generation of a fibroblast chemotactic factor in serum by activation of complement. *J Clin Invest.* 64:1379–1385.

Postlethwaite AE, Kang AH. (1980). Characterization of guinea pig lymphocyte-derived chemotactic factor for fibroblasts. *J Immunol.* 124:1462–1466.

Postlethwaite AE, Keski-Oja J, Kang AH. (1981). Induction of fibroblast chemotaxis by fibronectin. Localization of the chemotactic region to a 140,000 molecular weight. *J Exp Med.* 153:494–499.

Postlethwaite AE. (1983). Cell-cell interaction in collagen biosynthesis and fibroblast migration. In: Weissmann G, ed. *Advances in Inflammation Research.* New York: Raven Press, 27–55.

Postlethwaite AE, Kang AH. (1983). Induction of fibroblast proliferation by human mononuclear derived proteins. *Arthritis Rheum.* 26:22–27.

Postlethwaite AE, Lachman L, Mainardi CL, Kang AH. (1983). Stimulation of fibroblast collagenase production by human interleukin-1. *J Exp Med.* 157:801–806.

Postlethwaite AE, Lachman LB, Kang AH. (1984). Induction of fibroblast proliferation by interleukin-1 derived from human monocytic leukemia cells. *Arthritis Rheum.* 27:995–1001.

Postlethwaite AE, Keski-Oja J, Moses HL, Kang AH. (1987). Stimulation of the chemotactic migration of human fibroblasts by transforming growth factor β. *J Exp Med.* 165:251–256.

Postlethwaite AE, Kang AH. (1988). Fibroblasts. In: Gallin JI, Goldstein IM, Snyderman R, eds. *Inflammation: Basic Principles and Clinical Correlates.* New York: Raven Press; 577–597.

Prydze HA, Allison AC, Schlorlemner HU. (1977). Further link between complement activation and coagulation. *Nature.* 270:173–178.

Raftery AT. (1973a). Regeneration of parietal and visceral peritoneum. *Br J Surg.* 60:293–299.

Raftery AT. (1973b). Regeneration of parietal and visceral peritoneum in the immature animal. *Br J Surg.* 60:969–975.

Roberts AB, Anzano MA, Wakefield LM, Roche NS, Stern DF, Sporn MB. (1985). Type β transforming growth factor: a bi-directional regulation of cell growth. *Proc Natl Acad Sci USA.* 82:119–123.

Rodgers KE, diZerega GS. (1992). Modulation of peritoneal re-epithelialization by postsurgical macrophages. *J Surg Res.* (In press).

Ross R, Bowen-Pope DF. (1984). Platelet derived growth factor. *J Clin Endocrinol Metab.* 13:191–199.

Ryan GG, Grobety J, Majno G. (1973). Mesothelial injury and recovery. *Am J Pathol.* 71:93–112.

Samuelson B, Branstrom E, Greek K, Hamberg M, Hammerstrom S. (1971). Prostaglandins. *Annu Rev Biochem.* 44:669–692.

Sandy JD, Brown HLG, Lowther DA. (1978). Degradation of proteoglycan in articular cartilage. *Biochem Biophys Acta.* 543:536–544.

Scher CD, Shepard RC, Antoniades HN, Stiles CD. (1979). Platelet-derived growth factor and the regulation of the mammalian fibroblast cell cycle. *Biochem Biophys Acta.* 560:212–241.

Schmidt JA, Mizel SB, Cohen D, Green I. (1982). Interleukin-1, a potential regulator of fibroblast proliferation. *J Immunol.* 128:2177–2182.

Senior RM, Griffin GL, Mecham RP. (1982). Chemotactic responses of fibroblasts to tropoelastin and elastin-derived peptides. *J Clin Invest.* 70:614–618.

Senior RM, Griffin GL, Mecham RP, Wrenn DS, Prassad KU, Urry DW. (1984). Val-Gly-Val-Ala-Pro-Gly, a repeating peptide in elastin, is chemotactic for fibroblasts and monocytes. *J Cell Biol.* 99:870–874.

Senior RM, Huang JS, Griffin GL, Deuel TF. (1985). Dissociation of the chemotactic and mitogenic activities of platelet derived growth factor by human neutrophil elastase. *J Cell Biol.* 100:351–356.

Seppae H, Seppae S, Yamada KM. (1980). The cell binding fragment of fibronectin and platelet-derived growth factor are chemoattractants for fibroblasts. *J Cell Biol.* 87:323.

Seppae H, Grotendorst G, Seppae S, Schiffmann E, Martin GR. (1982). Platelet derived growth factor is chemotactic for fibroblasts. *J Cell Biol.* 92:584–588.

Shimokado K, Raines EW, Madtes DK, Barrett TB, Benditt EP, Ross R. (1985). A significant part of macrophage derived growth factor consists of at least two forms of PDGF cell. *Cell.* 43:277–286.

Simpson DM, R Ross. (1972). The neutrophilic leukocyte in wound repair. A study with anti-neutrophil serum. *J Clin Invest.* 51:2009–2023.

Sporn MB, Roberts AB, Shull JH, Smith JM, Ward JM, Sodik J. (1983). Polypeptide transforming growth factors isolated from bovine sources and used for wound healing in vivo. *Science.* 219:1329–1331.

Stiles CD, Capone GT, Scher CD, Antoniades HN, Van Wky JJ, Pledger WJ. (1979). Dual control of cell growth by somatomedins and platelet-derived growth factor. *Proc Natl Acad Sci USA.* 76:L279–L283.

Takemura R, Werb Z. (1984). Secretory products of macrophages and their physiological functions. *Am J Physiol.* 246:C1–C9.

Thalacker FW, Nilsen-Hamilton M. (1987). Specific induction of secreted proteins by transforming growth factor-β and 12-0-tetra-decanoyl phorbol-13-acetate. *J Biol Chem.* 262:2288–2290.

Tsukamoto Y, Helsen WE, Wahl SM. (1981). Macrophage production of fibronectin. A chemoattractant for fibroblast. *J Immunol.* 127:673–678.

Varga J, Jimenez SA. (1987). Stimulation of normal human fibroblast collagen production and processing by transforming growth factor-β and 12-0-tetradecanoyl phorbol-13-acetate. *J Biol Chem.* 262:2283–2287.

Wahl SM, Wahl LM, McCarthy JB. (1978). Lymphocyte-mediated activation of fibroblast proliferation and collagen production. *J Immunol.* 121:942–946.

Wahl SM, Wahl LM. (1985). Regulation of macrophage collagenase, prostaglandin, and fibroblast-activating factor production by anti-inflammatory agents: different regulatory mechanisms for tissue injury and repair. *Cell Immunol.* 92:302–312.

Wahl SM, McCartney-Francis N, Mergenhagen SE. (1989). Inflammatory and immunoregulatory roles of TGF-β. *Immunol Today.* 10:258–261.

Welgus HG, Campbell EJ, Bar-Shavit Z, Senior RM, Teitelbaum SL. (1985). Human alveolar macrophages produce a fibroblast-like collagenase and collagenase inhibitor. *J Clin Invest.* 76:219–224.

Woolley DE. (1984). Mammalian collagenases. In: Piez KA, Reddi AH, eds. *Extracellular Matrix Biochemistry.* New York: Elsevier; 119–157.

Wyler DJ, Rosenwasser LJ. (1982). Fibroblast stimulation in schistosomiasis. II. Functional and biochemical stimulating factor. *J Immunol.* 129:1706–1710.

Yamada KM, Kennedy DW, Kimata K, Pratt PM. (1980). Characteristics of fibronectin interactions with glycosaminoglycans and identification of active proteolytic fragments. *J Biol Chem.* 255:6055–6063.

5

Extracellular Matrix

FIBROBLASTS AND OTHER SPECIALIZED CONNECTIVE TISSUE CELLS SYN-
thesize extracellular matrix (ECM). Although the role of ECM in postsurgical repair is widely studied in epidermal injuries, little work has been
performed in peritoneal repair (Nishimura, Nakamura, & diZerega, 1983;
Nishimura & diZerega, 1984; Orita, Nakamura, & diZerega, 1985; Shimanuki & diZerega, 1985). In addition to their structural properties,
several matrix components possess important biological properties such
as mediation of inflammatory responses and tissue repair. Three components (collagens, fibronectin, and elastin) of the connective tissue matrix, as well as their degradation products, provide chemotactic signals
for fibroblasts (Postlethwaite, Snyderman, & Kang, 1979; Postlethwaite,
Keski-Oja, & Kang, 1981; Postlethwaite, 1983; Postlethwaite, Seyer, &
Kang, 1987a; Postlethwaite & Kang, 1988; Postlethwaite, Raghow, Stricklin, Poppleton, & Kang, 1988; Senior, Griffin, & Mecham, 1982; Senior
et al., 1984). Matrix components are degraded at sites of tissue injury
and the locally produced degradation products provide important signals
for repair. This chapter reviews the general nature of collagen and glycosaminoglycans derived primarily from studies of skin and superficial
wound repair. Correlates with peritoneal healing are summarized and
differences between peritoneal and skin repair are highlighted.

Collagen

Collagen is the most abundant protein, making up approximately one-
third of total body protein. It is the major protein that holds cells together
and provides the characteristic structure of organs. A feature common
to all collagens is that they contain triple-helical and globular domains
(Miller, 1985). Eleven distinct types of collagen are present in connective
tissue (Table 5.1). These collagens are composed of constituent polypeptide chains (α-chains), which come together to form a single collagen
molecule.

TABLE 5.1. Classification of the collagens.

Group	Characteristics	Common name	Function
1	Chain ≥95 kd, with continuous 300-nm-long helical domain	Type I	Structure, skin, bone, organs
		Type II	Structure, cartilage
		Type III	Structure, skin, organs
		Type V	Cytoskeleton
		Type XI	Chondrocyte cytoskeleton
2	Chain ≥95 kd, with helical and nonhelical domains	Type IV	Structure, basement membrane
		Type VI	Myofibril formation
		Type VII	Anchoring fibril
		Type VIII	Endothelial cell product function unknown
3	Chain <95 kd	Type IX	Unknown
		Type X	Structure, hypertrophic cartilage

Adapted from Miller, 1984.

Collagens can be subclassified into fibrillar and nonfibrillar types (Bornstein & Traub, 1979). Fibrillar collagens form the fibrils that provide the high tensile strength necessary to hold tissues and cells together. Nonfibrillar collagens form filtration barriers and scaffolding that allow for binding of tissue and cells (e.g., epithelial and endothelial cells).

The major fibrillar collagens are types I, II, and III (Table 5.1; Prockhop, Kivirikko, Tuderman, & Guzman, 1979). Type I collagen is found in most connective tissues and is the most abundant collagen (Seyer & Kang, 1985). Type III is present in most tissues that contain type I but in smaller amounts. Types I and III are the major collagens produced by fibroblasts. Type II is present in hyaline cartilage and is synthesized by chondrocytes (Seyer & Kang, 1985). The carbohydrate content is 1% or less in types I and III collagens. In collagen types I, II, III and IV, the carbohydrates are either the monosaccharide galactose or the disaccharide glycosylgalactose (Kivirikko & Myllyla, 1979).

Type I collagen, α-1(I), α-2(I), and α-1 CB5 peptide, as well as types II, III, and IV collagen, induce platelet aggregation (Beachey, Chiang, & Kang, 1979). In inflammatory reactions, type I collagen fibers are degraded by the action of collagenase. This degradation of extracellular matrix could expose type I collagen fibrils such that platelets released from damaged capillaries and blood vessels aggregate by interacting with the exposed collagen and collagenous peptides (Chiang, Beachey & Kang, 1975; Postlethwaite & Kang, 1988). In addition, solubilized collagens, α-chains, and collagenous peptides generated by the action of collagenase and proteinases provide chemotactic signals for monocytes and fibroblasts to migrate into the area of injury.

Proteoglycans

Proteoglycans are macromolecules that form the amorphous ground substance present in intercellular and interfibrillar spaces present in connective tissues (Aplin & Hughes, 1982). Although proteoglycans are mostly extracellular, there are both intracellular and cell-membrane associated forms (Heinegard & Paulson, 1984). Proteoglycans are complex molecules in which glycosaminoglycan (GAG) chains are linked covalently to a protein core. GAGs (hyaluronic acid, chondroitin sulfate, dermatan sulfate, heparan sulfate, heparin, and keratan sulfate) and long-chain, unbranched, carbohydrate polymers (-glycans) are composed of repeating disaccharide units (Figure 5.1; Hakomori, Fukuda, Sekiguchi, & Carter, 1984). One constituent of the unit is an amino sugar (glycosamino-), and the other is a hexuronic acid (glycurono-), with the exception of keratan sulfate, which contains galactose instead of hexuronic acid. Each proteoglycan molecule is composed of one or two different types of GAG, and the total number of GAG chains may vary from one or two to more than 100 (Postlethwaite & Kang, 1988). The molecular weights of proteoglycans are in the range of 50,000 to several million (Table 5.2). A still higher level of organization can be attained by the aggregation of some types of proteoglycans that have molecular weights greater than 100 million.

Hyaluronic Acid

Hyaluronic acid (HA) is the largest GAG. Its molecular weight can vary from a few hundred thousand to several million. HA is a negatively charged, high molecular weight glycosaminoglycan consisting of repeating disaccharide units of *N*-acetylglucosamine and glucuronate (Mason, 1981). It differs from other GAGs in its lack of sulfation and absence of covalently linked protein. HA is present in all connective tissues; fibroblasts in culture produce more HA than any other species of GAG (usually >50% of the total GAGs synthesized). HA may be bound to the cell surface, and specific receptors are present on liver cells, fibroblasts, chondrocytes; and macrophages (Solursh, Vaerewyck, & Reiter, 1974; Truppe, Basner, Von Figura, & Kresse, 1977).

A variety of cell types display a hyaluronate-dependent type of aggre-

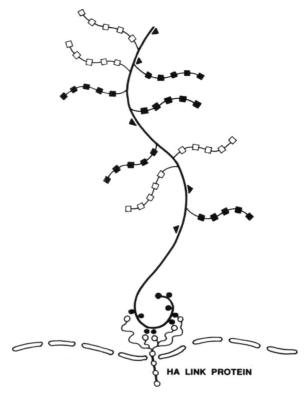

FIGURE 5.1. Proteoglycan molecule, depicting bottle-brush configuration and heterogeneity of the core protein with respect to attachment sites (▲) for chondroitin sulfate (■) and keratan sulfate (□); also shown is hyalurate-binding region (○;●). HA, hyaluronic acid.

gation. In the case of macrophages (Galindo, Myrvik, & Love, 1975; Love, Shannon, Myrvik, & Lynn, 1979), aggregation is induced by the addition of exogenous hyaluronate. For other cell types, such as fibroblasts, aggregation occurs spontaneously, being mediated by endogenous hyaluronate (Underhill & Toole, 1980). Hyaluronate cross-links the cells by interacting with a plasma-membrane receptor for hyaluronate. This aggregation can be prevented by the addition of hyaluronidase, which degrades the endogenous hyaluronate, or by high concentrations of hyaluronate, which saturate the receptors so cross-linking cannot occur (Underhill & Toole, 1981).

The hyaluronate receptor may also be involved in the macrophage disappearance reaction (Shannon, Love, & Myrvik, 1980). T cells release factors causing mesothelial cells lining the peritoneal cavity to increase their production of hyaluronate, which induces macrophage clumping

TABLE 5.2. The repeating disaccharide units of the glycosaminoglycans.

Glycosaminoglycan	Function	Number of disaccharide units	Disaccharide units
Hyaluronic acid	Retains water and regulates water flow in tissue; participates in proteoglycan aggregation	50–10,000	β-D-Glucuronic acid β-D-N-Acetylglucosamine
Chondroitin sulfate	Proteoglycan structure in cartilage, nucleus pulposus, and bone	20–60	β-D-Glucuronic acid β-D-N-Acetylgalactosamine
Dermatan sulfate	Proteoglycan structure in loose connective tissue (skin, sclera, cornea)	30–80	β-D-Glucuronic acid β-D-N-Acetylgalactosamine and α-L-iduronic acid β-D-N-Acetylgalactosamine
Heparin sulfate	Proteoglycan structure in basement membranes; binds to fibronectin; heparin proteoglycan from mast cells	10–60	β-D-Glucuronic acid α-D-N-Acetylglucosamine and α-L-iduronic acid α-D-N-Acetylglucosamine
Keratan sulfate	Proteoglycan structure, cartilage, pulposus	5–40	β-D-N-Acetylglucosamine β-D-Galactose

Compiled from information given by Heinegard and Paulson, 1984.

and epithelial attachment. Intraperitoneal injections of hyaluronate directly induce macrophage aggregation (Shannon & Love, 1980).

HA is thought to play a central role in regulating the flow and content of water in some tissues. It is also involved in the formation of proteoglycan aggregates in that it forms a "backbone" onto which other proteoglycans attach. HA appears to play a critical role in modulating cell differentiation (Toole, Jackson, & Gross, 1972; Toole, 1982a). HA can facilitate movement of cells by preventing cell-cell and cell-substrate interactions that immobilize the cells (Mason, 1981; Toole, 1982b). HA is produced in the early phases of tissue repair, promoting the migration of inflammatory cells and fibroblasts.

GAGs of mature vessels differ from those of newly formed capillary sprouts. At the migrating tip of a capillary sprout, the basal lamina contains HA, which may aid endothelial cell migration and provide a substrate for the mature lamina (Weigel, Fuller, & LeBoeuf, 1986). In the developing embryo HA plays a role in the formation of new blood vessels. HA and fibrin degradation products stimulate vascularization of the wound. Vascularization of the wound occurs during the period of active matrix remodeling and cell proliferation when these degradation products are produced (Figure 5.2). Hyaluronidase secreted into the wound matrix generates small breakdown products from the large polymeric HA.

Chondroitin Sulfate

Chondroitin sulfate is a sulfated GAG that contains ester sulfate groups that reside on carbon 4 or 6 of the *N*-acetylgalactosamine residue. It contains only one type of uronic acid, namely glucuronic acid. The number of repeat disaccharides within a preparation of chondroitin sulfate varies from 20 to 60 with an average molecular weight of approximately 20,000. Chondroitin sulfate is attached to the core protein by an O-glycosidic bond between serine and a xylose residue (Roden, 1980). This type of linkage is common to most GAGs. Very little chondroitin sulfate is found in fibrous connective tissue.

Dermatan Sulfate

Dermatan sulfate is structurally related to chondroitin sulfate. It contains an additional type of monosaccharide, L-iduronic acid (Heinegard & Paulson, 1984). The number of disaccharide units can vary in a dermatan sulfate molecule but is usually on the order of 50 to 60. Dermatan sulfate is found in fibrous connective tissues such as tendon and skin (Heinegard & Paulson, 1984). Dermatan sulfate can bind to, and interact with, several matrix components, including collagen (Toole & Lowther, 1968). Since dermatan sulfate can precipitate tropocollagen from solution causing fi-

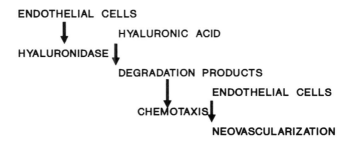

FIGURE 5.2. Vascularization of the wound occurs during the period of active matrix remodeling and cell proliferation when these degradation products are produced. Hyaluronidase secreted into the wound matrix generates small breakdown products from the large polymeric hyaluronic acid (HA).

bril formation in vitro, dermatan sulfate may facilitate collagen fiber formation (Mathews & Decker, 1969; Toole & Lowther, 1968).

Heparan Sulfate and Heparin

Heparan sulfate is synthesized by fibroblasts and other connective tissue cells, whereas heparin is synthesized by mast cells. Heparan sulfate is located on many cell surfaces and in certain fibrous connective tissues (Roden, 1980). Although its true physiologic functions are not known, it probably interacts with other matrix constituents, especially collagen. Heparin is found especially in the lungs and intestine. It is an efficient inhibitor of blood coagulation, but it also binds to a specific region of the fibronectin molecule and to a basic protein in granules of mast cells (Heinegard & Paulson, 1984).

Membrane-intercalated heparan sulfate proteoglycans are present on a variety of cells such as fibroblasts and endothelial cells (Norling, Glimelius, & Wasteson, 1981; Rapraeger & Bernfield, 1983). The intercalated heparan sulfate proteoglycans may serve as a link between the intracellular and extracellular fibers by interacting with fibronectin, laminin (a high molecular weight glycoprotein of basement membranes), or collagen fibers in the extracellular space.

Fibronectin

Fibronectin is a high molecular weight glycoprotein present in basement membranes, around primitive mesenchymal and smooth muscle cells, and in vascular walls (Linder, Stenman, Lehto, & Vaheri, 1978; Stenman & Vaheri, 1978). It is also present in soluble form in plasma (Mosher, 1984) and other body fluids (Mosesson & Amrani, 1980; Pearlstein, Gold, & Garcia-Pardo, 1980). Fibronectin is composed of two similar 250,000 molecular weight subunits. The subunits are joined near their C-termini by disulfide bonds. Each subunit has a series of tightly folded globular domains that have specialized binding characteristics (Figure 5.3; Ruoslahti, 1988). Fibronectin binds to collagen, proteoglycans (heparin, heparan sulfate, and hyaluronic acid), and cells, such as fibroblasts, and covalently cross-links these macromolecules, thereby facilitating matrix organization (Klebe, 1974; Kleinman, McGoodwin, & Klebe, 1976; Engvall & Ruoslahti, 1977; Yamada, Kennedy, Kimata, & Pratt, 1980; Ruoslahti, Engvall, & Hayman, 1981; Hynes & Yamada, 1982; Laterra & Culp, 1982; Oldberg & Ruoslahti, 1982).

Fibronectin in plasma and other body fluids promotes cell movement, attachment, spreading, and proliferation (Yamada, 1983a; Yamada, 1983b). Phagocytosis and clearance of cellular debris by the mononuclear phagocyte system are facilitated by the nonspecific opsonic activity of

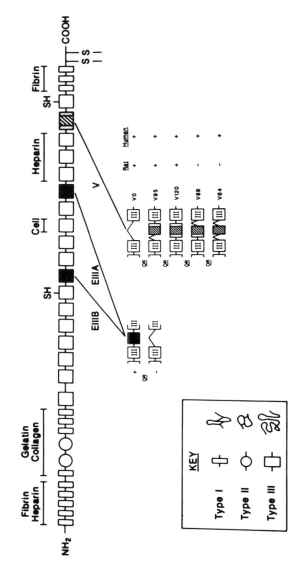

FIGURE 5.3. The general structure of the fibronectin polypeptide, location of its binding sites, and the alternatively spliced fibronectin variants. The key shows the disulfide bonding pattern of the type I and type II homology segments and a hypothetical folding of the type III segments (Hynes, 1987).

fibronectin (Yamada & Kennedy, 1984). This nonspecific opsonic activity of fibronectin is important in host defense and wound healing and is probably mediated by its ability to interact with fibrin and C1q component of complement (Ruoslahti & Vaheri, 1975; Kuusela, 1978; Zardi et al., 1979; Keski-Oja, Sen, & Todaro, 1980; Menzel, Smolen, Liotta, & Reid, 1981; Courtney, Simpson, & Beechey, 1983).

Fibronectin is a potent chemoattractant for fibroblasts and promotes attachment, spreading, and proliferation of fibroblasts. Fibronectin also promotes attachment and spreading of platelets on collagen fibers and cell attachment to fibrin clots (Grinnell, Hays, & Minter, 1977; Grinnell, 1983). Some intermediate fragments from fibronectin degradation retain biological activity, such as binding and chemotaxis. The differentiation and morphogenesis of certain types of cells is influenced by fibronectin. These properties of fibronectin facilitate repair to damaged connective tissue. For example, the promotion of adhesion and spreading of platelets on exposed collagen fibers and binding of circulating cells to fibrin clots and exposed collagen are important functions of fibronectin in hemostasis and wound repair.

Fibronectin is involved during the early phases of epidermal wound healing or tissue repair (Figure 5.4). Fibronectin can be cross-linked to fibrin through the action of plasma transglutaminase (blood coagulation

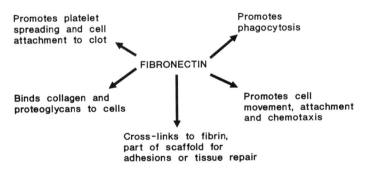

FIGURE 5.4. Fibronectin is involved during the early phases of epidermal wound healing or tissue repair. Fibronectin is a potent chemoattractant for fibroblasts and promotes attachment, spreading, and proliferation of fibroblasts. Fibronectin also promotes attachment and spreading of platelets on collagen fibers and cell attachment to fibrin clots (Grinnell et al., 1977; Grinnell, 1983). Some intermediate fragments from fibronectin degradation retain biologic activity, such as binding and chemotaxis. The differentiation and morphogenesis of certain types of cells is influenced by fibronectin. These properties of fibronectin facilitate repair to damaged connective tissue. For example, the promotion of adhesion and spreading of platelets on exposed collagen fibers and binding of circulating cells to fibrin clots and exposed collagen are important functions of fibronectin in hemostasis and wound repair.

factor XIII) (Mosher, 1975). Procollagen type III is found deposited in the fibronectin-containing immature matrix. Later, when collagenous proteins are organized into bundles, fibronectin and fibroblasts disappear. Thrombin stimulates the production of fibronectin by human fibroblasts (Mosher & Vaheri, 1978). Fibronectin intermixed with fibrin is a major component in the primary matrix formed during tissue repair, in cell-substrate interactions, and cell adhesion (Ruoslahti et al., 1981). The fibrin-fibronectin matrix offers a scaffolding into which fibroblasts and endothelial cell can invade and anchor.

A region of fibronectin termed the "cell-binding" region, interacts with the cell surface to mediate cell attachment and spreading on substrates (Pierschbacher, Hayman, & Ruoslahti, 1981; Hayashi & Yamada, 1983). A synthetic peptide from this region of fibronectin can mediate cell attachment to a plastic substrate (Pierschbacher et al., 1983). These molecules were found to be competitive, reversible inhibitors of fibronectin function, indicating that adhesive proteins have a dualistic nature depending on their concentrations and locations, i.e., in solution or bound to a substrate. Weakening of adhesive interactions might result from events that increase the local concentrations of soluble adhesive proteins, e.g., in certain disease states or possibly even at localized regions on the cell surface near the sites of secretion of such molecules.

Elastin

Elastin is found in high concentrations in the media of large blood vessels. It is present in relatively small, but important, amounts in peritoneum. Elastin has an unusual amino acid composition. Approximately one-third of its amino acid residues are glycine and 10% to 13% are proline, similar to collagen (Sandberg, Gray, & Franzblau, 1977). However, there is very little hydroxyproline and no hydroxylysine. The elastic property of tissue is due to elastin fibers present in the extracellular matrix. In addition, peptides generated by degrading elastin with pancreatic elastase are chemotactic for fibroblasts (Senior et al., 1982).

Integrins

The regulation of extracellular matrix assembly and cellular responses to these matrices are important in the control of wound healing. Proper adhesion of cells to a substrate is required for cell attachment and migration, maintenance of cellular polarity, and differentiation of cells. All of these functions are crucial in the repair of a wound (Chapter 3). Recently, a family of proteins was described that participates in the recognition between cells and the extracellular matrix that is referred to as

TABLE 5.3. Supergene family of related receptors.

β-Subunit (source)	α-Subunit	Receptor (α-β combination)
β_1 (avian integrin band 3,	α_0	Avian integrin (band 1)
fibronectin receptor, and	α_1	VLA 1
VLA)	α_2	VLA 2
	α_3	VLA 3 and avian integrin (band 2)
	α_4	VLA 4
	α_F	VLA 5 and mammalian fibronectin
β_2 (LFA-1/Mac-1 and p150,95)	α_L	LFA^{-1}
	α_M	Mac-1
	α_X	p150,95
β_3 (platelet glycoprotein IIIa and	α_{IIb}	Cytoadhesion glycoprotein IIb-IIIa
vitronectin receptor)	α_V	Vitronectin

The different α-chains are denoted by the nature of the ligand (e.g., α_F, fibronectin), the original cell type (e.g., α_L, leukocyte), or where no simple designation exists, by the subscript used by the original discoverer (e.g., α_1, VLA-1; Buck & Horwitz, 1987).

the integrin superfamily (Hynes, 1987). Integrins are a class of cell surface proteins that interact with specific proteins within the extracellular matrix. Vitronectin receptor on fibroblasts, Mac-1 on macrophages, GPIIIbIIa on platelets, and VLA antigens on lymphocytes are all members of the integrin superfamily.

Integrins are heterodimeric proteins containing α and β subunits. Integrins are divided into three families, each family is defined by a distinct β-subunit (all proteins within a family containing it complexes with a number of α-subunits) (Table 5.3; Buck & Horwitz, 1987). Members of the integrin family recognize an RGD sequence on the ligands to which they bind. For example, an integrin on platelets, GPIIIbIIa, recognizes fibrinogen and fibronectin (Phillips & Agin, 1977; Ginsberg, Forsyth, Lightsey, Chedrak, & Plow, 1983). There are sequences containing RGD in the proteins, fibrinogen, and fibronectin. Since peptides containing RGD can compete for the binding of fibrinogen and fibronectin to platelets, it was concluded that the RGD sequence contributes to the recognition of fibrinogen and fibronectin by GPIIIb/IIa (Ginsberg, Pierschbacher, Ruoslahti, Marguerie, & Plow, 1985). Although GPIIIbIIa can recognize multiple proteins, there are integrins, i.e., the fibronectin and vitronectin receptors that are specific for these extracellular matrix proteins (Pytela, Pierschbacher & Ruoslahti, 1985a; 1985b).

The mechanism by which adhesion of cells to extracellular matrix proteins is regulated is currently unknown, but can occur at many levels. The possible mechanisms for regulation include changes in receptor distribution, receptor concentrations, and posttranslational modifications of integrins.

Peritoneal Healing

Although few studies of ECM have been performed with peritoneum, some animal studies are available. Collagen and proteoglycans were extracted from rabbit peritoneum during postoperative mesothelial regeneration. Quantitation of these proteins was correlated with macroscopic observations of normal peritoneal re-epithelialization and/or postoperative adhesion formation (Nishimura et al., 1983; Nishimura & diZerega, 1984). As determined by recovered glycosamine and proline, a positive correlation was apparent between the severity of adhesion grade and formation of new glycosaminoglycans or collagens (Figures 5.5 and 5.6; Nishmura, Nakamura, & diZerega, 1984). A positive correlation existed between the formation of glycosaminoglycans and collagen in the site of uterine healing and the subsequent formation of adhesions.

The increase in the concentration of GAGs and collagen that occurs at the site of peritoneal trauma may originate in the serous exudate that is locally produced. Peritoneal tissue repair cells (TRCs; see Chapter 4) from rabbits incorporate the maximum amount of proline and glucosamine, indirect measures of collagen and GAG synthesis, on postsurgical days 5 to 7. TRCs had an eightfold greater rate of ^{14}C-proline incorporation (Figure 5.7; Orita et al., 1985) and a tenfold increase in ^{14}C-glucosamine incorporation compared to exudative cells (Figure 5.8; Orita et al., 1985). Previous studies of superficial skin wounds in rats reported the biosynthetic capacity of wound tissue for collagen and glycosaminoglycans reached an initial peak on postsurgical day 5 (Cohen, Moore, & Diegelman, 1979; Dolynchuk & Bowness, 1981).

TRCs maximally incorporated both radiolabeled precursors on postsurgical days 5 to 7, and then simultaneously decreased their incorporation to control levels by postsurgical day 10 (Fukasawa, Bryant & diZerega, 1988). Previous studies of superficial skin wounds in rats reported that the biosynthetic capacity of wound tissue for collagen and GAG production reached an initial peak on postsurgical day 5 (Dolynchuk & Bowness, 1981). The interval of enhanced incorporation of proline and glucosamine by TRCs was coincident with the interval of macrophage migration into the injured peritoneum after surgery (Fukasawa, Bryant, Orita, Campeau, & diZerega, 1989). These findings suggest that postsurgical macrophages may modulate the production of connective tissue matrix by TRCs, which provides the scaffolding to support mesothelial cell migration and proliferation required for peritoneal re-epithelialization. In addition, these TRC activities are modulated by the secretory products of peritoneal macrophages (Figures 5.9 and 5.10; Fukasawa et al., 1989).

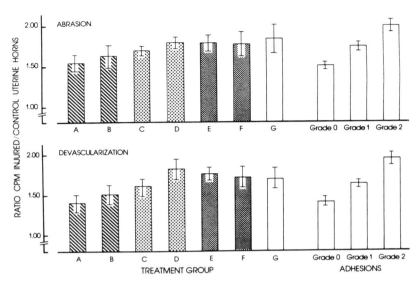

FIGURE 5.5. Glycosaminoglycan formation after abrasion (top) and devascularization (bottom) of rabbit uterine horns (mean ± SEM). Treatment groups: A,B: 70 mg/kg/day; C,D: 35 mg/kg/day; E,F: 17.5 mg/kg/day of ibuprofen; A,C,E: first postoperative dose 8 hours after surgery; B,D,F: first postoperative dose 12 hours after surgery. (From Nishimura et al., 1984. Reproduced by permission of Academic Press.)

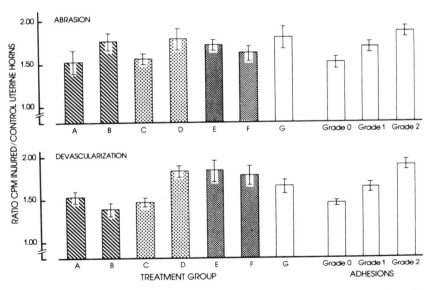

FIGURE 5.6. Collagen formation after abrasion (top) and devascularization (bottom) of rabbit uterine horns (mean ± SEM). Treatment groups: A,B: 70 mg/kg/day; C,D: 35 mg/kg/day; E,F: 17.5 mg/kg/day of ibuprofen; A,C,E: first postoperative dose 8 hours after surgery; B,D,F: first postoperative dose 12 hours after surgery (Nishimura et al., 1983).

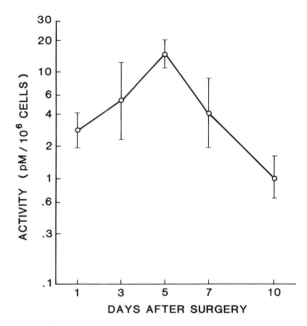

FIGURE 5.7. ^{14}C-proline incorporation by tissue repair cells after peritoneal abrasion. Each data point represents the geometric mean and 95% range of three experiments (Orita et al., 1985, with permission of the Forum on Fundamental Surgical Problems, American College of Surgeons).

Hyaluronic Acid in Coagulation and Wound Healing

Weigel et al. (1986) proposed that an activator (e.g. derived from a plasma precursor, platelets, or surrounding cells) is produced during the clotting reaction that stimulates blood cell types to synthesize and secrete HA into the clot-associated fibrin matrix. The new hyaluronic acid (HA)-fibrin matrix increases and stabilizes the volume and porosity of the clot and serves as a scaffold through which cells trapped in the clot or cells from the peripheral edge of the wound can migrate. The HA-fibrin matrix facilitates cell motility and activates leukocyte functions, including phagocytosis and chemotaxis. The secondary HA-fibrin matrix is then modified as cells continue to migrate into the wound, secreting hyaluronidase and plasminogen activator which degrade the HA and fibrin. These cells also secrete collagen and important regulatory molecules that control cellular functions involved in the inflammatory response and new blood vessel formation in the healing wound.

There appears to be a well-defined sequence of events in formation of granulation tissue: First, a matrix that contains large amounts of HA in

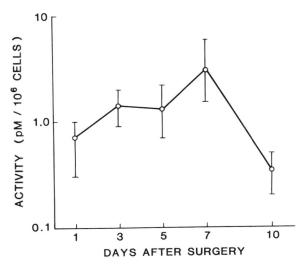

FIGURE 5.8. ^{14}C-glucosamine incorporation by tissue repair cells after peritoneal abrasion. Each data point represents the geometric mean and 95% range of three experiments (Orita et al., 1985, with permission of the Forum on Fundamental Surgical Problems, American College of Surgeons).

addition to other extracellular matrix proteins is laid down in a cell-poor space (Figure 5.11). Second, mesenchymal cell migration is stimulated and the HA matrix is infiltrated by cells migrating from the adjacent tissues. Third, cells within the HA matrix secrete both hyaluronidase, which degrades the HA, and sulfated glycosaminoglycans and collagen, which concomitantly replace the HA as the matrix is remodeled. In each of these stages the HA matrix is first synthesized and then degraded (Weigel, Fuller & LeBoeuf, 1986).

Rapidly (0 to 2 days) after the formation of the initial fibrin-based matrix, the blood clot is remodeled into a matrix that contains HA bound to the fibrin. Cells of various types are trapped within this clot. Fibrin polymers form a porous gel-like meshwork containing trapped or adsorbed plasma proteins such as plasminogen and fibronectin. Fibronectin is incorporated into the clot and distributed along the fibrin strands (Grinnell, Billingham, & Burgess, 1981).

Within a short time, 1 to 2 days, the HA content of the wound increases greatly as HA enters the fibrin matrix. HA specifically binds to fibrin, which facilitates and directs the assembly of HA into a three-dimensional matrix. Both fibrin and HA are macromolecules that can self-assemble into higher order structures. HA can hydrate a large amount of water to form a porous viscoelastic gel.

HA also enhances the phagocytic activity of monocytes (Ahlgren &

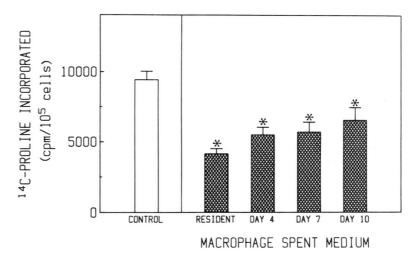

FIGURE 5.9. Tissue repair cells recovered from the site of injury 7 days after peritoneal abrasion in rabbits were incubated for 48 hours with 0.5 μCi ^{14}C-proline and spent medium from cultures of peritoneal exudate cells obtained from non-surgical (resident) peritoneal fluid or postsurgical peritoneal fluid (days 4 to 10). As the control, tissue repair cells were incubated with fresh Medium 199 and 3% fetal calf serum. Each data point represents the mean ± SEM (cpm/10^5 cells; *p <.05). (From Fukasawa et al., 1989. Reproduced by permission of Academic Press.)

Jarstrand, 1984) and also participates in the disappearance reaction displayed by peritoneal macrophages (Shannon et al., 1980). High, but not low, molecular weight fragments of HA inhibit phagocytosis in these cells (Forrester & Balazs, 1980). Cells secrete hyaluronidase and proteases, such as plasminogen activator, which degrade the HA and fibrin. Low molecular weight HA fragments will also stimulate the phagocytic activity of the macrophages responsible for clearing away the breakdown products and debris from the initial clot and the secondary HA-fibrin matrix.

Extracellular Matrix and Tissue Remodeling

The glycosaminoglycan component of the extracellular matrix may participate in modulating the deposition of collagen (reviewed in Bertolami, 1984). Although fibroblasts are known to synthesize both collagen and glycosaminoglycans, different mechanisms exist for controlling the production of each (Green & Goldberg, 1963; Green & Hamerman, 1964). Activated macrophages release soluble mediators that facilitate the directed migration of fibroblasts which then secrete collagen and glycosa-

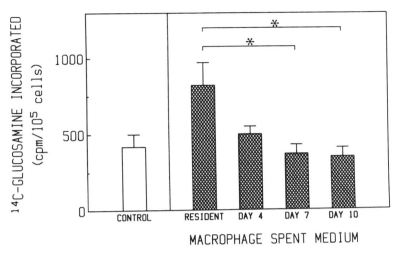

FIGURE 5.10. Tissue repair cells recovered from the site of injury 7 days after peritoneal abrasion in rabbits were incubated for 96 hours with 0.5 μCi ^{14}C-glucosamine and spent media from cultures of peritoneal exudate cells obtained from nonsurgical peritoneal fluid (resident) or postsurgical peritoneal fluid (days 4 to 10). As the control, fibroblasts were incubated with fresh Medium 199 and 3% FCS. Each data point represents the mean ± SEM (cpm/10[5] cells; *p < .05). (From Fukasawa et al., 1989. Reproduced by permission of Academic Press.)

minoglycans (Tsukamoto, Helsen, & Wahl, 1981; Adams & Hamilton, 1984; Graham et al., 1984).

Balazs and Halingrem (1950) reported that granulating wounds contained large amounts of nonsulfated glycosaminoglycans on postsurgical day 4 that were later replaced by sulfated mucopolysaccharides as healing progressed. These observations were supported by Bentley's (1967, 1968) observation of increased concentrations of chondroitin-4-sulfate and dermatan sulfate as tissues healed on days 5 through 17, whereas hyaluronic acid concentrations remained relatively unchanged. Dolynchuk and Bowness (1981) found that healing superficial wounds develop their maximum capacity to produce noncollagenous insoluble glycoproteins before their maximum capacity (wound days 4 to 5) for collagen biosynthesis.

Prostaglandins and Extracellular Matrix

Previous studies reported increased concentrations of prostaglandins, especially prostaglandins E_1 and E_2, in inflammatory exudate of damaged tissues. Palmoski and Brandt (1980) found that ibuprofen, but not indomethacin, inhibits net glycosaminoglycans synthesis in normal canine

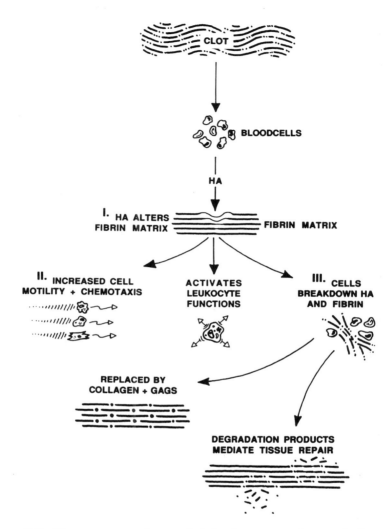

FIGURE 5.11. There appears to be a well-defined sequence of events in formation of granulation tissue: (I) a matrix rich in HA is laid down in a cell-poor space; (II) mesenchymal cell migration is stimulated and the HA matrix is infiltrated by cells migrating from the adjacent tissues; (III) cells within the HA matrix secrete both hyaluronidase, which degrades the HA, and sulfated glycosaminoglycans and collagen, which concomitantly replace the HA as the matrix is remodeled. In each of these stages, the HA matrix is first synthesized and then degraded.

articular cartilage in vitro in a concentration-dependent fashion. Although the rate of human articular cartilage glycosaminoglycan synthesis is variable, McKenzie reported a statistically significant depression in human articular cartilage synthesis of glycosaminoglycans with anti-inflammatory drugs, including ibuprofen, at doses commonly employed in rheumatology (McKenzie, Horsburgh, Ghosh & Taylor, 1976). Previously, we observed a reduction in postsurgical peritoneal adhesions, as well as collagen and glycosaminoglycan formation by cells collected from the site of peritoneal healing in rabbits treated with large doses of ibuprofen, a nonsteroidal anti-inflammatory drug (Nishimura et al., 1983, 1984).

Summary

After tissue damage occurs, platelets bind to exposed matrix via β_1 and β_2 integrins, including the $\alpha_2\beta_1$ collagen/laminin receptor, the $\alpha_5\beta_1$ fibronectin receptor, and the α_6/β_1 laminin receptor (Ginsberg, Loftus, & Plow, 1988). The activation of the blood coagulation cascade also generates thrombin, which activates platelet gpIIb/IIIa, and in turn promotes further platelet aggregation and granule release. A provisional wound matrix is thus formed that contains platelets, fibrinogen, fibrin, and fibronectin. At this point, an inflammatory reaction is initiated by the secretion of platelet granule contents (i.e., TGF-β), thrombin, and exposure of tissue factors. A cascade of endothelial cell and white blood cell activation, much like that occurring in an inflammatory reaction, ensues and results in the extravasation of white blood cells. Cytokines released by the activated white blood cells and platelets accumulate at the site of injury. These agents may then stimulate the up-regulation of integrins on macrophages and fibroblasts that promote their migration into the wound site (Heino & Massague, 1989). Epithelial cell migration over the fibro-

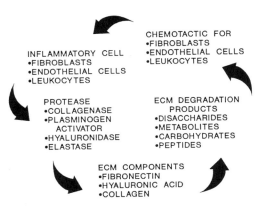

FIGURE 5.12. The involvement of the extracellular matrix in wound repair.

nectin-containing wound matrix may also be dependent on induction of new integrins (Toda, Tuan, Browh, & Grinnell, 1987).

The involvement of ECM in the process of tissue repair is summarized in Figure 5.12. Inflammatory cells at the site of injury release enzymes that degrade the components of the extracellular matrix. These degradation products are then released and these breakdown products are chemotactic for fibroblasts, endothelial cells, and leukocytes. Some studies also suggest that some degradation products can stimulate the activity of these cells. All these processes are necessary for the proper healing of a wound.

References

Adams DO, Hamilton TA. (1984). The cell biology of macrophage activation. *Rev Immunol.* 2:283–319.

Ahlgren T, Jarstrand C. (1984). Hyaluronic acid enhances phagocytosis of human monocytes in vitro. *J Clin Immunol.* 4:246–252.

Aplin JD, Hughes RC. (1982). Complex carbohydrates of the extracellular matrix. Structure, interactions and biological roles. *Biochim Biophys Acta.* 694:375–418.

Balazs A, Halingrem HJ. (1950). The basic dye-uptake and the presence of a growth inhibitory substance in the healing tissue of skin wounds. *Exp Cell Res.* 1:206–216.

Beachey EH, Chiang TM, Kang AH. (1979). Collagen platelet interaction. *Int Rev Connect Tissue Res.* 8:1–21.

Bentley JP. (1967). Rate of chondroitin sulfate formation in wound healing. *Ann Surg.* 165:186–192.

Bentley JP. (1968). Mucopolysaccharide synthesis in healing wounds. In: Dunphy JE, Van Winkle W Jr, eds. *Repair and Regeneration.* New York: McGraw-Hill; 151–160.

Bertolami CN. (1984). Glycosaminoglycan interactions in early wound repair. In: Hunt TK, Heppenstall RB, Pines E, Rovee D, eds. *Soft and Hard Tissue Repair.* New York: Praeger; 67–97.

Bitterman PB, Rennard SI, Hunninghake GW, Crystal RB. (1982). Human alveolar macrophage growth factor: regulation and partial characterization. *J Clin Invest.* 70:806–822.

Bornstein P, Traub W. (1979). The chemistry and biology of collagen. In: Newrath H, Hill RL, eds. *The Proteins.* New York: Academic Press; 4:411–432.

Buck CA, Horwitz AF. (1987). Cell surface receptors for extracellular matrix molecules. *Annu Rev Cell Biol.* 3:179–205.

Carpenter G. (1981). Vandate, epidermal growth factor and the stimulation of DNA synthesis. *Biochem Biophys Res Commun.* 102:1115–1121.

Carter WB, Hakomori S. (1981). A new cell surface, detergent-insoluble glycoproteins matrix of human and harvested fibroblasts. *J Biol Chem.* 256:6953–6960.

Chen AB, Mosesson MW, Solish GI. (1976). Identification of the cold-insoluble globulin of plasma in amniotic fluid. *Am J Obstet Gynecol.* 125:958–961.

Cheung HS, Story MT, McCarty DJ. (1984). Mitogenic effects of hydroxyopatite and calcium pyrophosphate dihydrate crystals on cultured mammalian cells. *Arthritis Rheum.* 27:668–674.

Chiang TM, Beachey EH, Kang AH. (1975). Interaction of a chick skin collagen fragment (alpha 1-CB 5) with human platelets. Biochemical studies during the aggregation and release reaction. *J Biol Chem.* 250:6916–6922.

Cohen IK, Moore CD, Diegelman RF. (1979). Onset and localization of collagen synthesis during wound healing in open rat skin wound. *Proc Soc Exp Biol Med.* 160:458–462.

Courtney HS, Simpson WA, Beachey EH. (1983). Binding of streptococcal lipoteichoic acid to fatty acid-binding sites on human plasma fibronectin. *J Bacteriol.* 153:763–770.

Dolynchuk KN, Bowness JM. (1981). The early metabolism of noncollagenous glycoproteins during wounds healing. *J Surg Res.* 31:218–224.

Engvall E, Ruoslahti E. (1977). Binding of soluble form of fibroblast surface protein, fibronectin, to collagen. *Int J Cancer.* 20:1–5.

Forrester JV, Balazs EA. (1980). Inhibition of phagocytosis by high molecular weight hyaluronate. *Immunology.* 40:435–442.

Fukasawa M, Bryant SM, diZerega GS. (1988). Incorporation of thymidine by fibroblasts; evidence for complex regulation by postsurgical macrophages. *J Surg Res.* 45:460–466.

Fukasawa M, Bryant SM, Orita H, Campeau JD, diZerega GS. (1989). Modulation of proline and glucosamine incorporation into tissue repair cells by peritoneal macrophages. *J Surg Res.* 46:166–171.

Galindo B, Myrvik QN, Love SH. (1975). A macrophage agglutinating factor produced during a pulmonary delayed hypersensitivity reaction. *J Reticuloendothel Soc.* 18:295–304.

Ginsberg MH, Forsyth J, Lightsey A, Chedrak J, Plow LF. (1983). Reduced surface expression and binding of fibronectin by thrombin stimulated thrombasthenic platelets. *J Clin Invest.* 71:619–624.

Ginsberg MH, Pierschbacher MD, Ruoslahti E, Marguerie G, Plow E. (1985). Inhibition of fibronectin binding platelet by proteolytic fragments and synthetic peptides which support fibroblast adhesion. *J Biol Chem.* 260:3931–3936.

Ginsberg MH, Loftus JC, Plow EF. (1988). Cytoadhesins, integrins, and platelets. *Thromb Haemost.* 59:1–6.

Graham MF, Diegelmann RF, Lindblad WJ, Gay S, Gay R, Cohen IK. (1984). Effects of inflammation on wound healing: in vitro studies and in vivo studies. In: Hunt TK, Heppenstall RB, Pines E, Rovee D, eds. *Soft and Hard Tissue Repair.* New York: Praeger; 361–379.

Green H, Goldberg G. (1963). Kinetics of collagen synthesis by established mammalian cell lines. *Nature.* 200:1097–1098.

Green H, Hamerman D. (1964). Production of haluronate and collagen by fibroblast clones in culture. *Nature.* 201:710–712.

Grinnell F, Hays DG, Minter D. (1977). Cell adhesion and spreading factor: partial purification and properties. *Exp Cell Res.* 110:175–190.

Grinnell F, Billingham RE, Burgess L. (1981). Distribution of fibronectin during wound healing in vivo. *J Invest Dermatol.* 76:181–189.

Grinnell F. (1983). Cell attachment and spreading factors. In: Guroff G, ed. *Growth and Maturation Factors.* New York: John Wiley; 267–292.

Hakomori S, Fukuda M, Sekiguchi K, Carter WB. (1984). Fibronectin, laminin, and other extracellular glycoproteins. In: Piez KA, Reddi AH, eds. *Extracellular Matrix Biochemistry*. New York: Elsevier; 229–275.

Hayashi M, Yamada KM. (1983). Domain structure of the carboxyl-terminal half of human plasma fibronectin. *J Biol Chem*. 258:3332–3340.

Heinegard D, Paulson M. (1984). Structure and metabolism of proteoglycans. In: Piez KA, Reddi AH, eds. *Extracellular Matrix Biochemistry*. New York: Elsevier; 277–328.

Heino J, Massague J. (1989). Transforming growth factor-β switches the pattern of integrins expressed in MG-63 human osteosarcoma cells and causes a selective loss of cell adhesion to laminin. *J Biol Chem*. 264:21806–21811.

Hynes RO, Yamada KM. (1982). Fibronectins: multifunctional modular glycoproteins. *J Cell Biol*. 95:369–377.

Hynes RO. (1985). Molecular biology of fibronectin. *Annu Rev Cell Biol*. 1:67–90.

Hynes RO. (1987). Integrins: a family of cell surface receptors. *Cell*. 48:579–558.

Keski-Oja J, Sen A, Todaro GH. (1980). Direct association of fibronectin and acting molecules in vitro. *J Cell Biol*. 85:527–533.

Kivirikko KI, Myllyla R. (1979). Collagen glycosyltransferases. *Int Rev Connect Tissue Res*. 8:23–72.

Klebe RU. (1974). Isolation of a collagen-dependent cell attachment factor. *Nature*. 250:248–251.

Kleinman HK, McGoodwin EB, Klebe RJ. (1976). Localization of the cell attachment region in types I and II collagen. *Biochem Biophys Res Commun*. 72:426–432.

Kuusela PC. (1978). Fibronectin binds to *Staphylococcus aureus*. *Nature*. 276:719–720.

Kuusela P, Vaheri A, Palo J, Ruoslahti E. (1978). Demonstration of fibronectin in human cerebrospinal. *J Lab Clin Med*. 92:595–601.

Laterra J, Culp LA. (1982). Differences in hyaluronate binding to plasma and cell surface fibronectin. *J Biol Chem*. 257:719–726.

Linder E, Stenmam S, Lehto V-P, Vaheri A. (1978). Distribution of fibronectin in human tissues and relationship to other connective tissue components. *Ann NY Acad Sci*. 312:151–189.

Love SH, Shannon BT, Myrvik QN, Lynn WS. (1979). Characterization of macrophage agglutinating factor as a hyaluronic acid protein complex. *J Reticuloendothel Soc*. 25:269–282.

McKenzie LS, Horsburgh BA, Ghosh P, Taylor TKF. (1976). Effect of anti-inflammatory drugs on sulphated glycosaminoglycan synthesis in aged human articular cartilage. *Ann Rheum Dis*. 35:487–493.

Mason MR. (1981). Recent advances in the biochemistry of hyaluronic acid in cartilage. In: Dyl Z, Adams M, eds. *Connective Tissue Research: Chemistry, Biology, and Physiology*. New York: Alan R. Liss; 87–112.

Mathews MB, Deckers L. (1969). The effect of acid mucopolysaccharide proteins on fibril formation from collagen solutions. *Biochem J*. 109:517–526.

Menzel EJ, Smolen JS, Liotta L, Reid KBM. (1981). Interaction of fibronectin with Clq and its collagen like fragment. *FEBS Lett*. 129:188–192.

Miller EJ. (1984). Chemistry of the collagens and their distribution. In: Piez KA, Reddi AH, eds. *Extracellular Matrix Biochemistry*. New York: Elsevier; 41–78.

Miller JM. (1985). The structure of fibril-forming collagens. *Ann NY Acad Sci.* 460:1–13.

Moses AC, Nissley SP, Rechler MM, Short A, Podskalny JM. (1979). The purification and characterization of multiplication stimulating activity (MSA) from media conditioned by a rat liver cell line. In: Geordano G, Van Wyk JJ, Minuto F, eds. *Somatomedins and Growth.* New York: Academic Press; 45–49.

Mosesson MW, Amrani DL. (1980). The structure and biologic activities of plasma fibronectin. *Blood.* 56:145–158.

Mosher DF. (1975). Cross-linking of cold-insoluble globulin by fibrin-stabilizing factor. *J Biol Chem.* 250:6614–6620.

Mosher DF, Vaheri A. (1978). Thrombin stimulates the production and release of a major surface-associated glycoprotein (fibronectin) in cultures of human fibroblasts. *Exp Cell Res.* 112:323–331.

Mosher DF. (1984). Physiology of fibronectin. *Annu Rev Med.* 35:561–575.

Muller R, Bravo R, Burckhardt J, Curran T. (1984). Induction of C-fos gene and protein by growth factors precedes activation of C-myc. *Nature.* 312:716–720.

Nishimura K, Nakamura RM, diZerega GS. (1983). Biochemical evaluation of postsurgical wound repair: prevention of intraperitoneal adhesion formation with ibuprofen. *J Surg Res.* 34:219–226.

Nishimura K, Nakamura RM, diZerega GS. (1984). Ibuprofen inhibition of postsurgical adhesion formation: a time- and dose-response biochemical evaluation. *J Surg Res.* 36:115–124.

Norling B, Glimelius B, Wasteson A. (1981). Heparan sulfate proteoglycan of cultured cells: demonstration of a lipid—and a matrix-associated from. *Biochem Biophys Res Commun.* 103:1265–1272.

Oldberg A, Ruoslahti E. (1982). Interaction between chondroitin sulfate proteoglycan, fibronectin and collagen. *J Biol Chem.* 257:4859–4863.

Orita H, Nakamura RM, diZerega GS. (1985). Kinetic analysis of postoperative peritoneal healing: incorporation of proline and glucosamine by exudative and tissue repair cells. *Surg Forum.* 36:467–469.

Palmoski MJ, Brandt KD. (1980). Effect of some nonsteroidal anti inflammatory drugs on proteoglycans metabolism and organization in canine articular cartilage. *Arthritis Rheum.* 23:1010–1020.

Pearlstein E, Gold LI, Garcia-Pardo A. (1980). Fibronectin: a review of its structure and biological activity. *Mol Cell Biochem.* 29:103–128.

Phillips DR, Agin P. (1977). Platelet plasma membrane glycoproteins. *J Biol Chem.* 252:2121–2126.

Pierschbacher MD, Hayman EG, Ruoslahti E. (1981). Location of the cell-attachment site in fibronectin with monoclonal antibodies and proteolytic fragments of the molecule. *Cell.* 26:259–267.

Postlethwaite AE, Snyderman R, Kang AH. (1976). The chemotactic attraction of human fibroblasts to a lymphocyte-derived factor. *J Exp Med.* 144:1188–1203.

Postlethwaite AE, Snyderman R, Kang AH. (1979). Generation of a fibroblast chemotactic factor in serum by activation of complement. *J Clin Invest.* 64:1379–1385.

Postlethwaite AE, Kang AH. (1980). Characterization of guinea pig lymphocyte-derived chemotactic factor for fibroblasts. *J Immunol.* 124:1462–1466.

Postlethwaite AE, Keski-Oja J, Kang AH. (1981). Induction of fibroblast chemotaxis by fibronectin. Localization of the chemotactic region to a 140,000 molecular weight. *J Exp Med.* 153:494–499.

Postlethwaite AE. (1983). Cell-cell interaction in collagen biosynthesis and fibroblast migration. In: Weissman G, ed. *Advances in Inflammation Research.* New York: Raven Press; 27–55.

Postlethwaite AE, Kang AH. (1983). Induction of fibroblast proliferation by human mononuclear derived proteins. *Arthritis Rheum.* 26:22–27.

Postlethwaite AE, Lachman L, Mainardi CL, Kang AH. (1983). Stimulation of fibroblast collagenase production by human interleukin-1. *J Exp Med.* 157:801–806.

Postlethwaite AE, Lachman LB, Kang AH. (1984). Induction of fibroblast proliferation by interleukin-1 derived from human monocytic leukemia cells. *Arthritis Rheum.* 27:995–1001.

Postlethwaite AE, Seyer JM, Kang AH. (1987a). Chemotactic attraction of human fibroblasts to type I, II and III collagens and collagen-derived peptides. *Proc Natl Acad Sci USA.* 75:871–875.

Postlethwaite AE, Keski-Oja J, Moses HL, Kang AH. (1987b). Stimulation of the chemotactic migration of human fibroblasts by transforming growth factor β. *J Exp Med.* 165:251–256.

Postlethwaite AE, Kang AH. (1988). Fibroblasts. In: Gallin JI, Goldstein IM, Snyderman R, eds. *Inflammation Basic Principles and Clinical Correlates.* New York: Raven Press; 577–597.

Postlethwaite AE, Raghow R, Stricklin GP, Poppleton H, Kang AH. (1988). Modulation of fibroblast functions by human recombinant interleukin-1 α and 1 β. *J Cell Biol.* 106:311–318.

Prockop DJ, Kivirikko KI, Tuderman L, Guzman NA. (1979). The biosynthesis of collagen and its disorders. *N Engl J Med.* 301:13–23,77–85.

Pytela R, Pierschbacher MD, Ruoslahti E. (1985a). Identification and isolation of a 140 kd cell surface glycoprotein with properties expected of a fibronectin receptor. *Cell.* 40:191–198.

Pytela R, Pierschbacher MD, Ruoslalhti E. (1985b). A 125/115 KDa cell surface receptor specific for vitronectin interacts with the arginine-glycine-aspartic acid adhesion sequence derived from fibronectin. *Proc Natl Acad Sci USA.* 82:5766–5770.

Rapraeger AC, Bernfield M. (1983). Heparan sulfate proteoglycans from mouse mammary epithelial cells. Putative membrane proteoglycan associates quantitatively with lipid vesicles. *J Biol Chem.* 258:3632–3636.

Roden L. (1980). Structure and metabolism of connective tissue proteoglycans. In: Lennarz WJ, ed. *The Biochemistry of Glycoproteins and Proteoglycans.* New York: Plenum; 267–371.

Ruoslahti E, Vaheri A. (1975). Interaction of soluble fibroblast surface antigen with fibronectin and fibrin, identity with cold in soluble globulin of human plasma. *J Exp Med.* 141:497–501.

Ruoslahti E, Engvall E, Hayman E. (1981). Fibronectin: Current concepts of its structure and function. *Coll Relat Res.* 1:95–128.

Ruoslahti E. (1988). Fibronectin and its receptors. *Ann Rev Biochem.* 57:375–413.

Sandberg LB, Gray WR, Franzblau C. (1977). *Elastin and Elastic Tissue.* New York: Plenum; 321–352.

Scher CD, Shepard RC, Antoniades HN, Stiles CD. (1979). Platelet-derived growth factor and the regulation of the mammalian fibroblast cell cycle. *Biochem Biophys Acta.* 560:212–241.

Schmidt JA, Mizel SB, Cohen D, Green I. (1982). Interleukin-1, a potential regulator of fibroblast proliferation. *J Immunol.* 128:2177–2182.

Senior RM, Griffin GL, Mecham KRP. (1982). Chemotactic responses of fibroblasts to tropoelastin and elastin-derived peptides. *J Clin Invest.* 70:614–618.

Senior RM, Griffin GL, Mecham RP, Lorenn DS, Prasad KU, Urry DW. (1984). Val-Gly-Val-Ala-Pro-Gly, a repeating sequence in elastin, is chemotactic for fibroblasts and monocytes. *J Cell Biol.* 99:870–874.

Seyer JM, Kang AH. (1985). Structural proteins: Collagen elastin and fibronectin. In: Kelley WN, Harris, Jr, ED, Ruddy S, Sledge CB, eds. *Textbook of Rheumatology.* Philadelphia: W.B. Saunders; 221–237.

Shannon BT, Love SH, Myrvik QN. (1980). Participation of hyaluronic acid in the macrophage disappearance reaction. *Immunol Commun.* 9:735–746.

Shimanuki T, diZerega GS. (1985). Prevention of postoperative peritoneal adhesions in rabbits with ibuprofen. *Semin Reprod Endocrinol.* 3:295–300.

Solursh M, Vaerewyck SA, Reiter RS. (1974). Depression by hyaluronic acid of glycosaminoglycan synthesis by chick cultured embryo chondrocytes. *Dev Biol.* 41:233–240.

Stenman S, Vaheri A. (1978). Distribution of a major connective tissue protein, fibronectin, in normal tissues. *J Exp Med.* 147:1054–1067.

Stiles CD, Capone GT, Scher CD, Antoniades HN, Van Wyk JJ, Pledger WJ. (1979). Dual control of cell growth by somatomedins and platelet-derived growth factor. *Proc Natl Acad Sci USA.* 76:L279–L283.

Toda K-I, Tuan T-L, Brown PJ, Grinnell F. (1987). Fibronectin receptors of human keratinocytes and their expression during cell culture. *J Cell Biol.* 105:3097–3104.

Toole BP, Lowther D. (1968). Dermatan sulfate protein: isolation from and interaction with collagen. *Arch Biochem.* 128:567–575.

Toole BP, Jackson G, Gross J. (1972). Hyaluronate in morphogenesis: inhibiton of chondrogenesis in vitro. *Proc Natl Acad Sci USA.* 69:1384–1389.

Toole BP. (1982a). Hyaluronate turnover during chondrogenesis in the developing chick limb and axial skeleton. *Dev Biol.* 29:321–330.

Toole BP. (1982b). Developmental role of hyaluronate. *Connect Tissue Res.* 10:93–101.

Truppe W, Basner R, Von Figura K, Kresse H. (1977). Uptake of hyaluronate by cultured cells. *Biochem Biophys Res Commun.* 78:713–719.

Tsukamoto Y, Helsen WE, Wahl SM. (1981). Macrophage production of fibronectin. A chemoattractant for fibroblast. *J Immunol.* 127:673–678.

Underhill CB, Toole BP. (1980). Physical characteristics of hyaluronate binding to the surface of simian virus 40-transformed 3T3 cells. *J Biol Chem.* 255:4544–4549.

Underhill CB, Toole BP. (1981). Receptors for hyaluronate on the surface of parent and virus transformed cell lines: binding and aggregation studies. *Exp Cell Res.* 131:419–423.

Wahl SM, Wahl LM, McCarthy JB. (1978). Lymphocyte-mediated activation of fibroblast proliferation and collagen production. *J Immunol.* 121:942–946.

Weigel PH, Fuller GM, LeBoeuf RD. (1986). A model for the role of hyaluronic acid and fibrin in the early events during the inflammatory response and wound healing. *J Theor Biol.* 119:219–234.

Woolley DE. (1984). Mammalian collagenases. In: Piez KA, Reddi AH, eds. *Extracellular Matrix Biochemistry.* New York: Elsevier; 119–157.

Wyler DJ, Rosenwasser LJ. (1982). Fibroblast stimulation in schistosomiasis. II. Functional and biochemical characteristics of egg granuloma-derived fibroblast stimulating factor. *J Immunol.* 129:1706–1710.

Yamada KM, Kennedy DW, Kimata K, Pratt PM. (1980). Characteristics of fibronectin interactions with glycosaminoglycans and identification of active proteolytic fragments. *J Biol Chem.* 255:6055–6063.

Yamada KM. (1983a). Cell surface interactions with extracellular materials. *Annu Rev Biochem.* 52:761–799.

Yamada KM. (1983b). Isolation of fibronectin from plasma and cells. In: Furthmayr H, ed. *Immunochemistry of the Extracellular Matrix.* Boca Raton, FL: CRC Press; 1:111–123.

Yamada KM, Kennedy DW. (1984). Dualistic nature of adhesive protein function: fibronectin and its biologically active peptide fragments can autoinhibit fibronectin function. *J Cell Biol.* 99:29–36.

Zardi L, Siri A, Carnemolla B, Santi L, Bardner WD, Hoch SO. (1979). Fibronectin: a chromatin-associated protein. *Cell.* 18:649–657.

6

Peritoneal Macrophages

CELLS COMPOSING THE MONONUCLEAR PHAGOCYTE SYSTEM SHARE A similar morphology, bone marrow origin, and avid phagocytic capacity. Cells currently assigned to the mononuclear phagocyte system are listed in Table 6.1 and include precursor cells in the bone marrow, and monocytes and macrophages present in the tissues and body cavities under normal conditions, inflammation, and postsurgical repair.

One mononuclear phagocyte, the macrophage, has received considerable attention in studies of peritoneal repair because of the multitude of functions this cell performs. This chapter reviews the ontogeny, physiology, and function of the macrophage with particular attention given to the role of the macrophage in the peritoneal cavity including postsurgical repair. Healing after peritoneal surgery involves a complex process of cellular migration, proliferation, differentiation, interaction, and secretion of extracellular matrix (discussed further in Chapters 3, 4, and 5). Macrophages play a pivotal role in these events.

Macrophage Life Cycle

Macrophages arise in two ways: differentiation of circulating monocytes following their emigration from the blood, and proliferation of precursors at a local site (van Furth & Diesselhoffden, 1970; Volkman, 1976). Although the rate of local production of macrophages is appreciable, under normal conditions most of the macrophage population in any given tissue appears to be of hematopoietic origin (see Mononuclear Phagocyte Kinetics, below).

Monocytes arise from precursor cells in the bone marrow (Volkman & Gowans 1965; van Furth & Cohn, 1968). The pool size of various mononuclear phagocytes under normal steady-state conditions is shown in Table 6.2. A stem cell gives rise to a monoblast which divides once, giving rise to two promonocytes. Each promonocyte also divides once, giving rise to two monocytes. Approximately 19 to 60 hours after they

TABLE 6.1. Cells composing the mononuclear phagocyte system.

Bone marrow
  Monoblasts
  Promonocytes
  Monocytes

Blood
  Monocytes

Tissues (macrophages in the following)
  Connective tissue (histiocytes)
  Skin (histiocytes; Langerhans cells)
  Liver (Kupffer cells)
  Spleen (red pulp macrophages)
  Lymph nodes (free and fixed macrophages; interdigitating cells)
  Thymus
  Bone marrow (resident macrophages)
  Bone (osteoclasts)
  Synovia (type A cell)
  Lung (alveolar and tissue macrophages)
  Mucosa-associated lymphoid tissue
  Gastrointestinal tract
  Genitourinary tract
  Endocrine organs
  Central nervous system (reactive macrophages, microglia; cerebrospinal
                          fluid macrophages)

Body cavities
  Pleural macrophages
  Peritoneal macrophages

Inflammation
  Exudate macrophages
  Epithelioid cells
  Multinucleated giant cells

From van Furth (1988), with permission.

are formed in man, monocytes are released in the G_1 phase into the blood where they circulate with a half-life of 8 to 71 hours (Whitelaw, 1972; Meuret, Bammert, & Hoffman, 1974; Nathan & Cohn, 1980). Monocytes are distributed over a circulating and marginating pool. They leave these pools either at random or via a process in which the older cells leave first (van Furth, 1988). Upon emigrating to tissues or body cavities, monocytes differentiate into macrophages.

The turnover time of tissue macrophages under normal conditions ranges from 20 to 60 days in rodents (Ebert & Florey, 1939). It is assumed that macrophages die in the tissues or body cavities or emigrate to yet another site before they die. Macrophages from the liver, lung and gut have been shown to migrate to nearby lymph nodes and it has been speculated that some die in these nodes.

TABLE 6.2. Pool size of various mononuclear phagocytes under normal steady-state conditions.

Site	Pool size
Bone marrow	
Monoblasts	0.25×10^6
Promonocytes	0.50×10^6
Monocytes	2.60×10^6
Peripheral blood	
Circulating monocytes	0.62×10^6
Marginating monocytes	0.92×10^6
Tissue	
Liver macrophages	9.0×10^6
Spleen macrophages	4.0×10^6
Lung macrophages	2.0×10^6
Peritoneal cavity macrophages	2.4×10^6

Adapted from van Furth (1988).

Macrophage Morphology and Physiology

Mononuclear phagocytes are irregularly shaped medium to large cells that have a single-lobed nucleus. An abundant cytoplasm surrounds a central or slightly eccentric reniform nucleus and contains numerous mitochondria, phase-lucent pinosomes, and phase-dense lysosomes. Numerous flanges, ruffles, and pseudopodia characterize the cytoplasm, particularly at the periphery. The cytoplasm contains a well-developed Golgi zone in the hof of the nucleus as well as actin filaments and microtubules. The complexity of the cytoplasm and its organelles increases with the maturation and activation of these cells (Nathan & Cohn, 1980; Adams & Hamilton, 1988).

The macrophage surface is endowed with a variety of proteins that allow it to maintain continual contact with its environment. Approximately 50 different types of proteins have been identified on the macrophage surface (Table 6.3). These surface proteins include immunoglobulin and fibrinogen-fibrin as well as those recognizing regulatory molecules, such as interferons, neuropeptides, and colony-stimulating factor-1.

The macrophage is active metabolically. Even in the absence of a phagocytic load, the equivalent of its entire surface area is interiorized about once every 33 minutes in the mouse (Steinman, Brodie & Cohn, 1976). Basal metabolic activities of the macrophage are supported by glycolysis and oxidative phosphorylation, although the primary energy source for the cell is dependent upon its origin (Axline, 1970). Many metabolic processes of the macrophage are increased upon stimulation with inflammatory and immune mediators. Studies included in this chapter describe

TABLE 6.3. Ligands for macrophage receptors.

Immunoglobulin and complement
  IgG1, IgG2b
  IgG2a
  IgG3
  IgG1, IgG3 monomers
  IgG complexes
  IgE
  C3b, C4b, C3bi, C3d, C5a

Other proteins
  Mannosyl-, fucosyl-, N-acetylglucosaminyl-terminal glycoproteins
  Alpha$_2$-macroglobulin-protease complex
  Fibronectin
  Fibrin
  Lactoferrin
  Colony-stimulating factors
  Migration inhibitory and macrophage-activation factors
  Insulin
  Factors VII, VIIa
  Interferons

Lipoproteins
  LDL and modified LDL
  Beta-VLDL

Peptides
  Neuropeptides (enkephalins, endorphins)
  Arginine vasopressin
  N-formylated peptides from bacteria, mitochondria

Polysaccharides
  Lipopolysaccharide endotoxin
  Carboydrates on certain cells
  Hyaluronic acid

Others
  Adrenergic agents
  Cholinergic agents
  Phorbol diesters
  Histamine

Modified from Nathan & Cohn (1980).

the effects of peritoneal surgery on the functional activity of peritoneal macrophages.

Pinosomes are rapidly formed in the macrophage and flow through the cytoplasm to the Golgi apparatus where many become filled with acid hydrolases and thus become primary lysosomes (Steinman, Mellman, Muller, & Cohn, 1983). There appears to be a recycling mechanism by which most of the pinocytosed fluid is expelled from the cell, and the vesicles reincorporate into the plasma membrane. The cytoskeleton of the macrophage consists of actin microfilaments and microtubular networks. Localized movements of the macrophage, such as ruffling and locomotion, are regulated by a complex network of actin microfilaments. The microtubular network appears to be responsible both for pinocytosis and for establishing the polarity of cell migration in response to chemotactic stimuli.

Macrophages are able to secrete at least 80 different products (Table 6.4). These include various components of the complement cascade, coagulation factors, proteases and antiproteases, and arachidonic acid metabolites (Unanue, 1986). Regulation of the macrophage's secretory ability differs from molecule to molecule, with most of the secretion being

TABLE 6.4. Secretory products of macrophages.

Enzymes	Additional proteins
Lysozyme	Transferrin
Plasminogen activator	Transcobalamin II
Collagenase	Fibronectin
Elastase	Apolipoprotein E
Angiotensin convertase	Tumor necrosis factor
Acid proteases	Interleukin-1
Acid lipases	Colony-stimulating factor
Acid nucleases	Erythropoietin
Acid phoshatases	Thymosin-β_4
Acid glycosidases	Serum amyloid A, P
Acid sulfatases	Haptoglobin
Arginase	Interferons alpha, beta
Lipoprotein lipase	Platelet-derived growth factor
Phospholipase A_2	Transforming growth factor-β
Enzyme inhibitors	Reactive oxygen intermediates
Alpha$_2$-macroglobulin	O_2^-
Alpha$_1$-antiprotease	H_2O_2
Lipocortin	OH·
Alpha$_1$-antichymotrypsin	
	Hypohalous acids
Coagulation factors	Lipids
Factors X, IX, VII, V	PGE$_2$, PGF$_{2\alpha}$
Protein kinase	Prostacyclin
Thromboplastin	Thromboxane A_2
Prothrombin	Leukotrienes B,C,D,E
Thrombospondin	Mono-HETES and di-HETES
Fibrinolysis inhibitor	Platelet activating factor
Complement cascade components	Small molecules
C1, C2, C3, C4, C5	Purines
Factors B,D	
Properdin	Pyrimidines
C3b inactivator	Gluthatione
Beta-1H	

From Adams and Hamilton (1988), with permission.

stimulated by receptor-ligand interaction. The secreted material is released via different routes, such as fusion of the vesicles with the membrane or by opening of the phagolysome to the surface.

Activation

Characteristic changes in the physiology of the cell occur upon activation of the macrophage. The precise definition of macrophage activation is still controversial. Most forms of activation include a down-regulation of certain physiologic characteristics along with an up-regulation of others. Historically, activation referred to the process by which macrophages gain the ability to destroy microbes and/or tumor cells. Others have defined activation more broadly to include the development of an enhanced potential to complete any complex function.

Mononuclear Phagocyte Kinetics

Leukocytes, especially macrophages, are essential to healing. During peritoneal trauma, leukocytes are both recruited into the site of injury and differentiated (Raftery, 1973; Orita, Campeau, Gale, Nakamura, & diZerega, 1986). The earliest leukocytes to respond to postsurgical trauma are polymorphonuclear leukocytes (i.e., neutrophils). In the absence of infection, these cells subside and do not appear to be involved in repair. Monocytes then enter the surgical site and rapidly differentiate into macrophages. The number of macrophages appears to peak 24 hours after the increase in neutrophils. Figure 6.1 illustrates the kinetics of cellular infiltration and accumulation in the peritoneal cavity of rabbits following reanastomosis of the ileum (Shimanuki, Nakamura, & diZerega, 1986). By postsurgical day 5, approximately 90% of the peritoneal exudate cells are macrophages. The kinetics of postsurgical cellular infiltration in the peritoneal exudate are similar to those observed at the site of injury following abrasion of the parietal peritoneum (Bryant, Fukasawa, Orita, Rodgers, & diZerega, 1988). Acute administration of tolmetin, a nonsteroidal anti-inflammatory drug (NSAID), that reduces postsurgical adhesion formation in a hyaluronic acid carrier, elevated leukocyte infiltration after surgery. Polymorphonuclear cell (PMN) infiltration was elevated within 6 to 12 hours after surgery, and macrophage infiltration was elevated 12 to 24 hours after surgery (Figures 6.2 and 6.3; Abe et al., 1990). Therefore, the kinetics and magnitude of the cell infiltration response can be modulated following instillations of tolmetin.

Blood Monocytes

The bone marrow contains only a limited reserve of preformed monocytes since monocytes typically enter blood circulation within 24 hours

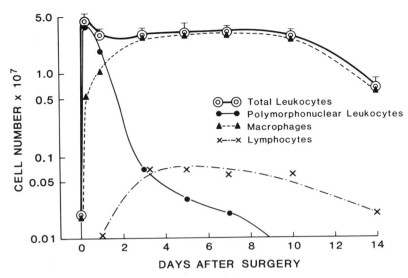

FIGURE 6.1. Kinetics of leukocyte infiltration and accumulation in peritoneal cavity of rabbits after reanastomosis of the ileum. Each point represents geometric mean and 95% range of six experiments. (From Shimanuki et al., 1986. Reproduced by permission of Academic Press.)

of their production (van Furth, 1988). Monocytes entering the circulation are distributed over a circulating and a marginating pool. In man, the marginating pool of monocytes represents approximately 75% of the total pool of cells (Meuret & Hoffmann, 1973). Monocytes enter tissues and body cavities from the circulating or marginating pools and the proportion of monocytes emigrating to various areas roughly corresponds to the size of the organ or cavity. Table 6.5 summarizes the results of labeling studies performed under normal steady-state conditions concerning the efflux of monocytes to various tissues and body cavities.

The kinetics of blood monocytes is altered by inflammation. Shortly after presentation of an inflammatory stimulus, monocyte production is dramatically increased. This increase is accomplished in several ways: expansion of the promonocyte pool, reduction in the promonocyte cycle time, and faster release of monocytes into circulation (Meuret, Detel, Kilz, Senn, & Van Lessen, 1975; van Furth, 1976). In these ways, the number of circulating monocytes is temporarily augmented two- to threefold relative to normal conditions in response to an inflammatory stimulus. The half-life of circulating monocytes is also reduced as part of the initial response to inflammation. Labeling studies in mice have shown that most of the increased monocytes in circulation emigrate to the site of inflammation (Nathan & Cohn, 1980).

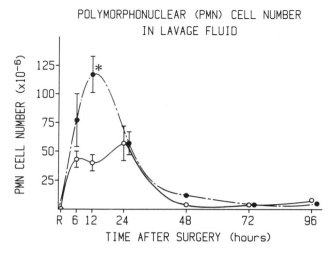

POLYMORPHONUCLEAR (PMN) CELL NUMBER
IN LAVAGE FLUID

FIGURE 6.2. Time course of white blood cell (WBC) number recovered in lavage fluid at various times following surgery. Each data point represents the mean ± SEM of 3 to 11 experiments. ○, control group (surgery alone); ●, treatment group (intraperitoneal administration of hyaluronic acid + tolmetin solution); R, WBC number from resident (nonsurgical rabbits). The values marked by * are significantly different compared to the other groups in each time point ($p < .01$). (From Abe et al., 1990. Reproduced by permission of Academic Press.)

Macrophages

The macrophage population is renewed both by the influx of circulating blood monocytes and by local production. As shown above for the stimulus of peritoneal surgery, the number of macrophages increases in response to inflammation (Figure 6.1). Calculations of the total monocyte influx and local macrophage production in response to various inflammatory stimuli indicate that the increased macrophage numbers are initially due to an augmented influx of monocytes. This occurs over the first 6 to 48 hours depending upon the stimulus employed. The contribution of stimulated local production, if any, is not evident until the second day after initiation of inflammation (van Furth, 1988).

The macrophage response to chronic inflammation can be divided into two types depending upon the inflammatory agent. Macrophage response to simple chronic inflammation is similar to that for acute inflammation—increased production of macrophages primarily due to an increased influx of circulating monocytes. A second response to chronic inflammation is granuloma formation (Spector, 1982). Granulomas typically form when the macrophage has difficulty digesting the irritant material. This type of response is typically seen around sutures or foreign bodies, such as talc or gauze fibers, left in the peritoneal cavity after surgery. They are com-

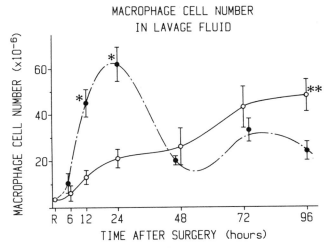

FIGURE 6.3. Time course of macrophage cell number recovered in lavage fluid at various times after surgery. Each data point represents the mean ± SEM of 3 to 8 rabbits. ○, control group (surgery alone); ●, treatment group (tolmetin-HA administration); R, macrophage number from resident nonsurgical) rabbits. The values marked by *(p <.05) and **(p <.01) are significantly different compared to the other group in each time point. (From Abe et al., 1990. Reproduced by permission of Academic Press.)

posed largely of macrophages recently recruited from the circulation. These macrophages take on the appearance of epithelioid cells and have a diminished vacuolar apparatus and increased rough endoplasmic reticulum. One striking feature of granulomas is the presence of multinucleated giant cells that are primarily the result of fusion of young, newly arrived monocytes and aging macrophages (Adams, 1983; Boros, 1986).

TABLE 6.5. Kinetics of macrophages at various tissues and body cavities.

Site	Monocytes leaving circulation (%)	Rate of monocyte influx (× 10³/hr)ᵃ	Rate of local production (× 10³/hr)ᵃ
Peritoneal cavity	6.7	4.2 (61%)	2.7 (39%)
Liver	71.8	93.3 (92%)	7.7 (8%)
Spleen	24.7	15.2 (55%)	12.2 (45%)
Lung	14.7	9.1 (67%)	4.4 (33%)

ᵃPercentages reflect the relative contribution made by influx and local production to the composition of the respective macrophage populations. (From van Furth (1988), with permission.)

Macrophage Function

Macrophages as Protective Cells

Macrophages are capable of destroying a wide range of prokaryotic and eukaryotic microorganisms as well as many different isogeneic and allogeneic cells (Nathan, 1986). The precise mechanisms involved in macrophage-mediated destruction depends upon the type of intruder and its stage of development, the state of the macrophage, and the engagement of other host inflammatory systems.

Macrophage-mediated destruction involves three general processes: recognition of the intruder as foreign material, decision regarding the means of intruder disposition, and destruction of the intruder (Nelson, 1982). During peritoneal surgery, macrophages are instrumental in elimination of bacterial contamination, tissue debris, and foreign bodies that enter during the surgical procedure.

Recognition of the intraperitoneal intruder most often involves cell-cell contact mediated by receptor-ligand interaction. The macrophage has various methods at its disposal to destroy an intruder. Intruders, particularly replicating cells such as tumor cells, can be retained at the macrophage surface (Edelson, 1982). The macrophage can endocytose the intruder either via pinocytosis, as in the case of viruses, or phagocytosis, as in the case of bacteria. Once endocytosis has occurred, the foreign material can either remain in the lysosomal compartment or can be passed into the cytosol. Little is currently known about the molecular mechanisms controlling the decision-making process in the macrophage. Macrophage-mediated destruction occurs via the secretion of lytic effector substances (Nathan, 1986). Secretion is typically triggered by receptor stimulation and occurs into the lysosomal compartment or into the extracellular space surrounding the macrophage and foreign intruder.

Antimicrobial Activity

Macrophages are a major defense against a variety of microorganisms, such as viruses, bacteria, fungi, and protozoa. Microorganisms are recognized by macrophages primarily through opsonins—molecules that bind to specific sites on the macrophage and microorganism. A variety of opsonins exist, including immunoglobulin and complement fragments. Once recognition occurs, the major antimicrobial activity of the macrophage is the production and intracellular release of reactive oxygen intermediates (ROI), such as O_2^-, H_2O_2 and $OH\cdot$ (Clark & Klebanoff, 1975; Klebanoff, 1975). There is a close correlation between the antimicrobial activity of a macrophage population and its ability to secrete ROI as well as between the ability of a microorganism to trigger ROI secretion during its ingestion and its susceptibility to macrophage destruction (Nathan & Root, 1977).

To determine the effect of peritoneal surgery on the differentiation of peritoneal macrophages, Fukasawa, Bryant, and diZerega (1988b) examined the release of O_2^- by peritoneal macrophages in response to phorbol myristate acetate (PMA) at various times after surgery (Figure 6.4). The potential to release O_2^- is greater for activated and elicited macrophages than for resident macrophages (Byrant, Lynch, & Hill, 1982). O_2^- release by macrophages rapidly increased after surgery, attaining peak levels at 6 hours, and then decreased by day 1. Activity gradually increased again, reaching peak levels by days 4 to 7 and returning to control levels by postoperative day 15. These data suggest that resident peritoneal macrophages are immediately primed by surgical insult. The peak in O_2^- activity at 6 hours postsurgery could correspond to either a rise in newly infiltrating macrophages or to the activity of these primed macrophages acting as scavenger cells in conjunction with neutrophils. In the absence of infection, this early priming stimulus abates. Later on, a new influx of macrophages and subsequent inflammatory stimulation may account for the second peak in O_2^- release.

A recent study by Kuraoka, Campeau, Nakamura, and diZerega (in press) showed that within 2 hours after peritoneal surgery, the secretion of O_2^- by peritoneal macrophages was elevated; this response peaked at

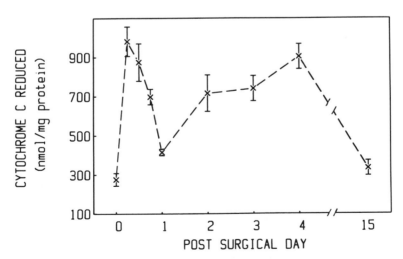

FIGURE 6.4. The release of superoxide anion by postsurgical macrophages recovered from the peritoneal cavity of rabbits at different days after surgery. Postsurgical macrophages were enriched using a Percoll discontinuous gradient. Each data point represents the mean ± SEM of three separate experiments. (From Fukasawa et al., 1988. Reproduced by permission of Academic Press.)

6 hours after surgery (Figure 6.5). Conditioned medium of PMN harvested 6 hours after surgery suppressed the production of O_2^- by early postsurgical macrophages. On the other hand, the production of O_2^- by early postsurgical macrophages was enhanced by conditioned medium of PMNs harvested 12 and 24 hours after surgery. These data taken together with the early peak and reduction in the production of O_2^- by postsurgical macrophages suggest that PMNs may be instrumental in the regulation of this early inflammatory response.

Studies have also shown that conditioned media of early postsurgical macrophage (2 to 24 hours after surgery) can modulate the respiratory burst of macrophages from nonsurgical rabbits (Kuraoka, Campeau, Rodgers, Nakamura, & diZerega, in review). At the earliest time point examined (2 hours), factors that modulate oxygen metabolism were secreted by postsurgical macrophages. Resident macrophages were maximally affected by the conditioned media from macrophages harvested from 6 hours after surgery. These data suggest that postsurgical macrophages can secrete factors that modulate macrophage function with kinetics similar to alterations in the respiratory burst of postsurgical macrophages.

The macrophage also appears capable of oxygen-independent antimicrobial activity (Nathan & Cohn, 1980). This antimicrobial activity appears to be the result of nitrogen metabolism to nitrite and nitrate (Stuehr

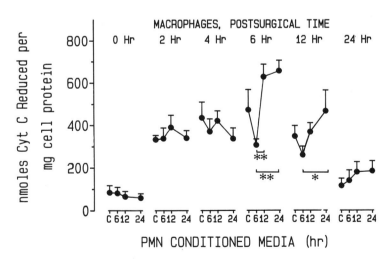

FIGURE 6.5. O_2^- of early postsurgical macrophages ± PMN conditioned media. Early postsurgical macrophage were harvested from the rabbit peritoneal cavity and exposed to conditioned media of PMN harvested at early postsurgical time points (Kuraoka et al., in press. Reproduced with the permission of Academic Press, Inc.).

& Marletta 1985, 1987). As murine macrophages differentiate, they acquire the capacity to convert L-arginine to nitrate and nitrite (Hibbs, Taintor, Varrin, & Rachlin, 1988). Under certain limited circumstances, opsonization may not be necessary for macrophage-mediated destruction of a microorganism. For example, if the microorganism expresses molecular characteristics on its surface that can be directly recognized by the macrophage, opsonization is not necessary.

Antitumor Activity

Macrophages have the ability to destroy tumor cells (Schreiber, 1984). The effect of peritoneal surgery on the tumoricidal activity of leukocytes was examined in the rat (Rodgers, Ellefson, Girgis, Scott, & diZerega, 1988). As early as 24 hours after surgery, there was a slight increase in the tumoricidal activity of rat macrophage (Figure 6.6). This elevation in tumoricidal activity was maximal by day 7 after surgery and had begun to return to control levels by day 14. This study also showed that acute administration of a cyclooxygenase inhibitor, tolmetin, at the time of surgery further elevated the tumoricidal activity of postsurgical macrophages.

The macrophage can injure a tumor cell by one of three distinct methods: inhibition of proliferation, tumor cytolysis, and antibody-mediated cellular cytotoxicity. Each of these methods differs with respect to target cell selectivity, the state of macrophage activation, the actual mechanism by which the tumor cell is destroyed and the time necessary for tumor cell destruction (Adams & Hamilton, 1988).

Inhibition of Proliferation

Macrophages have the ability to inhibit tumor cell division either through suppression or cytostasis (Adams & Hamilton, 1988). In certain stages of activation, macrophages can suppress the proliferation of lymphocytes in response either to specific antigens or to polyclonal mitogens. This suppression is relatively specific, requires few macrophages for activity, and probably acts by interfering with the initial mitogenic response (Allison, 1978). It has been proposed that suppression is mediated by arachidonic acid metabolites such as prostaglandin E_2 (PGE_2).

In contrast to suppression, macrophage-mediated cytostasis targets a broad spectrum of cells, including both neoplastic and normal cells, and requires a larger number of macrophages. Because of the relative lack of specificity, it is likely that the actual cytostatic effect is mediated by soluble factors that act upon all proliferating cells in a given local environment.

Potential cytostatic mediators include prostaglandins, thymidine, interferons, arginine, and tumor necrosis factor (TNF) (Gresser, Brouty-

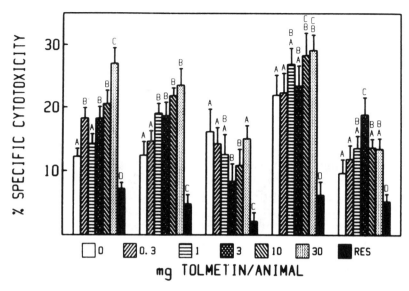

FIGURE 6.6. The rat peritoneal cells, 1.3 ml/well, were placed in 16-mm wells for 2 hours. Positive controls for tumoricidal activity were generated by preincubation of resident peritoneal adherent cells with 0.1 μg/ml lipopolysaccharide and lymphokine-containing supernatant. At the end of this time, each well was washed with PBS and 2.0×10^5 [^{3}H]thymidine–labeled TCMK, a SV-40 virus transformed cell line, cells were added to each well and incubated at 37 °C for 48 hours. A sample of the supernatant was then harvested and the amount of [^{3}H]thymidine released determined. The specific cytotoxicity for the positive control samples was between 48% and 65%. At all time points and doses, the positive controls were significantly different from all other groups. Each dose and time point result shown represents the mean and SE of five animals. The data were analyzed by one-way analysis of variance followed by Duncan's new multiple range test (α = 0.01). Bars with the same letter were considered statistically identical ($p <.01$) by this analysis. Reprinted with permission of the *International Journal of Immunopharmacology* 10:111–120, Rodgers et al., Effects of Tolmetin Sodium Dihydrate on Normal and Postsurgical Cell Function, © 1988, Pergamon Press plc.

Boye, Thomas, & Macierira-Cuelho, 1970; Samuelsson, Branstrom, Greer, Hamberg, & Hammerstrom, 1971; Calderon, Williams, & Unanue, 1974; Kung, Brooks, Jakway, Leonard, & Talmadge, 1977). One primary effect of such macrophage-derived mediators on the target cells seems to occur at the level of DNA synthesis by blocking movement of cells through the cell cycle. Cytostatic macrophages can inhibit proliferative responses even after they have been initiated in a target cell whereas macrophage-mediated suppression is effective only prior to target cell initiation.

Antibody-Independent Tumor Cytolysis

In certain stages of activation, macrophages have the ability to cytolyse tumor cells in the absence of a specific anti–target cell antibody (Alexander & Evans, 1971; Hibbs, Lambert, & Remington, 1972). Such cytolysis occurs over 1 to 3 days and it is contact-dependent, selective for neoplastic cells, and does not involve phagocytosis (Adams & Marino, 1984). Cytolysis involves two clearly definable steps: selective capture of tumor cells and binding to the macrophage surface, and secretion of toxic substances (Adams, Johnson, & Marino, 1982). The lytic substance(s) appears to be secreted into the limited space formed between the junction of the macrophage and the bound tumor cell. There is some evidence that a novel serine protease as well as TNF may serve as lytic substances (Adams and Nathan, 1983).

Antibody-Dependent Cellular Cytotoxicity (ADCC)

As with other leukocytes, macrophages have the ability to destroy target cells in the presence of specific antibodies. Since the selectivity of such macrophage-mediated cytotoxicity is based on the antibody, the reaction is not restricted to tumor cells. Macrophage recognition of the target cell is mediated by the interaction between Fab portions of immunoglobulins to surface antigens on the target cell and the Fc portions of the immunoglobulin to surface receptors on the macrophage (Somers, Johnson, & Adams, 1986). Following occupancy and cross-linking of the Fc receptor, a lytic attack occurs. ROI, and in particular H_2O_2, appears to play a major role in cytolysis by ADCC reaction.

There are two distinct variants of the ADCC reaction—rapid and slow. Evidence to date indicates that cytolysis follows the same fundamental sequence for both rapid and slow ADCC reactions. The difference lies in whether the target can be destroyed rapidly by relatively low amounts of H_2O_2 or whether prolonged incubation with H_2O_2 is necessary for destruction (Adams, Hall, Steplewski, & Koprowski, 1984; Johnson, Steplewski, Matthews, Koprowski, & Adams, 1986). Another distinction between rapid and slow ADCC reactions is that macrophages must be fully activated for the former reaction, whereas macrophages may be the responsive or primed state of development for the latter.

Arachidonic Acid Metabolites

Arachidonic acid metabolites are produced by PMNs and macrophages present at the site of inflammation (Shimanuki, et al., 1986). These secreted metabolites are thought to be involved in the mediation of inflammatory events. Selective increase in formation (synthesis) of 15-hydroxyeicosatetraenoic acid (15-HETE) and di-HETE formation beginning 24 hours after peritoneal surgery was observed along with a diminution of 5-HETE (Figure 6.7). This is indicative in the absence of infection. Thereafter, there was an additional increase in thromboxane B_2 and prostaglandin E_2 (PGE_2) on days 2 to 10 after surgery (Figure 6.8). These metabolites all undergo oxidation via the lipoxygenase and cyclooxygenase pathways. However, the activities and turnover times of these pathways are expressed differently following various stimuli.

Arachidonic acid metabolites produced by peritoneal exudate cells (PEC) from the postsurgical peritoneal cavity of rabbits reach peak values on day 3 and remain elevated until day 10 (Shimanuki, et al., 1986). In contrast, macrophages from the postsurgical peritoneal cavity harvested 3 to 7 days after surgery express a three- to fourfold greater potential to release O_2^- compared to resident macrophages, which thereafter gradually decrease to resident levels by postsurgical day 13. Thus, the time course of the secretion for various macrophage products from the peritoneal cavity of postsurgical rabbits varies depending upon the parameter examined. This dissociation between the different metabolic activities suggests that differentiative functions of the postsurgical macrophage are not uniform. The temporal dissociation between the different metabolic activities suggests that differentiation of macrophages from postsurgical rabbits is complex and under differential regulation.

Arachidonic acid metabolites are potent mediators of inflammatory responses and may therefore regulate many events that occur during wound repair, such as leukocyte chemotaxis. PGE_2 is proinflammatory and mediates events, such as edema formation, endothelial cell procoagulant activity, and vasodilation. Thromboxane B_2 is a potent stimulator

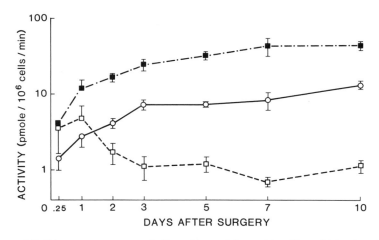

FIGURE 6.7. Lipoxygenase metabolites formed from [1-^{14}C]arachidonic acid by rabbit peritoneal exudative leukocytes in vitro. Each point represents the mean ± SEM of 5 to 10 experiments. ○, di-HETE; □, 5-HETE; ■, 15-HETE. (From Shimanuki et al., 1986. Reproduced by permission of Academic Press.)

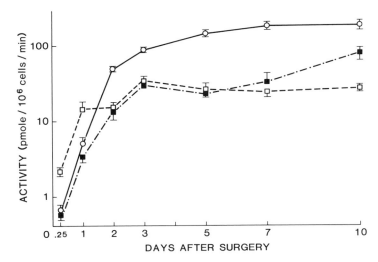

FIGURE 6.8. Cyclooxygenase metabolites formed in vitro from [1-^{14}C]arachidonic acid by rabbit peritoneal exudative leukocytes. Each point represents the mean ± SEM of 5 to 10 experiments. O, TxB$_2$; □, 6 keto-PGF$_{1\alpha}$; ■, PGE$_2$. (From Shimanuki et al., 1986. Reproduced by permission of Academic Press.)

of platelet aggregation and is chemotactic for PMNs. HETE metabolites inhibit the formation of arachidonic acid metabolites and lead to PMN infiltration. Therefore, an increase in arachidonic acid metabolism by PEC from postsurgical rabbits may contribute to the ongoing inflammatory and tissue repair processes.

Monokine Secretion

Interleukin-1 (IL-1) is one of several soluble proteins produced by macrophages in response to a variety of stimuli including endotoxin (lipopolysaccharide [LPS]) and phorbol esters (Table 6.4). IL-1 alters many of the biological activities of cells involved in peritoneal repair and is implicated in peritoneal healing (see Chapter 3). IL-1 was shown to stimulate the production of collagen, collagenase, and prostaglandin secretion by fibroblasts as well as endothelial cells in vitro (Postlethwaite, Lachman, Mainadri, & Kang, 1983). Bevilacqua, Schleef, Gimbrone, and Loskutoff (1986) reported that treatment of endothelial cells with IL-1 results in decreased production of tissue plasminogen activator (tPA), an increase in cell-associated procoagulant activity, and secretion of a PA inhibitor. Thus, exposure to IL-1 could result in a significant reduction in the fibrinolytic potential of endothelial cells. These complementary actions of IL-1 on procoagulant and fibrinolytic activities may, in turn, enhance the production and maintenance of fibrin.

Surgical injury of murine peritoneum enhances IL-1 secretion by peritoneal macrophages that reaches maximum levels on postsurgical day 10 (Abe, Rodgers, Ellefson, & diZerega, 1989). The kinetics of IL-1 secretion by unstimulated and LPS-PMA–stimulated macrophages from postsurgical animals are different. On postsurgical day 3, macrophages stimulated by LPS and PMA secrete maximum levels of IL-1. In contrast, the IL-1 levels from unstimulated macrophages remain low at this time (Abe et al., 1989).

Secretion of IL-1 by peritoneal macrophages from postsurgical rabbits also changes as a function of postsurgical time (Figure 6.9; Abe, Rodgers, Ellefson, & diZerega, 1991). In conditioned culture media from unstimulated macrophages from postsurgical rabbits, IL-1 levels are elevated on postsurgical day 14 compared to the level of IL-1 secreted on postsurgical day 3 and 7. Secretion of TNF, another monokine involved in inflammatory responses, by unstimulated macrophages from postsurgical rabbits peaks on day 1 and day 14 (Figure 6.10; Abe et al., 1991). The levels of TNF and IL-1 secreted by peritoneal macrophages from postsurgical rabbits are elevated during the latter phases of peritoneal healing. Responsiveness of macrophages from postsurgical rabbits to stimuli such as LPS and PMA changes during peritoneal repair. The maximum sensitivity of peritoneal exudate cells to this type of stimulation appears to occur on postsurgical days 3 to 4. In addition, the macrophage super-

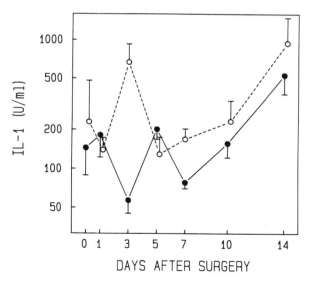

FIGURE 6.9. Interleukin-1 secretion in response to LPS and PMA stimulation (○) or no stimulation (●). Peritoneal surgery in rabbits modulated the secretion of IL-1 peritoneal macrophages such that it is maximum during the repair phase of healing. (From Abe et al., 1991. Reproduced by permission of Taylor & Francis.)

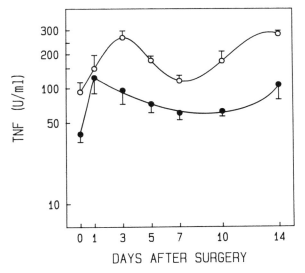

FIGURE 6.10. Tumor necrosis factor (TNF) secretion in response to LPS and PMA stimulation (O) or no stimulation (●). The secretion of TNF by rabbit peritoneal macrophages is modulated by peritoneal surgery. (From Abe et al., 1991. Reproduced by permission of Taylor & Francis.)

natant harvested in the early phase of peritoneal wound healing (post-surgical days 4 and 5) stimulates proliferation of epithelial cells recovered from the site of peritoneal injury (tissue repair cells [TRC]) more than supernatants from macrophages harvested in the later phases of perito-neal healing (Fukasawa, Bryant, Nakamura, & diZerega, 1987; Fukasawa, Bryant, & diZerega, 1988a).

IL-1 is a pleiotropic cytokine that could modulate peritoneal repair at many levels (described more fully in Chapter 3). IL-1 induces changes in endothelial cells and fibroblasts, which are central to the repair of wounds. IL-1 can stimulate the proliferation of both fibroblasts and en-dothelial cells, but not peritoneal tissue repair cells. IL-1 also modulates the secretion of components of the extracellular matrix and proteases that degrade and remodel these matrices. Therefore, IL-1 may be essential in the remodeling of repaired tissue.

Influence of Postsurgical Macrophages on TRC Proliferation

Fibroblasts contain a larger number of membrane receptors for IL-1 than other cell types (Dower et al., 1985). Therefore, IL-1 may act as a mediator between TRC and macrophages. Schmidt, Mizel, Cohen, and Green

(1982) showed that IL-1 augmented the replication of skin fibroblasts stimulated in serum, but not serum-free, cultures, but only when other growth factors, such as platelet-derived growth factor (PDGF) or macrophage-derived growth factor (MDGF), were present in culture (Leibovich & Ross, 1976; Estes, Pledger, & Gillespie, 1984; Bitterman, Wewers, Rennard, Adelberg, & Crystal, 1986). Since TRCs harvested from the site of peritoneal injury do not proliferate in response to recombinant IL-1, IL-1 may not provide a primary signal for TRC replication, but rather augment the signal response of TRC (Fukasawa, Yangihara, Rodgers, & diZerega, 1989b).

Levels of IL-1 produced by unstimulated macrophages harvested during the early phase after surgery are lower than in the later phases (Abe et al., 1989). Growth factor(s) for fibroblast proliferation in macrophage conditioned media from the early phase may therefore be other than IL-1. IL-1 directly increases collagen synthesis and stimulates synthesis of hyaluronate by fibroblasts, which provide essential matrix for repair (Matsushima, Bano, Kidwell, & Oppenheim, 1985; Bronson, Bentiolami, & Siebert, 1987). IL-1 and TNF also stimulate the release of PGE_2 which inhibits fibroblast replication and macrophage activation, both of which are important in the remodeling phase (Ko, Page, & Narayanan, 1977; Schnyder, Dewald, & Baggiolini, 1981; Zucali et al., 1986; Phan, McGarry, Loeffler, & Kunkel, 1987). Korn, Halushka, and LeRoy (1980) reported that supernatants of human peripheral monocytes suppress fibroblast proliferation and this inhibition of growth parallels the increase in PGE synthesis by the fibroblast. In addition, this inhibition is reversed by inhibitors of PGE synthesis (indomethacin, etc.) and is reproduced by addition of exogenous PGE_2 to fibroblast cultures. Elias, Rossman, Zurier, and Daniela (1985) reported the same result using the supernatant of human alveolar macrophages. Thus, IL-1 secretion by macrophages from postsurgical animals may play a role, through several different mechanisms, in the later phases of repair after peritoneal surgery.

Endometriosis is associated with increased levels of monokines and growth factors in the peritoneal space. Fakih et al. (1987) found IL-1 in the peritoneal fluid of patients with endometriosis but not in that of controls. In addition a study was conducted of TNF secretion by human peritoneal macrophages following exposure to the exotoxin responsible for toxic shock (TSST-1) or LPS (Halme, White, Kauma, Estes, & Haskell, 1988; Buyalos, Rutanem, Tsui, & Halme, 1991). Enhanced secretion of TNF-α by macrophages obtained from patients with endometriosis was observed compared to macrophages obtained from women without endometriosis after stimulation with TSST-1 or LPS. These data suggest that the peritoneal environment is modulated by endometriosis.

Summary

The susceptibility of peritoneal macrophages from postsurgical rabbits to stimuli such as LPS and PMA changes during postsurgical repair. The maximum sensitivity to this type of stimulation appears to occur when the number of macrophages in the peritoneal cavity is greatest. It is conceivable that the cellular mechanisms necessary for monocytes to migrate into the wound site preclude responsiveness to LPS and PMA stimuli. The increase in the number of macrophages (which continues until postsurgical day 3) is probably due to emigration of blood monocytes from the intravascular space into the peritoneal cavity perhaps at the site of trauma and not through proliferation of resident peritoneal macrophages. However, if monocytes, emigrated from the blood, are more sensitive to stimuli immediately after emigration, then the sensitivity of macrophages harvested on postsurgical day 1 should be more than was found. Therefore, to attain sensitivity to this type of stimulation, macrophages from postsurgical rabbits must undergo differentiation within the peritoneal cavity. Other studies have shown that exposure of macrophages to a stimulus, such as IL-1, causes them to become refractory to additional stimulation by this same agent in vitro. It is therefore conceivable that macrophages harvested from the peritoneal cavity at early postsurgical intervals were exposed to stimuli that caused them to become refractory to further in vitro stimulation.

Regulation of Macrophage Function

Induction of Functional Competence

Macrophages retain considerable potential for development after their maturation. The cytotoxic and cytostatic properties of macrophages discussed above are acquired functions. Not all macrophages are equally responsive to activation for a given functional competence. For example, resting tissue macrophages are relatively insensitive to activating stimuli (Adams & Hamilton, 1988).

Competence for a specific function appears to be acquired in discrete steps and to require the presence of activating signals, such as lymphokines and bacterial products. The process involved in the induction of competence for antibody-independent cytolysis has been described (Adams & Hamilton, 1988). Responsive macrophages (e.g., young cells at inflammatory sites) become primed following interaction with macrophage-activating factors. One of the most well-characterized of these activating factors is interferon-γ (Schreiber, 1984). Primed macrophages are then sensitive to a second signal, such as bacterial lipopolysaccharide (LPS). Upon exposure to this second signal they become activated and have acquired full competence for antibody-independent tumor cytolysis. Each signal alone, if present in sufficiently high enough concentrations, is able to fully activate the macrophage (Meltzer, Ruco, Boraschi, & Nacy, 1979). As macrophages acquire tumoricidal competence, they lose their ability to perform other functions, such as multiplication. Competence for cytostasis also requires exposure to interferon-γ and LPS. Although activation appears somewhat related to antibody-independent tumor cytolysis, the events regulating competence for ADCC are poorly understood (Adams & Hamilton, 1988).

Signal Transduction

There is only a rudimentary understanding of how signals produced by external stimuli are transduced into altered cellular behavior. A schematic model of the process underlying macrophage activation has recently been proposed (Adams & Hamilton, 1988). As shown in Figure 6.11, the interaction of interferon-γ with its receptor on the macrophage surface likely induces generation of an as yet unidentified immediate second messenger(s) (Adams & Hamilton, 1987). Although the existence of immediate second messengers are unknown, interferon-γ has been shown to induce changes in the intracellular metabolism of Ca^{2+} as well as alterations in the potential activity of protein kinase C in macrophages.

Little is known about how the macrophage perceives a signal from

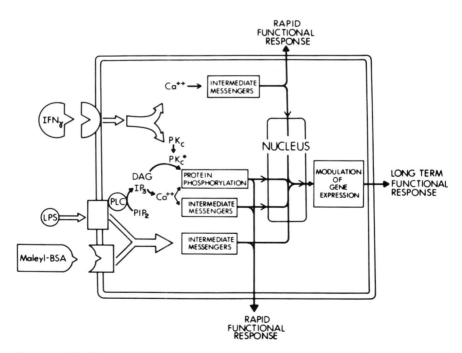

FIGURE 6.11. Schematic model of signal transduction mechanism in macrophages by interferon-γ and LPS. (From Adams & Hamilton, 1988. Reproduced by permission of Raven Press.)

lipopolysaccharide (LPS) (Adams & Hamilton, 1987). Breakdown products of phosphatidylinositol metabolism, such as various isomers of inositol triphosphate (IP_3) and diacylglycerol (DAG), have been implicated as early second messengers of LPS in macrophages. Rapid increases in intracellular Ca^{2+} levels and changes in protein phosphorylation are induced by LPS, as are other early effects that are independent of polyphosphoinositol hydrolysis and that result in protein synthesis. These actions in response to interferon-γ and LPS can result in immediate functional responses, such as the respiratory burst and secretion of arachidonic acid metabolites, as well as in modulation of gene expression, leading to the generation of products necessary for functional competence.

The schematic model shown in Figure 6.11 illustrates the potential for cooperation between activating signals. For example, previous modulation of protein kinase C by interferon-γ can enhance LPS-induced phosphorylation via protein kinase C. Additionally, cooperation between the transductional signals can also regulate gene expression, which, in turn, regulates the expression of surface proteins or secretion proteins by the macrophage (Adams & Hamilton, 1987).

Suppression of Functional Competence

Because of the potent destructive ability of the macrophage, mechanisms for suppressing macrophage function have evolved. A number of agents present at inflammatory sites have the potential to suppress certain macrophage functions (Table 6.6; Steeg, Johnson, & Oppenheim, 1982; Esparza, Green, Schreiber, 1983). Some of these same agents, under specific conditions, can also enhance many macrophage functions.

The macrophage itself also has the potential to secrete suppressive agents. One of these is antiprotease alpha$_2$-macroglobulin (α_2-m). When α_2-m interacts with a protease in an inflammatory site, it undergoes a conformational change. This change exposes a binding site that is recognized by a specific receptor on the macrophage surface (Feldman, Gon-

TABLE 6.6. Suppressive factors interacting with macrophages.

Factor	Effect
Lipopolysaccharide (endotoxin)	Decrease expression of Ia Decrease Fc receptor function
Immune complexes	Decrease antitumor function and expression of Ia
Corticosteroids	Decrease expression of Ia and activity of phospholipase A_2
Alpha$_2$-macroglobulin	Decrease secretion of H_2O_2, proteases, tumor cytolysis and Ia
Prostaglandin E series	Decrease expression of Ia and tumor cytolysis

From Adams & Hamilton (1988), with permission.

ias, & Pizzo, 1985). Interaction of the α_2-m–protease complex with the macrophage receptor results in suppression of tumor cytolytic activity, neutral and cytolytic protease secretion, respiratory burst activity, and macrophage induction of Ia antigen (Feldman et al., 1985). Prostaglandins, in particular PGE_2, secreted by the macrophage can also suppress antitumor activity and the ability of the macrophage to present antigen. Exposure of peritoneal macrophages to an inhibitor of cyclooxygenase at the time of surgery enhanced the tumoricidal activity of postsurgical macrophages (Figure 6.6; Rodgers et al., 1988).

Macrophage-Induced Tissue Injury

The array of destructive molecules produced by macrophages such as ROI, hydrolytic enzymes, and proteases, makes it inevitable that damage to normal tissue will occur in certain circumstances. For example, necrosis is frequently apparent with epithelioid granulomas. Regulation of the destructive ability of the macrophage is controlled at several levels:

the time of secretion since secretion of toxic molecules must be triggered by specific signals;
the point of secretion, since this is regulated, at least in part, by phagosomes;
the presence or absence of suppressive factors;
the presence or absence of endogenous inhibitors of the toxic molecules in the tissue.

Macrophage-induced damage to normal tissue can also occur indirectly (Adams & Hamilton, 1988). Secretion of ROI and arachidonic acid metabolites can cause genomic injury to bystander cells which can, in turn, promote mutagenesis.

Terminology for Mononuclear Phagocytes Participating in Inflammatory Reactions

A variety of terms are often used interchangeably to refer to mononuclear phagocytic cells participating in an inflammatory reaction, and often, little distinction is made between the developmental stage and functional state of the cells. Therefore, the following definitions have been proposed (van Furth, 1988):

Resident macrophage: a macrophage occurring at any site in the absence of an inflammatory stimulus.
Exudate macrophage: a specific developmental stage of macrophage, consisting of cells occurring in exudate and identified by specific markers

and cell-kinetic analysis. This has almost the same characteristics as a monocyte.

Exudate-resident macrophage: transitional form between resident and exudate macrophage. It can be characterized only via electron microscopy after staining for peroxidatic activity.

Activated macrophage: a macrophage with increased functional activity induced by a specific stimulus.

Elicited macrophage: a macrophage attracted to a given site by a specific substance. This term does not refer to a specific developmental stage or functional state, as elicited populations are typically heterogeneous for both.

Proliferation: the increase in cell number due to division of cells.

Accumulation: the increase in cell number due to migration of nondividing cells.

Macrophage-Mediated Regulation of Extracellular Matrix Degradation and Deposition

Macrophages have been implicated in the degradation of the extracellular connective tissue matrix at inflammatory sites. Degradation of rat vascular smooth muscle cell matrix by thioglycolate-elicited macrophages was shown to be dependent both on the length of incubation and the number of macrophages plated (Jones & Werb, 1980; Werb, Banda, & Jones, 1980a). The ability of the macrophage to degrade is related to the secretion of neutral proteinases, including plasminogen activator, elastase, and collagenase. Each of these proteinases digests a different component of the extracellular matrix. Plasmin, the result of an interaction between plasminogen activator and plasminogen, is a potent proteinase that degrades the insoluble glycoprotein components of the extracellular matrix. The matrix components elastin and collagen are principally degraded by the enzymes elastase and collagenase, respectively.

The effects of surgery on the secretion of plasminogen activator (PA) by macrophages is more fully discussed in Chapter 7. The time course for postsurgical macrophage secretion of PA following bowel reanastomosis was described by Orita et al. (1986) and Fukasawa et al. (1989c). Increasing levels of PA activity is evident 3 to 7 days after surgery, with peak levels occurring on postsurgical day 10; thereafter, activity levels gradually decline to preoperative values by day 21 (Figure 6.12). The activity levels of PA secreted by postsurgical macrophages during the first 5 days postsurgery are lower than the activity levels expressed by nonsurgical peritoneal macrophages. Plasminogen activator cleaves plasminogen to the active enzyme, plasmin, which is the primary fibrolytic enzyme. Thus, inhibition of PA activity in the early stages of wound repair may facilitate the deposition of fibrin. Enhanced production of PA in the

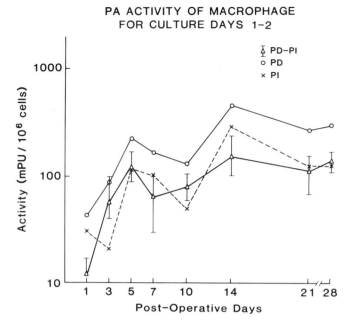

FIGURE 6.12. Plasminogen activator activity in spent media from culture days 1 to 2 from rabbit peritoneal exudative cells after reanastomosis of small intestine. At early postsurgical time points the level of PA activity secreted by peritoneal exudate cells is reduced and is elevated at later time points after surgery. Each data point represents the geometric mean and 45% range of three experiments. ○, plasminogen-dependent (PD) activator activity; x, plasminogen-independent (PI) activator activity; △, specific plasminogen activator activity (PD-PI). (From Orita et al., 1986. Reproduced by permission of Academic Press.)

later stages of wound repair may be important in the remodeling of the tissue matrix and in moderating fibrin deposition.

Although plasmin has no direct elastinolytic activity, it indirectly facilitates the degradation of elastin by removing the glycoprotein coat that surrounds this protein. Following glycoprotein depletion, the rate of elastin degradation by macrophage elastase is enhanced. Jones and Werb (1980) found that, in the thioglycolate-elicited rat vascular smooth muscle cell macrophage, both the rate of total matrix digestion and the amount of elastin digested by macrophages are dependent upon the extent of prior glycoprotein depletion. Their studies suggest that collagen depletion by macrophage collagenase is also stimulated by glycoprotein depletion.

In addition to its indirect facilitatory effect on elastase and collagenase activity, plasmin appears to influence the activation of collagenase to its active form (Diegelmann, Cohen, & Kaplan, 1981). The collagenase synthesized by the macrophage is in a latent form and must be activated before it is capable of digesting collagen. Plasmin is among the molecules that are capable of activating latent collagenase.

The role of the various proteinases in matrix degradation by macrophages was further illustrated by the addition of different proteinase inhibitors to the cell medium (Table 6.7). Inhibitors of plasmin, collagenase, and/or elastase, such as alpha$_2$-macroglobulin, alpha$_1$-proteinase inhibitor, and ethylenediaminetetraacetic acid (EDTA), all reduce the percentage of the matrix solubilized. In contrast, pepstatin, an inhibitor of lysosomal cathepsin D, is without effect on macrophage-mediated matrix degradation in this model (Werb, Bainton, & Jones, 1980b).

In a series of experiments aimed at determining the localization of macrophage-mediated degradation of the connective tissue matrix, Werb and colleagues (1980b) demonstrated that extracellular, pericellular and lysosomal events are involved. Live macrophages appear to degrade connective tissue matrix by extracellular proteolysis followed by degradation of the fragments to amino acids and oligopeptides within the lysosome.

A membrane location for plasminogen activator activity in human alveolar macrophages was shown (Chapman, Stone, & Vavrin, 1984). Activation of plasmin appears to be localized to the cell surface. These findings explain why matrix degradation can occur even in the presence of serum proteinase inhibitors. Chapman and colleagues reported that when alveolar macrophages are in contact with fibrin, matrix digestion occurs despite the presence of proteinase inhibitors. Activation of plasmin probably occurs at the site of cell-surface–expressed plasminogen activator. The close juxtaposition of the macrophage to fibrin attenuates the binding of plasmin to antiplasmin. Plasmin binds to fibrin, thereby initiating the proteolytic process. These same researchers also observed elastinolytic activity in the presence of proteinase inhibitors when macrophages are in contact with elastin.

TABLE 6.7. Effect of proteinase inhibitors on matrix digestion by thioglycolate-elicited smooth muscle cell macrophages.[a]

Inhibitor	Radioactivity solubilized (%)	
	With plasminogen	Without plasminogen
None	32.0	4.5
FBS (10%)	12.1	2.5
Alpha$_2$-macroglobulin (25 μg/mL)	10.3	1.8
Alpha$_1$-proteinase inhibitor (100 μg/mL)	8.3	5.8
EDTA (0.5 mM)	17.3	1.5
Pepstatin (1 μg/mL)	30.8	5.1

[a]Macrophages (5×10^5/well) were plated on [^{3}H]proline-labeled smooth muscle cell matrix with added inhibitors in the presence or absence of 10 μg bovine plasminogen/mL. Radioactivity solubilized was measured at 48 hours. Adapted from Werb et al. (1980b).

Macrophages are heterogeneous in their ability to degrade the extracellular matrix. Pyran copolymer-elicited macrophages secrete substantial amounts of plasminogen activator but little elastase, whereas thioglycolate- and periodate-elicited macrophages secrete abundant amounts of both enzymes. Resident and endotoxin-elicited macrophages were the least active with respect to matrix digestion in these experiments, and the amount of matrix components solubilized by the other macrophages was related to their abilities to secrete the various proteinases.

The ability of various macrophage populations to digest collagen was augmented by the addition of fibroblasts to the macrophage culture (Laub, Huybrechts-Godin, Peeters-Joris, & Vaes, 1982). As shown in Figure 6.13, the extent of collagen degradation in coculture of macrophages and fibroblasts was greater than the sum of degradation observed with either two cell populations alone. Enhanced collagen degradation was observed when only a small number of fibroblasts ($\leq 1\%$ of total cell number) were cultured with macrophages. Synergy between fibroblasts and macrophages with respect to glycoprotein depletion was also demonstrated by

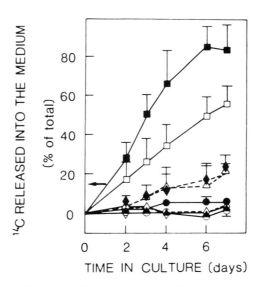

FIGURE 6.13. Interactions in collagen degradation between mouse peritoneal macrophages and either mouse or rabbit fibroblasts when cocultured. The extent of collagen degradation in coculture of macrophages and fibroblasts is greater than the sum of degradation observed with the two-cell population alone. Thioglycolate-elicited (●) or resident (○) macrophages; skin fibroblasts from either mouse (▲) or rabbit (△); mouse fibroblasts are either elicited (■) or resident (□) macrophages. Each point is the mean of three cultures; the vertical bars correspond to 1 SD. Arrow indicates maximal release of ^{14}C achieved by trypsin (50 μg/well). (From Laub et al., 1982. Reproduced by permission of Elsevier Science.)

these researchers, but this effect was less obvious because of the high rate of glycoprotein digestion achieved by either cell type alone.

Fibronectin

Fibronectin is a glycoprotein produced by several cells, including fibroblasts and endothelial cells. It is important in peritoneal healing and participates in a variety of reactions related to this process, such as adhesion and spreading of platelets on collagen, promoting neutrophil and monocyte migration to the injury and promoting opsonization reactions in phagocytic cells (Kleinman, Klebe, & Martin, 1981; Grinnell, 1984).

Fibronectin also influences fibroblast function during healing. Fibronectin is chemotactic for fibroblasts and promotes fibroblast adhesion (Grinnell, 1984). Following their migration to the wound region, fibroblasts secrete an extensive fibronectin matrix. Fibroblasts and fibronectin were shown to be among the first substances present at the inflammatory site (Kurkinen, Vaheri, Roberts, & Stenman, 1980). Their presence was followed by the appearance of type III collagen; as the collagen became organized into bundles and type I collagen predominated, fibroblasts and fibrinogen disappeared from the wound area. These researchers and others (e.g., Gay, Viljanto, Raekallio, & Penttinen, 1978; Dolynchuk & Bowness, 1981) hypothesized that the fibronectin matrix may provide a scaffolding onto which invading fibroblasts anchor and on which collagen can be organized.

Fibronectin also appears crucial to macrophage binding of fibrin (Hormann, Richter, & Jelinic, 1987). In a series of experiments, the N-terminal region of the fibronectin subunit chain was shown to mediate binding of radiolabeled fibrin to guinea pig peritoneal macrophages. This binding appeared to involve a transamidase-catalyzed reaction. Macrophages themselves possess this enzyme and the expression of transamidase was shown to be the likely rate-limiting step for binding of fibrin to macrophages in the presence of fibronectin.

Not surprisingly, growth factors can alter fibronectin synthesis. The expression of the fibronectin gene as well as deposition of fibronectin into the pericellular matrix was enhanced by transforming growth factor-β_1 (TGF-β_1) (Keski-Oja, Raghow, Sawdwy, & Loskutoff, 1988). Expression of the fibronectin cell adhesive receptor was also stimulated by TGF-β_1 (Roberts, Birkenmeier, McQuillan, & Sporn, 1988); fibroblasts interact with fibronectin via this receptor.

Peritoneal Fibronectin

Altered fibronectin activity is implicated in diseases involving enhanced fibrinogen production, such as endometriosis and peritoneal adhesion formation. The concentration of fibronectin in the peritoneal fluid was substantially less in patients undergoing surgery for endometriosis (mean = 59 μg/mL) or tubal occlusions and/or adhesions (mean = 60 μg/mL) than in fertile controls (mean = 80 μg/mL) (Kauma, Clark, White, & Halme, 1988). Peritoneal fluid fibronectin concentration was not correlated with peritoneal fluid volume, concentration of macrophages in the peritoneal fluid, or the synthesis of fibronectin by peritoneal macrophages in this study. These researchers postulated that the reduced fibronectin concentration in patients with endometriosis or tubal occlusions and/or adhesions was related to an augmentation in fibronectin deposition at the inflammatory site. This increased deposition may serve as an additional chemoattractant to fibroblasts, which in turn may eventually result in increased production of extracellular matrix. Interestingly, fibronectin production by peritoneal macrophages was significantly enhanced in patients with endometriosis relative to fertile controls (55.2 versus 18.8 ng/ 2.5×10^5 cells); fibronectin production by patients with tubal occlusions and/or adhesions (19.1 ng/2.5×10^5 cells) was similar to that in controls (Kauma et al., 1988).

Role of Postsurgical Macrophages in Tissue Repair

Following surgical insult to the peritoneum, tissue repair cells (TRC) at the wound surface proliferate and secrete extracellular matrix (discussed more fully in Chapter 4). Fukasawa and colleagues (1989b) demonstrated that the TRC collected from the injured rabbit peritoneum following peritoneal abrasion initially contained a mixture of cell types, including macrophages and fibroblasts, but by postsurgical day 4 >95% of the TRC were adherent fibroblast-like cells. Despite their morphological and immunohistochemical similarity to fibroblasts, TRC collected from injured peritoneum have different characteristics from other established fibroblast cell lines. For example, TRCs respond to a variety of growth factors differently than do normal rat kidney fibroblasts (Fukasawa et al., 1989b; see Chapter 3).

Available data suggest that TRCs harvested from the site of peritoneal injury can change their functional characteristics in response to macrophage-mediated secretory products during the process of postsurgical peritoneal re-epithelialization. TRCs are activated to proliferate when co-cultured with postsurgical macrophages. As shown in Figure 6.14, incorporation of [³H]thymidine into TRCs recovered from the injured rabbit peritoneum 7 days after peritoneal abrasion was significantly greater when the cells were incubated with spent media from postsurgical macrophages (Fukasawa, Campeau, Yanagihara, Rodgers, & diZerega, 1989a). Furthermore, TRC proliferation was greater with exposure to postsurgical macrophages compared to nonsurgical macrophage culture

POSTSURGICAL DAY7 FIBROBLASTS
AFTER ABRASION

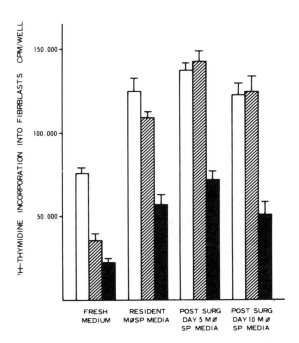

FIGURE 6.14. Incorporation of [³H]thymidine into TRCs was determined. TRCs were cultured for various time (□, 4 days; [/], 8 days; ■, 12 days) prior to the assay and incubated with spent media from macrophages collected from various postsurgical days. The incorporation of ³H-thymidine into TRCs recovered from the injured rabbit peritoneum was greater when incubated with spent media from postsurgical macrophages. Data represent means ± SEM (cpm/well). (From Fukasawa et al., 1989a. Reproduced by permission of Taylor & Francis.)

media. Collagen and glycosaminoglycan production (as indicated by [³H]proline and [³⁵S]sulfate incorporation in TRC, respectively) were also shown to be stimulated by macrophage-spent media (Fukasawa et al., 1989a). However, this stimulation appeared to be related to the enhanced proliferation of TRCs induced by postsurgical macrophages.

In the above studies, TRC cells were incubated with postsurgical macrophage media for 48 hours. Other studies indicate that postsurgical macrophages recovered from peritoneal exudate initially suppress (first 48 hours of incubation) and later enhance (>48 hours of incubation) incorporation of [³H]thymidine into fibroblasts (Fukasawa et al., 1988a). The suppression of fibroblast proliferation by postsurgical macrophages, however, was substantially less than that observed with nonsurgical macrophages. Thus, macrophage-mediated modulation of TRC proliferation following peritoneal surgery is a complex process that involves both suppression and stimulation. The fibroproliferative activity of postsurgical macrophages was shown to be reduced to the level of resident macrophages on postsurgical day 28 (Fukasawa et al., 1987). Accordingly, postsurgical macrophages appear to revert to resident-like macrophages after cessation of mesothelial repair.

The occurrence of macrophages at the surgical site precedes that of fibroblasts; thus, it is conceivable that macrophages may facilitate the migration of fibroblasts by secretion of a chemotactic factor(s). Fibroblasts recovered from peritoneal injury sites in rabbits were shown to undergo a morphologic change when cultured with macrophage-spent media (Bryant et al., 1988). The change in the fibroblast from a flat oval shape to a more spindly appearance coincided with the timing of macrophage-mediated inhibition of fibroblast proliferation. Interestingly, the morphological change was more pronounced in postsurgical day 4 fibroblasts than in postsurgical day 8 cells, despite the fact that the mitotic activity of day 4 fibroblasts in the presence of macrophage spent media was less than that of day 8 fibroblasts. Bryant and colleagues proposed that the alteration in the morphology of fibroblasts indicates a change in cell metabolism to maximize the potential for migration.

Thus, postsurgical activated macrophages appear to be able to induce both the migration and the proliferation of TRC at the peritoneal wound surface. Macrophages are presumed to influence migration and proliferation of TRCs through secretion of a variety of factors. Furthermore, other cellular components actively involved in wound repair, namely fibroblasts and platelets, also secrete substances that can affect the growth and function of TRCs. Fukasawa and colleagues (1989b) evaluated the effects of a number of growth factors on [^{3}H]thymidine incorporation in TRCs collected on postsurgical day 5 from the peritoneum of rabbits that had undergone peritoneal abrasion. As shown in Chapter 3, epidermal growth factor (EGF) and fibroblast growth factor (FGF) stimulated TRC proliferation, whereas transforming growth factor-β (TGF-β) inhibited it. Interleukin-1 (IL-1) and platelet-derived growth factor (PDGF) had little to no effect in this study. TRC responses to these growth factors increased during the postsurgical period, with postsurgical day 10 having the greatest response. PDGF and IL-1 may not have had a discernible effect on TRC proliferation in this study because they act as initiation factors that induce the movement of cells from the G_0 stage. Since TRCs are already in an active proliferative phase, they may not show as great a response to these two factors. Conversely, EGF and FGF may act as competence factors and facilitate the movement of cells from the G_0 to S phase. TGF-β stimulates fibroblast-induced production of extracellular matrix (collagen and fibronection) (e.g., Roberts et al., 1985). Thus, TGF-β may induce TRCs to enter a functional or secretory stage rather than to proliferate.

In a clinical study, macrophage-derived growth factor (MDGF) secretion by human peritoneal macrophages from 55 women was examined. Macrophages from 23 women released MDGF. When compared to the status of the patients, 28% of macrophages from women with normal pelvic anatomy released significant MDGF activity and 68% of macrophages from women with endometriosis released MDGF. This finding suggests that MDGF secretion by peritoneal macrophages is associated with endometriosis (Halme et al., 1988).

Conclusions

Recent studies clearly demonstrate that the ability of the macrophage to secrete soluble substances is at least as important as its phagocytic ability. The secretory products released by the macrophage are more numerous and diverse than those recognized for any other cell of the immune system and allow the macrophage to have pro- as well as anti-inflammatory effects and to regulate the function of other cells. Peritoneal wound healing represents one process in which the macrophage appears to be crucial. They are specifically recruited to the peritoneal cavity following injury. Through secretion of a variety of factors, macrophages appear capable of influencing the entirety of the healing process, from fibroblast proliferation to extracellular matrix formation and tissue remodeling.

References

Abe H, Rodgers KE, Ellefson D, diZerega GS. (1989). Kinetics of interleukin-1 secretion by murine macrophages recovered from the peritoneal cavity after surgery. *J Surg Res.* 47:178–182.

Abe H, Rodgers KE, Campeau D, Girgis W, Ellefson DD, diZerega GS. (1990). The effect of intraperitoneal administration of sodium tolmetin-hyaluronic acid on the postsurgical cell infiltration in vivo. *J Surg Res.* 49:322–327.

Abe H, Rodgers KE, Ellefson D, diZerega GS. (1991). Kinetics of interleukin-1 and tumor necrosis factor secretion by rabbit macrophages recovered from the peritoneal cavity after surgery. *J Invest Surg.* 4:141–151.

Adams DO, Johnson WJ, Marino PJ. (1982). Mechanisms of target recognition and destruction in macrophage mediated tumor cytotoxicity. *Fed Proc* 41:134.

Adams DO. (1983). The biology of the granuloma. In: Ioachim H, ed. *Pathology of Granulomas.* New York: Raven Press; 1–20.

Adams DO, Nathan CF. (1983). Molecular mechanisms in tumor-cell killing by activated macrophages. *Immunol Today.* 4:166–170.

Adams DO, Hall T, Steplewski Z, Koprowski H. (1984). Tumor undergoing rejection induced by monoclonal antibodies of the IgG$_2\alpha$ isotype contain increased numbers of macrophages activated for a distinctive form of antibody-dependent cytolysis. *Proc Natl Acad Sci USA.* 81:3506–3510.

Adams DO, Marino P. (1984a). Activation of mononuclear phagocytes for destruction of tumor cells as a model for the study of macrophage development. In: Gordon AS, Silver R, LoBue J, eds. Contemporary Topics in Hematology-Oncology. New York: *Plenum Press;* 69–136.

Adams DO, Hamilton TA. (1987). Molecular basis of signal transduction in macrophage activation induced by IFN-γ and by second signals. *Immunol Rev.* 97:1–27.

Adams DO, Hamilton TA. (1988). Phagocytic cells: cytotoxic activities of macrophages. In: Gallin JI, Goldstein IM, Synderman R, eds. *Inflammation: Basic Principles and Clinical Correlates.* New York: Raven Press; 471–492.

Alexander P, Evans R. (1971). Endotoxin and double stranded RNA render macrophages cytotoxic. *Nature.* 232:76–79.

Allison AC. (1978). Mechanisms by which activated macrophages inhibit lymphocyte responses. *Immunol Rev.* 40:3–27.

Axline S. (1970). Functional biochemistry of the macrophages. *Semin Hematol.* 7:142–150.

Bevilacqua MP, Schleef RR, Gimbrone MA, Loskutoff DJ. (1986). Regulation of fibrinolytic system of cultured human vascular endothelium by interleukin 1. *J Clin Invest.* 73:587–591.

Bitterman PB, Wewers MD, Rennard SI, Adelberg S, Crystal RG. (1986). Modulation of alveolar macrophages-derived fibroblast proliferation by alternative macrophage mediators. *J Clin Invest.* 77:700–713.

Boros DL. (1986). Immunoregulation of granulomatous formation in murine schistosomiasis mansoni. *Ann NY Acad Sci.* 465:313–323.

Bronson RE, Bentiolami CN, Siebert EP. (1987). Modulation of fibroblast growth and glycosaminoglycan synthesis by interleukin-1. *Collagen Rel Res.* 7:323–332.

Bryant SM, Lynch RE, Hill HR. (1982). Kinetic analysis of superoxide anion production by activated and resident murine peritoneal macrophages. *Cell Immunol.* 96:46–58.

Bryant SM, Fukasawa M, Orita H, Rodgers KE, diZerega GS. (1988). Mediation of post-surgical wound healing by macrophages. *Growth Factors and Other Aspects of Wound Healing: Biological and Clinical Implications.* New York: Alan R. Liss; 263–290.

Buyalos RP, Rutanem E-M, Tsui E, Halme J. (1991). Release of tumor necrosis factor alpha by human peritoneal macrophages in response to toxic shock syndrome toxin-1. *Obstet Gynecol.* 78:182–186.

Calderon J, Williams RT, Unanue ER. (1974). An inhibitor of cell proliferation released by cultures of macrophages. *Proc Natl Acad Sci USA.* 71:4273–4277.

Chapman HA, Stone OL, Vavrin Z. (1984). Degradation of fibrin and elastin by intact human alveolar macrophages in vitro. *J Clin Invest.* 73:806–815.

Clark RA, Klebanoff SJ. (1975). Neutrophil-mediated tumor cell cytotoxicity: role of the peroxidase system. *J Exp Med.* 141:1442–1457.

Diegelmann RF, Cohen IK, Kaplan AM. (1981). The role of macrophages in wound repair: a review. *Plast Reconstr Surg.* 68:107–113.

Dolynchuk KN, Bowness JM. (1981). The early metabolism of noncollagenous glycoproteins during wound healing. *J Surg Res.* 31:218–224.

Dower SK, Kronheim SR, March CJ, Conlon PJ, Hopp TP, Gillis S, Urdal DL. (1985). Detection and characterization of high affinity plasma membrane receptors for human interleukin 1. *J Exp Med.* 162:501–517.

Ebert RH, Florey HW. (1939). The extravascular development of the monocyte observed in vivo. *Br J Exp Pathol.* 20:342–351.

Edelson PJ. (1982). Intracellular parasites and phagocytic cells: Cell biology and pathophysiology. *Rev Infect Dis.* 4:124–156.

Elias JA, Rossman MD, Zurier RB, Daniele RP. (1985). Human alveolar macrophage inhibition of lung fibroblast growth. A prostaglandin-dependent process. *Am Rev Respir Dis.* 131:94–99.

Esparza I, Green R, Schreiber RD. (1983). Inhibition of macrophage tumoricidal activity by immune complexes and altered erythrocytes. *J Immunol.* 131:2117–2123.

Estes JE, Pledger WJ, Gillespie GY. (1984). Macrophage derived growth factor for fibroblasts and interleukin-1 are distinct entities. *J Leukoc Biol.* 35:115–128.

Fakih H, Baggett B, Holtz G, Tsang KY, Lee JC, Williamson HO. (1987). Interleukin-1: a possible role in the infertility associated with endometriosis. *Fertil Steril.* 47:213–217.

Feldman SR, Gonias SL, Pizzo SV. (1985). A model of α_2-macroglobulin structure and functions. *Proc Natl Acad Sci USA.* 82:5700–5704.

Fukasawa M, Bryant SM, Nakamura RM, diZerega GS. (1987). Modulation of fibroblast proliferation by postsurgical macrophages. *J Surg Res.* 43:513–520.

Fukasawa M, Bryant SM, diZerega GS. (1988a). Incorporation of thymidine by fibroblasts: evidence for complex regulation by postsurgical macrophages. *J Surg Res.* 45:460–466.

Fukasawa M, Bryant SM, diZerega GS. (1988b). Superoxide anion production by postsurgical macrophages. *J Surg Res.* 45:382–388.

Fukasawa M, Campeau JD, Yanagihara DL, Rodgers KE, diZerega GS. (1989a). Mitogenic and protein synthetic activity of tissue repair cells: control by the postsurgical macrophage. *J Invest Surg.* 2:169–180.

Fukasawa M, Yanagihara DL, Rodgers KE, diZerega GS. (1989b). The mitogenic activity of peritoneal tissue repair cells: control by growth factors. *J Surg Res.* 47:45–51.

Fukasawa M, Campeau D, Girgis W, Bryant SM, Rodgers KE, diZerega GS. (1989c). Production of protease inhibitors by postsurgical macrophages. *J Surg Res.* 16:256–261.

Gay S, Viljanto J, Raekallio J, Penttinen R. (1978). Collagen types in early phases of wound healing in children. *Acta Chir Scand.* 144:205–211.

Gresser J, Brouty-Boye K, Thomas MG, Macierira-Cuelho A. (1970). Interferon and cell division I. Inhibition of the multiplication of mouse leukemia C12 106/B in vitro by interferon preparations. *Proc Natl Acad Sci USA.* 66:1052–1058.

Grinnell F. (1984). Fibronectin and wound healing. *J Cell Biochem.* 26:107–116.

Halme J, White C, Kauma S, Estes J, Haskell S. (1988). Peritoneal macrophages from patients with endomtriosis release growth factor activity in vitro. *J Clin Endocrinol Metab.* 66:1044–1048.

Hibbs JB, Lambert LH, Remington JS. (1972). In vitro nonimmunologic destruction of cells with abnormal characteristics by adjuvant activated macrophages. *Proc Soc Exp Biol Med.* 139:1049–1055.

Hibbs JB, Taintor RR, Varrin Z, Rachlin EM. (1988). Nitric oxide: a cytotoxic activated macrophage effector molecule. *Biochem Biophys Res Commun.* 157:87–94.

Hormann H, Richter H, Jelinic V. (1987). The role of fibronectin fragments and cell-attached transamidase on the binding of soluble fibrin to macrophages. *Thrombosis Res.* 46:39–50.

Johnson WJ, Steplewski Z, Matthews TJ, Koprowski H, Adams DO. (1986). Characterization of lytic conditions and requirements for effector activation. *J Immunol.* 136:4704–4713.

Jones PA, Werb Z. (1980). Degradation of connective tissue matrices by macrophages. III. Influence of matrix composition on proteolysis of glycoprotein, elastin and collagen by macrophages in culture. *J Exp Med.* 152:1527–1536.

Kauma S, Clark MR, White C, Halme J. (1988). Production of fibronectin by peritoneal macrophages and concentration of fibronectin in peritoneal fluid from patients with or without endometriosis. *Obstet Gynecol.* 72:13–18.

Keski-Oja J, Raghow R, Sawdey M, Loskutoff DJ. (1988). Regulation of mRNAs for type I plasminogen activator inhibitor, fibronectin, and type I procollagen by transforming growth factor-β. *J Biol Chem.* 263:3111–3115 .

Klebanoff SJ. (1975). Antimicrobial mechanisms of neutrophilic polymorphonuclear leukocytes. *Semin Hematol.* 12:117–124.

Kleinman HK, Klebe RJ, Martin GR. (1981). Role of collagenous matrices in the adhesion and growth of cells. *J Cell Biol.* 88:473–485.

Ko SD, Page RC, Narayanan AS. (1977). Fibroblast heterogenesity and prostaglandin regulation of subpopulation. *Proc Natl Acad Sci USA.* 74:3429–3440.

Korn JH, Halushka PV, LeRoy EC. (1980). Mononuclear cell modulation of connective tissue function: suppression of fibroblast growth by stimulation of endogenous prostaglandin production. *J Clin Invest.* 65:543–554.

Kung JT, Brooks SB, Jakway JB, Leonard LL, Talmadge DW. (1977). Suppression of in vitro cytotoxic response by macrophages due to induced arginase. *J Exp Med.* 146:665–680.

Kuraoka S, Campeau JD, Rodgers KE, Nakamura RM, diZerega GS. (1992). Effects of interleukin-1 (IL-1) on postsurgical macrophage secretion of protease and protease inhibitor activities. *J Surg Res.* 52:71–78.

Kuraoka S, Campeau JD, Nakamura RM, diZerega GS. (in press.) Modulation of postsurgical macrophage function by early postsurgical polymorphonuclear leukocytes. *J Surg Res.*

Kuraoka S, Campeau JD, Rodgers KE, Nakamura RM, diZerega GS. (in review). Modulation of cytotoxic activity of resident macrophages by postsurgical macrophages.

Kurkinen M, Vaheri A, Roberts PJ, Stenman S. (1980). Sequential appearance of fibronectin and collagen in experimental granulation tissue. *Lab Invest.* 43:47–51.

Laub R, Huybrechts-Godin G, Peeters-Joris C, Vaes G. (1982). Degradation of collagen and proteoglycan by macrophages and fibroblasts. *Biochim Biophys Acta.* 721:425–433.

Leibovich SJ, Ross R. (1976). A macrophage-dependent factor that stimulates the proliferation of fibroblast in vitro. *Am J Pathol.* 84:501–508.

Matsushima K, Bano M, Kidwell WR, Oppenheim JJ. (1985). Interleukin-1 increases collagen type IV production by murine mammary epithelial cells. *J Immunol.* 134:904–909.

Meltzer MS, Ruco LP, Boraschi D, Nacy CA. (1979). Macrophage activation for tumor cytotoxicity: analysis of intermediary reaction. *J Reticuloendothel Soc.* 26:403–416.

Meuret G, Hoffmann G. (1973). Monocyte kinetic studies in normal and disease states. *Br J Haematol.* 24:275–285.

Meuret G, Bammert J, Hoffman G. (1974). Kinetics of human monocytopoiesis. *Blood.* 44:801–806.

Meuret G, Detel U, Kilz HP, Senn HJ, Van Lessen H. (1975). Human monocytopoiesis in acute and chronic inflammation. *Expt Hematol.* 54:328–334.

Nathan CF, Root KA. (1977). Hydrogen peroxide release from mouse peritoneal macrophages dependence on sequential activation and triggering. *J Exp Med.* 146:1648–1662.

Nathan CF, Cohn ZA. (1980). Cellular components of inflammation: monocytes and macrophages. In: Kelley W, Harris E, Ruddey S, Hedge R, eds. *Textbook of Rheumatology.* Philadelphia: WB Saunders; 144–169.

Nathan CF. (1986). Mechanisms of macrophage antimicrobial activity. *Trans R Soc Trop Med Hyg.* 77:620–630.

Nelson DS. (1982). Macrophages as effector of cell-mediated immunity. In: Laskin AI, LeChevalier H, eds. *Macrophages and Cellular Immunity.* Cleveland: CRC Press; 45–76.

Orita H, Campeau JD, Gale JA, Nakamura RM, diZerega GS. (1986). Differential secretion of plasminogen activator activity by postsurgical activated macrophages. *J Surg Res.* 41:569–573.

Phan SH, McGarry BM, Loeffler KM, Kunkel SL. (1987). Regulation of macrophage derived fibroblast growth factor release by arachidonate metabolites. *J Leukoc Biol.* 42:106–113.

Postlethwaite AE, Lachman LB, Mainadri CL, Kang AH. (1983). Interleukin-1 stimulation of collagenase production by cultured fibroblasts. *J Exp Med.* 157:801–806.

Raftery AT. (1973). Regeneration of parietal and visceral peritoneum: An electron microscopical study. *J Anat.* 115:375–392.

Roberts AB, Anzano MA, Wakefield LM, Roche NS, Stern DF, Sporn MB. (1985). Type B transforming growth factor: a bifunctional regulatory of cellular growth. *Proc Natl Acad Sci USA.* 82:119–123.

Roberts CJ, Birkenmeier TM, McQuillan JJ, Sporn MB. (1988). Transforming growth factor B stimulates the expression of fibronectin and of both subunits of the human fibronectin receptor by cultured human lung fibroblasts. *J Biol Chem.* 263:4586–4592.

Rodgers KE, Ellefson D, Girgis W, Scott L, diZerega GS. (1988). Effects of tolmetin sodium dihydrate on hormal and postsurgical cell function. *Int J Immunopharmacol.* 10:111–120.

Samuelsson B, Branstrom E, Greer K, Hamberg M, Hammerstrom S. (1971). Prostaglandins. *Anu Rev Biochem.* 44:669–694.

Schmidt JA, Mizel SB, Cohen D, Green I. (1982). Interleukin-1, a potential regulator of fibroblast proliferation. *J Immunol.* 128:2177–2192.

Schnyder J, Dewald B, Baggiolini M. (1981). Effects of cyclooxygenase inhibitors and prostaglandin E_2 on macrophage activation in vitro. *Prostaglandins.* 22:411–419.

Schreiber R. (1984). Identification of γ-interferon as murine macrophage activating factor for tumor cytotoxicity. *Comtemp Top Immunobiol.* 13:174–199.

Shimanuki T, Nakamura RM, diZerega GS. (1986). A kinetic analysis of peritoneal fluid cytology and arachidonic acid metabolism after abrasion and reabrasion of rabbit peritoneum. *J Surg Res.* 41:245–251.
Somers SD, Johnson WJ, Adams DO. (1986). Destruction of tumor cells by macrophages: mechanisms of recognition and lysis and their regulation. In: Herberman R, ed. *Basic and Clinical Tumor Immunology.* New York: Marcel-Dekker; 68–130.
Spector WG. (1982). Experimental granulomas. *Pathol Res Pract.* 175:110–117.
Steeg PS, Johnson HM, Oppenheim JJ. (1982). Regulation of murine macrophage I-A antigen expression by an immune interferon-like lymphokine: inhibitory effect of endotoxins. *J Immunol.* 129:2402–2408.
Steinman RM, Brodie SE, Cohn ZA. (1976). Membrane flow during pinocytosis: a stereologic analysis. *J Cell Biol.* 68:665–671.
Steinman RM, Mellman IS, Muller WA, Cohn ZA. (1983). Endocytosis and the recycling of plasma membrane. *J Cell Biol.* 96:1–27.
Stuehr DJ, Marletta MA. (1985). Mammalian nitrite biosynthesis: mouse macrophages produce nitrite and nitrate in response to *Escherichia coli* lipopolysaccharide. *Proc Natl Acad Sci USA.* 82:7738–7742.
Stuehr DJ, Marletta MA. (1987). Induction of nitrite/nitrate synthesis in murine macrophages by, BCG infection, lymphokines or interferonγ. *J Immunol.* 139:518–523.
Unanue ER. (1986). Secretory function of mononuclear phagocytes. *Am J Pathol.* 83:396–417.
van Furth R, Cohn ZA. (1968). The origin and kinetics of mononuclear phagocytes. *J Exp Med.* 128:415–435.
van Furth R, Diesselhoff-den MC. (1970). The kinetics of promonocytes and monocytes in the bone morrow. *J Exp Med.* 132:813–828.
van Furth R. (1976). Origin and kinetics of mononuclear phagocytes. *Ann NY Acad Sci.* 278:161–188.
van Furth R. (1988). Phagocytic cells: development and distribution of mononuclear phagocytes in normal steady-state and inflammation. In: Gallin JI, Goldstein IM, Synderman R, eds. *Inflammation: Basic Principles and Clinical Correlates.* New York: Raven Press; 281–295.
Volkman A, Gowans JL. (1965). The origin of macrophages from bone marrow in the rat. *Br J Exp Pathol.* 46:62–70.
Volkman A. (1976). Disparity in origin of mononuclear phagocyte populations. *J Reticuloendothel Soc.* 19:249–253.
Werb Z, Banda MJ, Jones PA. (1980a). Degradation of connective tissue matrices by macrophages. I. Proteolysis of elastin, glycoproteins and collagen by proteinases isolated from macrophages. *J Exp Med.* 152:1340–1357.
Werb Z, Bainton DF, Jones PA. (1980b). Degradation of connective tissue matrices by macrophages. II. Morphological and biochemical studies on extracellular, pericellular and intracellular events in matrix proteolysis by macrophages in culture. *J Exp Med.* 152:1537–1553.
Whitelaw DM. (1972). Observations on human monocyte kinetics after pulse labelling. *Cell Tissue Kinet.* 5:311–317.
Zucali JR, Dinarello CA, Oblon DJ, Gross MA, Anderson L, Weiner RS. (1986). Interleukin 1 stimulates fibroblasts to produce granulocyte-macrophage colony-stimulating activity and prostaglandin E_2. *J Clin Invest.* 77:1857–1863.

7

Fibrinolysis

FIBRINOLYSIS, WHICH REPRESENTS THE END STAGE OF COAGULATION, was defined by Dastre in 1893 as the dissolution of polymerized fibrin. Todd (1959) reported the presence of fibrinolytic activity in serosal cells derived from human peritoneum and pleura. Astrup and Allbrechtsen (1957) demonstrated plasminogen activator in extracts of serosa from the human fallopian tube and parietal peritoneum of the rat uterus. These studies were confirmed by others who demonstrated fibrinolytic activity and plasminogen activator in parietal pleura, pericardium, and peritoneum (Myhre-Jensen, Larsen, & Astrup, 1969; Porter, McGregor, Mullen, & Silver, 1969; Porter, Ball, & Silver, 1971; Raftery, 1979; Merlo, Fausone, Barbero, & Castagna, 1980). Pugatch and Poole (1969) subsequently reported the presence of fibrinolysis-inhibiting agents in bovine parietal peritoneum. Plasmin, the major enzyme involved in fibrinolysis, is formed from the inactive precursor, plasminogen, by the action of plasminogen activators (PA). PAs are found in urine, tissues, and blood. Normally, coagulation and fibrinolysis are in balance such that no net fibrin deposition occurs.

The formation of fibrin is part of a hemostatic process by which the extravasation of blood after an injury is prevented. Fibrin also aids in tissue repair by becoming a matrix for migrating fibroblasts and the formation of connective tissue. Thus, the processes by which the formation and resolution of fibrin occur have major physiologic significance. Deposition of fibrin is a prerequisite for normal tissue repair but the ultimate removal and resolution of the deposit is necessary for reestablishment of preoperative conditions. Disturbance in the balance between these two processes results in excess fibrin deposition, which can lead to thrombotic events and adhesion formation (see Chapter 9). Alterations can occur through modulation in the rate of fibrin deposition or the rate of fibrinolysis through changes in the levels of fibrinolytic enzymes or inhibitors of these enzyme. Surgery or bacterial peritonitis can disrupt the balance between coagulation and fibrinolysis, thus leaving excess polymerized fibrin in the peritoneal cavity. This excess fibrin then provides the scaffold upon which adhesions form (Ellis, Harrison, & Hugh, 1965; Hau, Payne, & Simmons, 1979; Raftery 1979).

Fibrinolytic System

The individual components of the fibrinolytic system, including plasminogen, plasmin, plasminogen activator (PA), and inhibitors of fibrinolysis (Table 7.1), are more fully discussed in Chapter 8. Plasminogen is a β-globulin of 85 kd that is present at concentrations between 0.2 and 0.3 g/L in plasma (Deutsch & Mertz, 1970). Plasminogen is activated to plasmin via agents appropriately called activators (Figure 7.1). This process includes conformational changes and cleavage of peptide bonds at Arg-Val and a disulfide bond between two peptide fragments. Plasmin is the active proteolytic enzyme in the fibrinolytic system. However, proteolytic enzymes other than plasmin can be involved in fibrinolysis (Moroz & Gilmore, 1976).

Fibrin is the major substrate for plasmin, but fibrinogen can be cleaved in vitro (Ratnoff, 1953). Plasmin can also digest coagulation factors II, V, and VIII, glucagon, ACTH, and growth hormone. Plasmin can interfere with the complement and kinin systems. Due to the potential for havoc that circulating functional plasmin could cause, the formation and activity of plasmin is highly regulated. The activation of plasminogen to plasmin is controlled by the plasminogen activators (PA) and PA inhibitors. Two separate PAs are known: tissue (tPA) and urokinase (uPA). They are secreted by a variety of cell types and tissues under different physiologic conditions.

Tissue PA specifically binds to fibrin, which then enhances subsequent fibrinolytic activity. Binding affinity to fibrin facilitates tPA's therapeutic efficacy, even after systemic administration. tPA exists in two forms: single-chain or two-chain. Both of these forms contain the same fibrin-

TABLE 7.1. Major proteins involved in fibrinolyses.

Name	Molecular Weight (d)	Function
Plasminogen	85,000	Inactive precursor to plasmin
Plasmin	81,000	Active enzyme in fibrinolysis
Plasminogen activators		Cleaves plasminogen to plasmin
Tissue type	65,000	
Urokinase	55,000	
	33,000	
Alpha$_2$-macroglobulin	700,000	Nonspecific protease inhibitor
Alpha$_2$-antiplasmin	70,000	Inhibitor of plasmin
PA1-1	40–50,000	Plasminogen activator inhibitors
PAI-2	47–48,000	

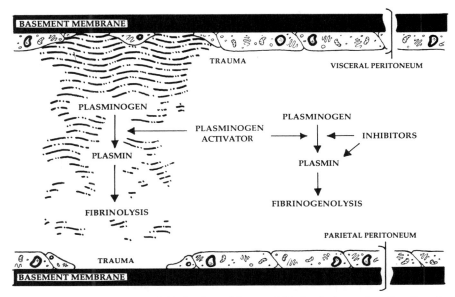

FIGURE 7.1. Mechanism of fibrin deposition and fibrinolysis at the site of peritoneal injury. Adhesion formation occurs when opposing peritoneal surfaces are denuded and fibrin is deposited. Fibrinolytic enzymes resolve the deposited clot, and inhibitors of fibrinolysis allows the maintenance of fibrin deposition.

olytic and plasminogen activating activities. Single-chain tPA was isolated from a melanoma cell line and is a glycoprotein of 65 kd; it was cloned from the cDNA melanoma cells. Two-chain tPA is formed by enzymatic cleavage of single-chain tPA. Recombinant tPA is used clinically in coronary thrombolysis after acute myocardial infarction (Grossbard, 1987). Research as to the utility of recombinant tPA in the prevention of peritoneal adhesions is an area of active laboratory research (Doody, Dunn, & Buttram, 1989; Menzies & Ellis, 1989; Orita, Girgis, & diZerega, 1991) and is reviewed in Chapter 10.

Release of tPA can be provoked by venous occlusion, trauma, surgery, and stress (Andersson, Nilson, & Olow, 1962; Chakrabarti, Hocking, & Fearnley, 1969; Nilsson & Pandolfi, 1970; Engqvist & Winther, 1972; Innes & Sevitt, 1974; Rennie, Bennett, & Ogston, 1977). Regulation of tPA secretion is partially understood. Secretion of tPA is modulated by catecholamines and corticosteroids. Inflammatory cytokines, such as interleukin-1 (IL-1) and tumor necrosis factor (TNF), can inhibit the secretion of tPA by endothelial cells.

Urokinase, a PA produced by the kidneys, is most abundant in urine. Cells such as peritoneal macrophages secrete urokinase-type PA. These cells also contain membrane localized receptors for uPA that can bind uPA as it is produced. Even in contact with the matrix to be degraded, macrophages can degrade fibrin and elastin only in the presence of plasminogen (Chapman, Stone, & Vavrin, 1984). PA bound to the cell membrane is relatively resistant to inactivation by soluble proteinase inhibitors.

Inhibitors of Fibrinolysis

The fibrinolytic balance is maintained not only by the need to convert plasminogen to plasmin, but also by inhibitors of both PA and plasmin. Plasmin contains three kinds of inhibitors. Alpha$_2$-macroglobulin is a nonspecific proteinase inhibitor that can rapidly inhibit plasmin along with other proteases and growth factors. Another inhibitor of plasmin is slow-reacting alpha$_1$-antitrypsin. Alpha$_2$-antiplasmin, which is a specific inhibitor of plasmin, is probably the most important inhibitor of plasmin activity in vivo.

Inhibitors of PA are also known. These proteins are released by a variety of cells including platelets (PAI-1), macrophages (PAI-2), and endothelial cells (PAI-1) (Donse, Dupuy, & Bodevin, 1978; Esnard, Dupuy, Dosne, & Bodevin, 1982; Emeis, Van Hinsbergh, Verheijen, & Wijngaards, 1983; Loskutoff, Van Mourik, Erickson, & Lawrence, 1983; Levin, 1983; Erickson, Ginsberg, & Loskutoff, 1984; Philips, Juul, & Thorsen, 1984; Sprengers, Verheijen, Van Hinsbergh, & Emeis, 1984; Ny, Bjersing, Hsuek, & Loskutoff, 1985; Booth, Anderson & Bennett, 1985; Laug, 1985). PAI-1 reacts with both tPA and uPA to form a detergent-stable complex of a molecular mass 40 to 50 kd larger than PA (Kruithof, Tran-Thang, Ransijn, & Bachmann, 1984; Thorsen & Philips, 1984). PAI-1 is synthesized in an active form and is rapidly inactivated in vitro. Reactivation can occur through exposure to protein denaturants. PAI-2 was originally isolated from human placenta, but subsequently found to be produced by macrophages (which may be the source in the placenta). PAI-2 is an inhibitor of both high and low molecular weight uPA, and tPA, especially two-chain tPA. This PA inhibitor was found to have a molecular mass of 47 to 48 kd. Protease nexin I is an inhibitor with broad specificity including uPA, tPA, and plasmin. It is produced by a variety of anchorage-dependent cells: fibroblasts, heart, muscle, and kidney epithelium.

The secretion of inhibitors is also highly regulated. PAI-1 in blood plasma behaves as an acute phase reactant protein. PA-inhibitory activity rapidly increases after surgery and myocardial infarction, as well as after infusion of bacterial endotoxin or interleukin-1. This increase is also observed after endothelial cells are cocultured with these stimulants in vitro. Long-term administration of synthetic anabolic steroids to humans decreases levels of plasma PA-inhibitory activity (Engqvist & Winther, 1972). However, this treatment does not affect the decline in fibrinolytic activity that occurs after surgery. A recent study showed that when human peritoneum was harvested at the time of surgery, PAI-1 was not detectable in control peritoneum, but was present in inflamed tissue (Figure 7.2; Vipond, Whawell, Thompson, & Dudley, 1990).

Tumor Necrosis Factor Modulation of Fibrinolysis

Tumor necrosis factor (TNF) has been shown to be a crucial factor in the initiation of microvascular thrombosis in patients with septicemia, and it leads to activation of coagulation and fibrinolysis in cancer patients (Bauer et al. 1989; Silverman, Goldsmith, Spitzer, Rehmus, & Berger, 1990). During septicemia, there is an activation of the coagulation cascade that is accompanied by a biphasic change in the fibrinolytic system

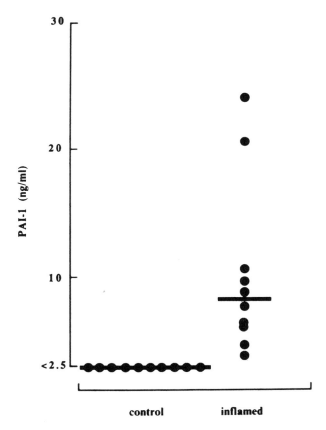

FIGURE 7.2. Concentration of plasminogen activator inhibitor-1 (PAI-1) in control and inflamed human peritoneum is shown. PAI-1 concentrations are elevated in inflamed peritoneum. This elevation may contribute to resultant adhesion formation. (From Vipond et al., 1990. Reproduced by permission of Lancet.)

(Brandtzaeg, Joo, Brusletto, Kierulf, 1990). A recent study of the fibrinolytic system following infusion of TNF was performed (van der Poll et al., 1991). TNF induced a brief increase in PA activity and in uPA and tPA levels in the serum of treated persons with a peak at 1 hour (Figure 7.3). A rise in PAI-1 antigen correlated with a decrease in PA activity.

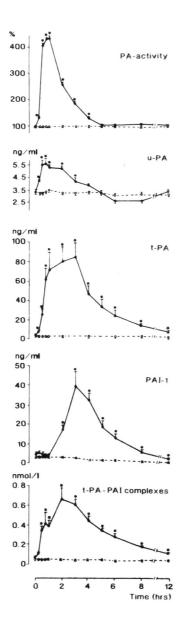

FIGURE 7.3. Mean (± SEM) plasma levels of indexes of stimulation and inhibition of plasminogen activation after intravenous bolus injections of recombinant human TNF (50 μg/m²; filled circles) or an equivalent volume of isotonic saline (open circles) to human volunteers. PA activity, uPA antigen, tPA antigen, PAI-1 antigen, and tPA–PAI-1 complexes were the parameters tested. Asterisks indicate statistical significance for the comparison of TNF with saline ($p < .05$ by Newman-Keul's test for multiple comparison). (From van der Poll et al., 1991. Reproduced by permission of Rockefeller University Press.)

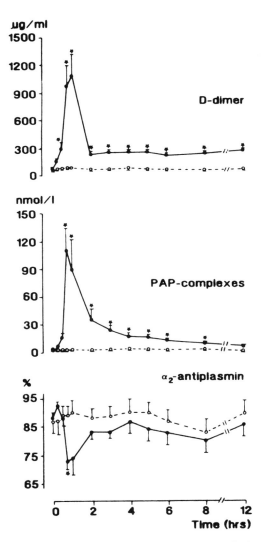

FIGURE 7.4. Mean (± SEM) plasma levels of indexes of plasmin activity and inhibition after intravenous bolus injections of recombinant human TNF (50 μg/m², filled circles) or an equivalent volume of isotonic saline (open circles) to human volunteers. The parameters measured were D-dimer, PAP complexes, and α^2-antiplasmin activity. Asterisks indicate statistical significance for the comparison of TNF with saline ($p < .05$ by Newman-Keul's test for multiple comparison). (From van der Poll et al., 1991. Reproduced by permission of Rockefeller University Press.)

Plasmin activity was also rapidly elevated after TNF infusion (Figure 7.4). A reduction in plasmin activity was reflected in an increase in plasmin–α_2-plasmin (PAP) complexes. These studies show that TNF causes a rapid, transient increase in fibrinolytic activity peaking at 1 hour followed by a rapid inhibition. In addition there was a sustained activation of the coagulation system. These studies confirm the findings of the in vitro studies that TNF can modulate cellular functions in such a way as to favor fibrin deposition (discussed below and in Chapter 3).

Tissue Distribution of Fibrinolytic Activity

An assay to measure the fibrinolytic potential of various tissues in vitro was developed by Astrup and Albrechtsen (1957) (Table 7.2). In humans, the uterus, adrenals, lymph nodes, prostate, and thyroid all have high fibrinolytic activity. Lung, ovary, peritoneum, pituitary, kidney, and skeletal muscles all have somewhat lower activity. Heart and brain have low activity, and little or no activity was found in testes, liver, and spleen (Albrechtsen, 1957a; Ende & Auditore, 1961). In general, animal organs contain less fibrinolytic activity than their human counterparts (Table 7.3; Albrechtsen, 1957b).

Endometrial fibrinolytic activity varies throughout the human menstrual cycle (Albrechtsen, 1956). Little or no fibrinolytic activity is present in the intima and media of the human aorta, however, higher levels of activity are present in the adventitia (Table 7.4; Astrup & Claassen, 1957;

TABLE 7.2. Plasminogen activator in human organs.

Organ	Average	Range
Uterus	720	450–900
Adrenals	410	63–1,278
Lymph nodes	378	16–1,278
Prostate	334	81–630
Thyroid	325	189–504
Lung	223	38–648
Ovary	210	40–378
Pituitary	140	77–288
Kidney	119	0–342
Muscle	110	14–324
Heart	82	27–144
Brain	35	8–65
Testis	25	0–68
Spleen	20	0–99
Liver	0	0–6

Concentration in units per gram fresh tissue as determined from an arbitrary standard obtained from rat tissue. (Albrechtsen, 1957a).

TABLE 7.3. Plasminogen activator in some animal species.

	Brain	Lung	Heart	Uterus	Muscle	Prostate	Adrenals	Testis	Ovary
Pig	44	0	216	145	24	5	55	0	173
Horse	73	61	32	138	85	161	18	32	28
Ox	68	0	28	3	0	4	38	12	12
Dog	9	14	0	41	0	133	37	12	29
Rabbit	+	+	0	48	0	0	0	0	22
Guinea pig	24	15	39	45	0	—	6	15	—
Cat	0	13	0	22	0	0	20	0	6
Mouse	4	212	0	2	0	—	—	—	—
Rat	25	238	20	10	+	—	60	—	61

All samples of liver and spleen: 0 or +. (0, no measured activity; +, slight digestion of the substrate.) Units per gram fresh tissue as determined by comparison against an arbitrary standard obtained from rat tissue. Averages calculated after Albrechtsen (1957b).

Astrup, Albrechtsen, Claassen, & Rasmussen, 1959). A striking difference was found between the fibrinolytic activity of veins and arteries (Todd, 1958, 1959, 1960; Coccheri & Astrup, 1961). Both types of vessels contain activity in the adventitial layer. The venous, but not arterial intima, was active.

Peritoneal Fibrinolytic Activity

Unkeless, Gordon, and Reich (1974) showed that stimulated peritoneal macrophages promote active plasminogen-dependent fibrinolysis in vitro for several days. The morphologic changes noted in the fibrin filaments over the 2-day period suggest a long-term production and release of plasminogen activator by stimulated macrophages in the peritoneal cavity.

Ryan, Grobety, and Majno (1973) correlated the changes in the fibrin-

TABLE 7.4. Plasminogen activator in the coats of normal and arterioscleortic human aorta.

	Intima		Media		Adventitia	
Patient	Normal	Pathol.	Normal	Pathol.	Normal	Pathol.
F 36	0	0	0	+	74	384
M 38	0	0	0	22	180	749
M 45	0	0	0	0	138	368
M 58	0	0	0	+	154	526
F 64	0	0	0	0	200	478
(Behind plaque)	—	0	—	0	—	1,188
F 70	0	0	0	0	324	984

Units per gram fresh tissue as determined by comparison against an arbitrary standard obtained from rat tissue. After Astrup and Claassen (1957).

olytic activity of visceral peritoneum covering the cecum of rats with the histologic changes that accompany re-epithelialization. Injury was induced by a stream of compressed CO_2 blowing over the peritoneum for 5 minutes. Fibrinolytic activity was measured using the fibrin slide technique. Initially fibrinolytic activity rapidly declined and began to return by postsurgical day 3. By day 5 the extent of fibrinolytic activity exceeded that of presurgical controls. This increased fibrinolytic activity remained relatively unchanged for an additional 2 to 3 weeks before declining. At 2 months fibrinolytic activity was still greater than the levels of presurgical controls.

Porter et al. (1971) showed that mesothelial tissue contains large amounts of PA activity. They evaluated the fibrinolytic activity of pleura, pericardium, and peritoneum obtained from patients undergoing various surgical procedures. Fibrinolytic activity was determined by their ability to lyse fibrin gels. Peritoneum and pericardium exhibited the same amount of lysis, which was reduced by 30% after abrasion. Further, they found large amounts of fibrin-split products as well as fibrinolytic activity in drainage fluids from these mesothelial tissues. However, this study did not clarify if the activity originated from the submesothelial vascular endothelium or from mesothelial cells. A further study examining a single layer of mesothelial cells from human peritoneum showed fibrinolytic activity in all areas, but there were differences between sites. For example, the fibrinolytic activity of the serosa obtained from different areas of the sigmoid colon had different amounts of PA activity (Figure 7.5). In this study the fibrinolytic activity of the omentum was found to be the highest (Merlo et al., 1980).

Species Difference

Species difference in the level of fibrinolytic activity in the peritoneal mesothelium were observed. The mesothelium of rats and guinea pigs, but not rabbits, has fibrinolytic activity (Myhre-Jensen et al., 1969). A study by Whitaker, Papadimitriou, and Walters (1982) reported that pure cultures of mesothelial cells were able to induce fibrinolysis.

A comparative survey of fibrinolysis and qualitative determination of plasminogen activator activity was made by Myhre-Jensen et al. (1969). A comparative survey of fibrinolytic and plasminogen activator activities was made in parietal and visceral peritoneum of rats, guinea pigs, and rabbits. Using the fibrin slide technique, none of the samples produced lysis of plasminogen-free fibrin. Consequently, all of the fibrinolytic activity was considered to be dependent upon plasminogen activator. The three species showed differences in the rate of fibrinolysis by peritoneal mesothelium: rats 10 to 50 minutes, guinea pigs 30 to 90 minutes, rabbits minimal to no activity at 240 minutes. In all three species, fibrinolytic

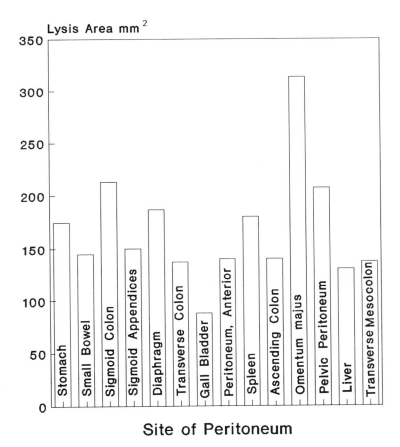

FIGURE 7.5. PA activity of human serosal peritoneum. Biopsies of serosal peritoneum were obtained from various sites during peritoneal surgery. The level of fibrinolytic activity of the human peritoneum is depicted here. (From Merlo et al., 1980. Reproduced by permission of S. Karger AG.)

activity was relatively weak in mesothelial tissue in comparison to endothelial or vascular tissue.

Porter et al. (1969) biopsied human mesothelium and resected 5-mm segments of peritoneum, pleura, and pericardium from dogs. All tissues produced a similar amount of lysis on fibrin plates. The fibrinolysis was destroyed by heat. Mechanical abrasion reduced by 25% the fibrinolytic activity of human mesothelium. Raftery (1981b) developed a semiquantitative fibrin plate assay that was useful for measuring fibrinolytic activity in a single layer of cells. He found parietal peritoneum of the rat contained considerable fibrinolytic activity, which decreased 35% by stripping from the abdominal cavity (Figure 7.6). Visceral peritoneum removed from

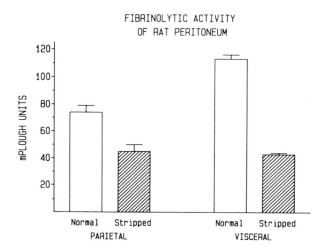

FIGURE 7.6. The effect of peritoneal injury on the fibrinolytic activity of a single layer of cells in a semiquantitative fibrin plate assay in mPlough units of plasminogin activator activity. The fibrinolytic activity of visceral and parietal peritoneum was reduced by surgical injury. (From Raftery, 1981b. Reproduced by permission of British Medical Association.)

the rat cecum was found to contain relatively more fibrinolytic activity, which decreased 65% by abrasion. Fibrinolytic activity of visceral peritoneum appeared to be even greater than that of parietal peritoneum.

Surgical Injury

Gervin, Puckett, and Silver (1973) demonstrated fibrinolytic activity (presumably plasminogen activator) in canine serosa removed from various parts of the gastrointestinal tract including the descending colon, ileum, stomach and omentum after different types of surgical injuries. After abrasion of the peritoneum these authors noted a 20% to 100% decrease in fibrinolytic activity. After abrasion of the midportion of the ileum, a 50% decrease was found in fibrinolytic activity, which was accompanied by severe adhesions. Few or no adhesions were seen in the other five dogs; fibrinolytic activity was decreased less than 50% in these dogs.

Raftery (1981a) determined the changes in peritoneal fibrinolytic activity in rats following four types of trauma: (1) excision of parietal peritoneum, (2) grafting of free peritoneum, (3) electrocoagulation, and (4) ischemia (Figure 7.7). Immediately after each procedure there was a reduction in fibrinolytic activity. In the case of the unsutured defect, free peritoneal graft, and ischemic bowel, the activity was further reduced over the next 24 hours. In the case of electrocautery, fibrinolytic activity

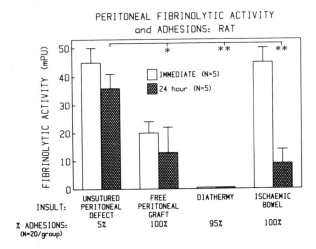

FIGURE 7.7. Effect of various types of peritoneal trauma on peritoneal fibrinolytic activity immediately and 24 hours after surgery in rats. Free peritoneal grafts, diathermy coagulation, and ischemic bowel resulted in a reduction in fibrinolytic activity and were associated with a significantly higher incidence of adhesion formation. (Adapted from Raftery, 1981a. Reproduced by permission of S. Karger AG.)

was completely abolished and remained suppressed for 24 hours. The unsutured peritoneal defects showed the smallest reduction in fibrinolytic activity and these defects were associated with the lowest incidence of adhesion formation. Free peritoneal grafting, electrocoagulation, and ischemic bowel resulted in a significant reduction in fibrinolytic activity compared with the unsutured defect, and were associated with a significantly higher incidence of adhesion formation. A general correlation was apparent between suppression of peritoneal fibrinolytic activity by abrasion and the extent of subsequent adhesion formation.

These data were confirmed and extended by Buckman, Maj, Buckman, Hufnagel, and Gervin (1976). The fibrinolytic activity of normal peritoneum was compared with the fibrinolytic activity of peritoneal defects or peritoneal grafts (Figure 7.8). Peritoneal grafting inhibited the fibrinolytic activity. In addition, the effect of biopsies of tissue from areas of peritoneal defects or from peritoneal grafts on the fibrinolytic activity of normal peritoneum was examined (Figure 7.9). Incubation of normal peritoneum with a biopsy from a peritoneal defect resulted in significantly elevated fibrinolytic activity. However, a biopsy of a peritoneal graft with normal peritoneum resulted in reduced fibrinolytic activity.

The fibrinolytic activity of human peritoneum, both control and inflamed peritoneum, was recently characterized (Vipond et al., 1990). In

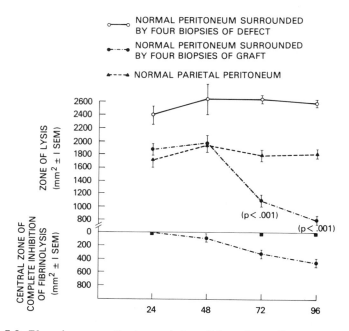

FIGURE 7.8. Plasminogen activator activity of deperitonealized surfaces versus activity of peritoneal grafts. The fibrinolytic activity of a peritoneal defect is similar to the control. However, a peritoneal graft results in reduced fibrinolytic activity. Each point represents the mean of duplicate observations in five animals. (From Buckman et al., 1976. Reproduced by permission of Academic Press.)

this study, antibodies specific for tPA inhibited the activation of fibrinolytic activity by homogenates of human peritoneum. The PA activity of the inflamed peritoneum was much lower than control tissue, which resulted from an increase in PAI-1 production rather than a decrease in tPA antigen (Figure 7.10).

Mesothelial cells from human peritoneum produce tPA along with PAI-1 and PAI-2 (van Hinsbergh, Kooistra, Scheffer, van Bockel, & van Muijen, 1990). PAI-1 antigen was present in the culture medium of mesothelial cells, whereas PAI-2 antigen remained cell-associated. Upon exposure of the mesothelial cultures to TNF, the level of tPA antigen was reduced, whereas levels of both PAI-1 and PAI-2 antigens were elevated. Therefore, inflammatory cytokines, such as TNF, can modulate the fibrinolytic activity of human mesothelial cells. In general, inflammation or surgery suppress intraperitoneal cell-associated or -secreted fibrinolytic activity (Fukasawa et al., 1989; van Hinsbergh et al., 1990).

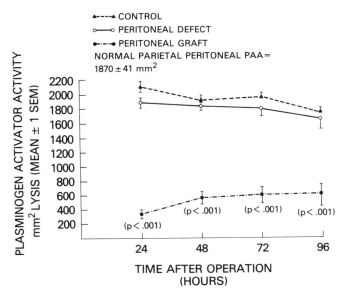

FIGURE 7.9. Inhibition of normal fibrinolysis by biopsies of peritoneal grafts. Deperitonealized surfaces augmented normal fibrinolytic activity. However, peritoneal grafts reduced fibrinolytic activity of normal peritoneum. Each point represents the mean of duplicate observations in five animals. (From Buckman et al., 1976. Reproduced by permission of Academic Press.)

Implications of Fibrinolysis in Peritoneal Surgery

The role of peritoneal fibrinolysis in the removal of fibrin after surgery and the relative suppression of fibrinolysis leading to postsurgical adhesion formation were unified into a testable hypothesis by Buckman et al. (1976). They found that plasminogen activator activity in rat cecal peritoneum was suppressed for 48 hours and 96 hours after crush and abrasion injuries, respectively. Plasminogen activator activity was more severely suppressed after ischemia produced by an avascular graft (Figures 7.8 and 7.9). This suppression persisted for the entire 96-hour study interval although partial recovery became measurable after 48 hours.

Bleeding can be associated with increased fibrinolysis. Bleeding complications during surgery are often associated with hyperfibrinolysis (Macfarlane, 1937) perhaps involving catecholamines (Britton, Giddings, Brooks, & Bloom, 1977). Some investigators reported that stress and anesthesia can activate the fibrinolytic system (Engqvest & Winther, 1972; Pike, Turner, Manohitharajah, & Deverall, 1975). In addition, there is a normal diurnal alteration in fibrinolytic activity in the blood (Korsan-Bengtsen, Wilhelmsen, & Tibblin, 1973). In patients that develop throm-

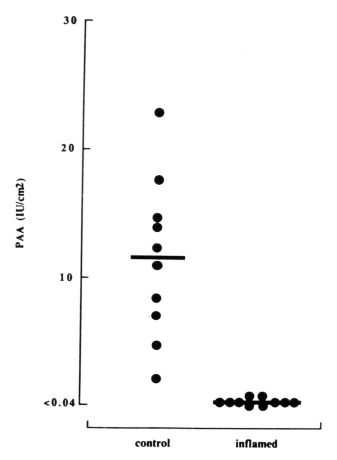

FIGURE 7.10. Plasminogen activating activity (PAA) of control and inflamed human peritoneum. The level of PAA is decreased in inflamed peritoneum. This decrease may result from increased levels of PAI-1 (see Figure 7.2). (From Vipond et al., 1990. Reproduced by permission of Lancet.)

bosis, PA antigen does not decrease but inhibitor activity increases, lasting 7 to 10 days. The significance of this increased inhibitory activity is a risk for thrombotic complications and adhesion formation.

Certain surgical procedures within the peritoneum are more likely to result in excessive bleeding due to activation of fibrinolysis. These include surgery to organs rich in PA, such as pancreas, or extensive surgery to the liver. Studies by Hau et al. (1979) showed that surgery alone partially inhibited fibrinolytic activity in the peritoneal cavity. However, induction of fibrinopurulent peritonitis by the creation of an ischemic portion of the ileum abolished fibrinolytic activity almost completely. Since peritoneal infection is known to lead to adhesion formation, these data are consistent with the finding that adhesion formation is inversely correlated with fibrinolytic activity. To reduce the risk of hemorrhage during or after surgery, antifibrinolytic therapy may be instituted (Andersson, 1964; Hedlund, 1969).

On the other hand, thrombosis and adhesion formation are complications that are due to a relative reduction in fibrinolytic activity after surgery. Excess fibrin deposition that is not resolved can lead to the formation of adhesions (Figure 7.11). Dextran, which facilitates fibrinolysis, was shown to suppress adhesion formation (Wallenbeck & Tangen, 1975; Markwardt & Klocking, 1977; Jespersen & Astrup 1983; Mayer et al., 1988). Further, intraperitoneal administration of recombinant tPA reduces adhesion formation in animal models. Tolmetin, a nonsteroidal anti-inflammatory drug that prevents adhesion formation in animal models, elevates the fibrinolytic activity of the peritoneum in traumatized animals and reduces PA-inhibitory activity in early postsurgical peritoneal fluid (further discussed in Chapter 10).

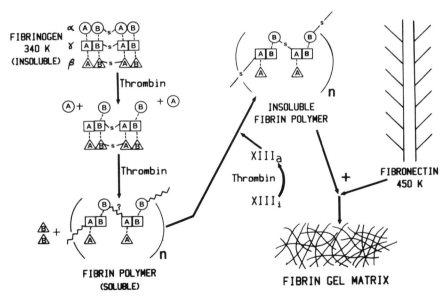

FIGURE 7.11. Schematic representation of fibrin gel matrix formation. Insoluble fibrinogen deposited on the surface of injured peritoneum interacts with thrombin to become the soluble polymer fibrin, which is further modified to an insoluble form. Together with fibronectin, the insoluble fibrin polymer and cellular debris form the fibrin gel matrix, which provides the scaffolding for intraperitoneal adhesion formation.

Several studies were conducted on the effects of tolmetin on protease activity in macrophage conditioned medium and lavage fluid from rabbits that had undergone peritoneal surgery (Rodgers, 1990; Abe et al., 1990; Rodgers et al., in press). In vitro exposure of postsurgical macrophages to tolmetin suppressed collagenase and elevated elastase activities at early time points after surgery (Rodgers, 1990). The level of PA inhibitory activity was reduced either through in vitro exposure of postsurgical macrophages to tolmetin or exposure of cell-free culture media from postsurgical macrophages to tolmetin. These latter data were confirmed by addition of tolmetin to postsurgical peritoneal lavage fluid. This inhibition of PA inhibitor activity may allow increased PA activity and hence, increased fibrinolysis. In vivo administration of tolmetin to rats after surgical trauma increased the level of fibrinolytic activity of the injured peritoneum in an in vitro assay. These data suggest that tolmetin can alter the protease–protease inhibitor balance such that increased fibrinolysis is possible at early postsurgical time points.

Summary

The balance between coagulation and fibrinolysis is required to maintain homeostasis. Although fibrin deposition after peritoneal surgery is necessary for hemostasis and tissue repair, fibrin resolution is necessary for the return of preoperative conditions. The fibrinolytic system is under tight control, both at the level of plasmin formation from plasminogen by PA and the inhibition of plasmin and PA activities by inhibitors. Thus, multiple modes of control interplay to regulate fibrinolysis. Bleeding can be a complication of increased fibrinolysis that may occur through an enhanced conversion of plasminogen to plasmin, a facilitated availability of plasmin for substrate, or a reduction in PA inhibitor production. Conversely, thrombosis can be the result of reduced fibrinolysis. Persistence of fibrin or enhanced fibrin deposition on surfaces of damaged peritoneum that opposes an adjacent peritoneal surface leads to adhesion formation.

References

Abe H, Rodgers KE, Campeau JD, Girgis W, Ellefson D, diZerega GS. (1990). The effect of intraperitoneal administration of sodium tolmetin-hyaluronic acid on the postsurgical cell infiltration in vivo. *J Surg Res.* 49:322–327.

Albrechtsen OK. (1956). The fibrinolytic activity of the human endometrium. *Acta Endocrinol.* 23:207–218.

Albrechtsen OK. (1957a). The fibrinolytic activity of human tissues. *Br J Haematol.* 3:284–291.

Albrechtsen OK. (1957b). The fibrinolytic activity of animal tissues. *Acta Physiol Scand.* 39:284–290.

Andersson L, Nilsson IM, Olow B. (1962). Fibrinolytic activity in man during surgery. *Thromb Diath Haemorrh.* 7:392–403.

Andersson L. (1964). Antifibrinolytic treatment with epsilon-amino-caproic acid in connection with prostatectomy. *Acta Chir Scand.* 127:552–559.

Astrup T, Albrechtsen OK. (1957). Estimation of the plasminogen activator and the trypsin inhibitor in animal and human tissues. *Scand J Clin Lab Invest.* 9:233–243.

Astrup T, Albrechtsen OK, Claassen M, Rasmussen J. (1959). Thromboplastic and fibrinolytic activity of human aorta. *Circ Res.* 7:969–974.

Astrup T, Claassen M. (1957). Fibrinolytic activity of the peritoneum. Trans. 6th Congr. European Soc. Haematol., Copenhagen. Basel; Karger; 455–459.

Bauer KA, ten Cate H, Barzegar S, Spriggs DR, Sherman ML, Rosenberg RD. (1989). Tumor necrosis factor infusions have a procoagulant effect on the hemostatic mechanism of humans. *Blood.* 74:165–177.

Booth NA, Anderson JA, Bennett B. (1985). Platelet release protein which inhibits plasminogen activators. *J Clin Pathol.* 38:825–830.

Brandtzaeg P, Joo GB, Brusletto B, Kierulf P. (1990). Plasminogen activator inhibitor 1 and 2, α_2-antiplasmin, plasminogen, and endotoxin levels in systemic meningococcal disease. *Thromb Res.* 57:271–275.

Britton BJ, Giddings JC, Brooks L, Bloom AL. (1977). Fibrinolytic, factor VIII and pulse rate responses to repeated adrenaline infusion followed by haemorrhagia. *Thromb Haemost.* 37:527–534.

Buckman RF Jr., Maj MC, Buckman PD, Hufnagel HV, Gervin AS. (1976). A physiologic basis for the adhesion-free healing of deperitonealized surfaces. *J Surg Res.* 21:67–76.

Chakrabarti R, Hocking ED, Fearnley GR. (1969). Reaction pattern to three stresses—electroplexy, surgery and myocardial infarction—of fibrinolysis and plasma fibrinogen. *J Clin Pathol.* 22:659–662.

Chapman HA Jr, Stone OL, Vavrin Z. (1984). Degradation of fibrin and elastin by intact human alveolar macrophages in vitro. Characterization of a plasminogen activator and its role in matrix degradation. *J Clin Invest.* 73:806–815.

Coccheri S, Astrup T. (1961). Thromboplastic and fibrinolytic activities of large human vessels. *Proc Soc Exp Biol Med.* 108:369–372.

Dastre A. (1893). Fibrinolyse dans le sang. *Arch Physiol Norm Pathol.* 5:661–663.

Deutsch DG, Mertz ET. (1970). Plasminogen purification from human plasma by affinity chromatography. *Science.* 170:1095–1096.

Donse AM, Dupuy E, Bodevin E. (1978). Production of a fibrinolytic inhibitor by cultured endothelial cells derived from human umbilical vein. *Thromb Res.* 12:377–387.

Doody KJ, Dunn RC, Buttram VC. (1989). Recombinant tissue plasminogen activator reduces adhesion formation in a rabbit uterine horn model. *Fertil Steril.* 51:509–512.

Ellis H, Harrison W, Hugh TB. (1965). The healing of peritoneum under normal and pathologic conditions. *Br J Surg.* 52:471–476.

Emeis JJ, Van Hinsbergh VWM, Verheijen JH, Wijngaards G. (1983). Inhibition of tissue-type plasminogen activator by conditioned medium from cultured human and porcine vascular endothelial cells. *Biochem Biophys Res Commun.* 110:392–398.

Ende N, Auditore J. (1961). Fibrinolytic activity of human tissues and dog mast cell tumors. *Am J Clin Pathol.* 36:16–24.

Engqvist A, Winther O. (1972). Variations of plasma cortisol and blood fibrinolytic activity during anaesthetic and surgical stress. *Br J Anaesth.* 44:1291–1297.

Erickson LA, Ginsberg MH, Loskutoff DJ. (1984). Detection and partial characterization of an inhibitor of plasminogen activator in human platelets. *J Clin Invest.* 74:1465–1472.

Esnard F, Dupuy E, Dosne AM, Bodevin E. (1982). Partial characterization of a fibrinolytic inhibitor produced by cultured endothelial cells derived from human umbilical vein. *Thromb Haemost.* 47:128–131.

Fukasawa M, Campeau JD, Girgis W, Bryant SW, Rodgers KE, diZerega GS. (1989). Production of protease inhibitors by postsurgical macrophages. *J Surg Res.* 46:256–261.

Gervin AS, Puckett CL, Silver D. (1973). Serosal hypofibrinolysis. A cause of postoperative adhesions. *Am J Surg.* 125:80–88.

Grossbard EB. (1987). Recombinant tissue plasminogen activator: a brief review. *Pharmacol Res.* 4:375–378.

Hau T, Payne D, Simmons RL. (1979). Fibrinolytic activity of the peritoneum during experimental peritonitis. *Surg Gynecol Obstet.* 148:415–418.

Hedlund PO. (1969). Antifibrinolytic therapy with cyklokapron in connection with prostatectomy. *Scand J Urol Nephrol.* 3:177–182.

Innes D, Sevitt S. (1974). Coagulation and fibrinolysis in injured patients. *J Clin Pathol.* 17:1–13.

Jespersen J, Astrup TA. (1983). Study of the fibrin plate assay of fibrinolytic agents. *Haemostasis.* 13:301–315.

Korsan-Bengtsen K, Wilhelmsen L, Tibblin G. (1973). Blood coagulation and fibrinolysis in relation to degree of physical activity during work and leisure time. *Acta Med Scand.* 193:73–77.

Kruithof EKO, Tran-Thang C, Ransijn A, Backmann F. (1984). Demonstration of a fast-acting inhibitor of plasminogen activators in human plasma. *Blood.* 64:907–913.

Laug WE. (1985). Vascular smooth muscle cells inhibit plasminogen activator secreted by endothelial cells. *Thromb Haemost.* 53:165–169.

Levin EG. (1983). Latent tissue plasminogen activator produced by human endothelial cells in culture: evidence for an enzyme-inhibitor complex. *Proc Natl Acad Sci USA.* 80:6804–6808.

Loskutoff DJ, Van Mourik JA, Erickson LA, Lawrence D. (1983). Detection of an unusually stable fibrinolytic inhibitor produced by bovine endothelial cells. *Proc Natl Acad Sci USA.* 80:2956–2961.

Macfarlane RG. (1937). Fibrinolysis following operation. *Lancet.* 1:10.

Markwardt F, Klocking HP. (1977). Heparin-induced release of plasminogen activator. *Haemostasis.* 6:370–374.

Mayer M, Yedgar S, Hurwitz A, Palti Z, Finzi Z, Milwidsky A. (1988). Effect of viscous macromolecules on peritoneal plasminogen activator activity: potential mechanism for their ability to reduce postoperative adhesion formation. *Am J Obstet Gynecol.* 159:957–963.

Menzies D, Ellis H. (1989). Intra-abdominal adhesions and their prevention by topical tissue plasminogen activator. *J R Soc Med.* 82:534–535.

Merlo G, Fausone G, Barbero C, Castagna B. (1980). Fibrinolytic activity of the human peritoneum. *Eur Surg Res.* 12:433–438.

Moroz LA, Gilmore NJ. (1976). Fibrinolysis in normal plasma and blood: evidence for significant mechanisms independent of the plasminogen-plasmin system. *Blood.* 48:531–545.

Myhre-Jensen O, Larsen SB, Astrup T. (1969). Fibrinolytic activity in serosal and synovial membranes. *Arch Pathol.* 88:623–630.

Nilsson IM, Pandolfi M. (1970). Fibrinolytic response of the vascular wall. *Thromb Diath Haemorrh Suppl.* 40:231–242.

Ny T, Bjersing L, Hsuek AJW, Loskutoff DJ. (1985). Cultured granulosa cells produce two plasminogen activators and an antiactivator, each regulated differently by gonadotropins. *Endocrinology.* 116:1666–1668.

Orita H, Girgis W, diZerega GS. (1991). Inhibition of postsurgical adhesions in a standardized rabbit model: intraperitoneal administration of tissue plasminogen activator. *Int J Fert.* 36:172–177.

Philips M, Juul AG, Thorsen S. (1984). Human endothelial cells produce a plasminogen activator inhibitor and a tissue-type plasminogen activator-inhibitor complex. *Biochim Biophys Acta.* 802:99–110.

Pike GJ, Turner RL, Manohitharajah SM, Deverall PB. (1975). Fibrinolysis in cyanotic and acyanotic children before and after open intracardiac operations with the Bentley temptrol oxygenator. *J Thorac Cardiovosc. Surg.* 69:922–926.

Porter JM, McGregor FH, Mullen DC, Silver D. (1969). Fibrinolytic activity of mesothelial surfaces. *Surg Forum.* 20:80–82.

Porter JM, Ball AP, Silver D. (1971). Mesothelial fibrinolysis. *J Thorac Cardiovasc Surg.* 62:725–730.

Pugatch EM, Poole JC. (1969). Inhibitor of fibrinolysis from mesothelium. *Nature.* 221:269–270.

Raftery AT. (1979). Regeneration of peritoneum: a fibrinolytic study. *J Anat.* 129:659–664.

Raftery AT. (1981a). Effect of peritoneal trauma on peritoneal fibrinolytic activity and intraperitoneal adhesion formation. *Eur Surg Res.* 13:397–401.

Raftery AT. (1981b). A method for measuring fibrinolytic activity in a single layer of cells. *J Clin Pathol.* 34:625–629.

Ratnoff OD. (1953). Studies on a proteolytic enzyme in human plasma. IX. Fibrinogen and fibrin as substrated for the proteolytic enzyme of plasma. *J Clin Invest.* 32:473–479.

Rennie JAN, Bennett B, Ogston D. (1977). Effect of local exercise and vessel occlusion on fibrinolytic activity. *J Clin Pathol.* 30:350–352.

Rodgers KE. (1990). Nonsteroidal anti-inflammatory drugs (NSAIDs) in the treatment of postsurgical adhesion. In: diZerega GS, Malinak LR, Diamond MD, Linsky CL, eds. *Treatment of Postsurgical Adhesions* (Progress in Clin Biol Res). New York: Wiley-Liss Press; 358:119–130.

Rodgers KE, Abe H, Campeau JD, Ellefson DD, Girgis W, diZerega GS. (in press). In vivo administration of tolmetin in hyaluronic acid modulates protease secretion by postsurgical macrophages. *J Invest Surg.*

Ryan GB, Grobety J, Majno G. (1973). Mesothelial injury and recovery. *Am J Pathol.* 71:93–112.

Silverman P, Goldsmith GH Jr., Spitzer TR, Rehmus EH, Berger NA. (1990). Effect of tumor necrosis factor on the human fibrinolytic system. *J Clin Oncol.* 8:468–472.

Sprengers ED, Verheijen JH, Van Hinsbergh VWM, Emeis JJ. (1984). Evidence for the presence of two different fibrinolytic inhibitors in human endothelial cell conditioned medium. *Biochim Biophys Acta.* 801:163–170.

Thorsen S, Philips M. (1984). Isolation of tissue-type plasminogen activator-inhibitor complexes from human plasma. Evidence for a rapid plasminogen activator inhibitor. *Biochim Biophys Acta.* 802:111–118.

Todd AS. (1958). Fibrinolysis autographs. *Nature.* 181:495–496.

Todd AS. (1959). The histological localisation of fibrinolysis activator. *J Pathol Bacteriol.* 78:281–283.

Unkeless JC, Gordon S, Reich S. (1974). Secretion of plasminogen activator by stimulated macrophages. *J Exp Med.* 139:834–850.

van der Poll T, Levi M, Buller HR, van Deventer SJA, de Boer JP, Hack CE, ten Cate JW. (1991). Fibrinolytic response to tumor necrosis factor in healthy subjects. *J Exp Med.* 175:729–732.

van Hinsbergh VWM, Kooistra T, Scheffer MA, van Bockel JH, van Muijen GNP. (1990). Characterization and fibrinolytic properties of human omental tissue mesothelial cells. Comparison with endothelial cells. *Blood.* 75:1490–1497.

Vipond MN, Whawell SA, Thompson JN, Dudley HAF. (1990). Peritoneal fibrinolytic activity and intra-abdominal adhesions. *Lancet.* 335:1120–1122.

Wallenbeck IAM, Tangen O. (1975). On the lysis of fibrin formed in the presence of dextran and other macromolecules. *Thromb Res.* 6:75–86.

Whitaker D, Papadimitriou JM, Walters N-I. (1982). The mesothelium: its fibrinolytic properties. *J Pathol.* 136:295–299.

8

Proteinases and
Proteinase Inhibitors

THE PERITONEAL CAVITY IS WELL ENDOWED WITH PROTEINASES BOTH
in the parietal and viseral peritoneum as well as in the peritoneal fluid.
Proteinases have a major role in activating and modulating the complement, coagulation, kinin, fibrinolytic, and extracellular matrix remodeling
systems, and thus are critical components of the peritoneal response to
inflammation and tissue injury. Inflammation or trauma initiate proteinase release from a number of cells, including neutrophils, platelets,
and macrophages. Proteinase inhibitor proteins are part of the regulatory
mechanisms controlling the activity of proteolytic enzymes. Like proteinases, inhibitor proteins are ubiquitous, making up 10% of the total
proteins in human plasma. Most inhibitors are relatively specific for a
particular proteinase. The balance of activity between proteinases and
proteinase inhibitors contributes to the final resolution of fibrin after
tissue injury. This chapter summarizes information on proteinases and
proteinase inhibitors that are implicated in peritoneal response to injury.

Fibrinolytic System

Plasmin

As was discussed more extensively in Chapter 7, fibrinolysis, which represents the end stage of coagulation, was defined by Dastre in 1893 as
the dissolution of polymerized fibrin. Plasmin, the major enzyme involved in fibrinolysis, is formed from the inactive precursor, plasminogen, by the action of plasminogen activators (PA). Proteolytic enzymes
other than plasmin can be involved in fibrinolysis (Moroz & Gilmore,
1976). Fibrin is the major substrate for plasmin, although fibrinogen can
be cleaved in vitro (Ratnoff, 1953). Plasmin can also digest coagulation
factors II, V, and VIII, glucagon, ACTH, and growth hormone. Plasmin
can interfere with the complement and kinin systems.

    The formation of fibrin is part of a hemostatic process by which the extravasation of blood after an injury is prevented. Fibrin also aids in tissue repair by becoming a matrix for migrating fibroblasts and the formation of connective tissue. Thus, the processes by which the formation and resolution of fibrin occur have important physiologic and clinical significance. Deposition of fibrin is a prerequisite for normal tissue repair, but the ultimate removal and resolution of the deposit is necessary for the reestablishment of presurgical conditions (further discussed in Chapter 7). Disturbance of this balance can occur through modulation in the rate of fibrin deposition or the rate of fibrinolysis through changes in the levels of fibrinolytic enzymes or inhibitors of these enzyme. Surgery or bacterial peritonitis can disrupt the balance between coagulation and fibrinolysis, thus leaving excess polymerized fibrin in the peritoneal cavity. This excess fibrin then provides the scaffold upon which adhesions are formed (Ellis, Harrison, & Hugh, 1965; Hau, Payne, & Simmons, 1979; Raftery 1979).

Plasminogen Activator

Plasminogen is a β-globulin with a molecular weight of 85 kd that is present at concentrations between 0.2 and 0.3 g/L in plasma (Deutsch & Mertz 1970). Plasminogen is activated to plasmin via agents appropriately called activators, which involves conformational changes and cleavage of peptide bonds at the Arg-Val bond near the carboxyl terminus and a disulfide bond between two peptide fragments. Individual components of the fibrinolytic system are summarized in Chapter 7. Two biochemically and immunologically distinct forms of plasminogen activator are known—tissue plasminogen activator (tPA) and urokinase (urine-derived) plasminogen activator (uPA), which are the products of separate genes. Multiple molecular forms of these activators, consisting of single- and two-chain versions, exist in the plasma. tPA and uPA are secreted by a variety of cell types and tissues under many physiologic conditions. The tissue distribution of fibrinolytic activity is discussed later in this chapter and more fully in Chapter 7.

Tissue PA specifically binds to fibrin and its activity is enhanced. This unique characteristic allows tPA to be an effective therapeutic agent, even after systemic administration. Recombinant tPA is being used to treat coronary thrombosis following acute myocardial infarction (Grossbard, 1987). Research as to the utility of recombinant tPA in the prevention of peritoneal adhesions is reviewed in Chapter 10 (Doody, Dunn, & Buttram, 1989; Menzies & Ellis, 1989; Orita, Girgis, & diZerega, 1991). Release of tPA can be provoked by venous occlusion, trauma, surgery, and stress (Andersson, Nilsson, & Olow, 1962; Chakrabarti, Hocking, & Fearnley, 1969; Engqvist & Winther, 1972; Innes & Sevitt, 1974; Nilsson & Pandolfi, 1970; Rennie, Bennett, & Ogston, 1977). Inflammatory cytokines, catecholamines and corticosteroids are capable of modulating the secretion of tPA by a variety of cell types.

Urokinase is a PA produced by the kidneys and peritoneal macrophages that also contain receptors for uPA and therefore are able to bind uPA as it is produced. Since macrophages degrade fibrin and elastin only in the presence of plasminogen and membrane-bound PA is relatively resistant to inactivation by soluble proteinase inhibitors, it is believed that cell surface proteases are involved in the degradation of matrix by macrophages.

Peritoneal trauma, including that resulting from abrasion and ischemia, is associated with a depression of local fibrinolytic activity (Figure 8.1). Plasminogen activator activity (PAA) of both parietal (Figure 8.2) and serosal (Figure 8.3) peritoneum is depressed following peritoneal trauma or ischemia (e.g., Thompson et al., 1989; Vipond, Whawell, Thompson, & Dudley, 1990), and depression of PAA may be the principal factor resulting in postsurgical intraperitoneal adhesion formation (Menzies & Ellis, 1989; discussed further in Chapter 7). Supporting this hypothesis are experimental findings of diminished intraperitoneal adhesion formation after topical administration of recombinant tissue plasminogen activator at the surgical site (Doody et al., 1989; Menzies & Ellis, 1989; Orita et al., 1991).

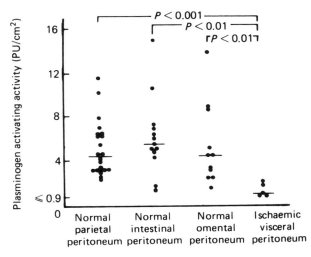

FIGURE 8.1. The plasminogen activating activity of normal parietal, intestinal (including appendix), and omental peritoneum compared with ischemic visceral peritoneum (bars show median values). The activities are shown in Plough units (PU) compared to a standard. Ischemia reduces the fibrinolytic activity of visceral peritoneum. (From Thompson et al., 1989. Reproduced by permission of Butterworth Scientific.)

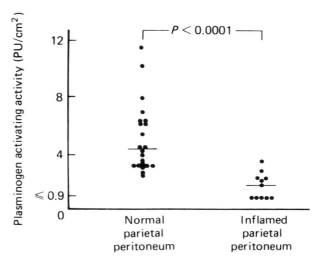

FIGURE 8.2. The plasminogen activating activity of normal and inflamed parietal peritoneum (bars show median values). Inflammation reduces the fibrinolytic activity of parietal peritoneum. (From Thompson et al., 1989. Reproduced by permission of Butterworth Scientific.)

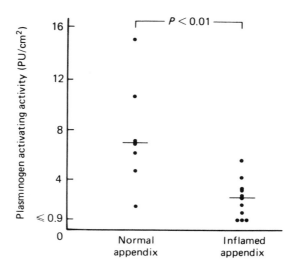

FIGURE 8.3. The plasminogen activating activity of normal and inflamed appendix serosa (bars show median values). Inflammation reduces the fibrinolytic activity of visceral peritoneum. (From Thompson et al., 1989. Reproduced by permission of Butterworth Scientific.)

Plasminogen Activator Gene

Tissue PA produced by endothelial cells has a high specific binding affinity for fibrin, whereas uPA does not. uPA binds to a variety of cells, including monocytes and human epidermoid carcinoma cells. Specific binding of uPA to the cell may be important in localizing proteolysis (i.e., plasmin activity) to the cell surface in much the same way that tPA binding to fibrin localizes fibrinolytic activity.

The uPA gene was isolated and its nucleotide sequence identified for the mouse, human, and pig (Degen, Heckel, Reich, & Degen, 1987; Riccio, Grimaldi, & Verde, 1985; Nagamine, Pearson, Altus, & Reich, 1984, respectively). The uPA genes from these three species are remarkably similar in that their exon size, nucleotide sequence, corresponding amino acid sequence, and the localization of intervening sequences with respect to nucleotide and amino acid sequence are highly conserved between the species. Furthermore, the level of intron sequence identity approaches that of the exon sequence identity in the three species when one excludes recognizable repetitive DNA sequences. All three genes are relatively small, between 5,852 base pairs (porcine) and 6,710 base pairs (murine). The exon sequences compose between 34.7% (murine) and 40.8% (porcine) of the gene. Table 8.1 compares the murine, human, and porcine uPA genes.

Plasminogen Activator Secretion

Fibroblasts

Human synovial fibroblasts produce uPA (Hamilton & Slywka, 1981; Medcalf & Hamilton, 1986) and uPA is elevated in rheumatoid synovial fluid (Mochan & Uhl, 1984). Leizer and Hamilton (1989) demonstrated the presence of a novel monokine (Mr of 25,000 to 34,000), which they termed synovial activator, in media conditioned by synovial mononuclear cells. This synovial activator stimulated secretion of uPA but not prostaglandin E_2. Moreover, this monokine was distinguished from other cytokines found in the conditioned media (i.e., interleukin-1α, interleukin-1β, and tissue necrosis factor-α) by immunologic, biochemical, and functional criteria.

Endothelial Cells

Endothelial cells are thought to be a major source of plasminogen activator. Endothelial cells producing plasminogen activator differ in their levels of expression and the molecular forms of plasminogen activator they produce. Macro- and microvascular endothelial cells from the renal circulation were shown to produce only high levels of single-chain uPA, whereas omental microvascular and umbilical vein endothelial cells produced tPA almost exclusively (Table 8.2; Wojta, Hoover, & Daniel, 1989).

TABLE 8.1. Comparison of the murine, human, and porcine uPA genes.

	Size (bp)			Sequence identity (%)			
				Mouse/Human		Porcine/ Human	
Exon/intron	Mouse	Human	Porcine	DNA	Protein	DNA	Protein
Exon							
1	71	88	85	55.7	—[a]	55.7	—[a]
2	87	88	88	71.6	52.6	85.2	78.9
3	31	28	34	32.3	20.0	67.6	54.5
4	108	108	108	79.6	69.4	88.9	77.8
5	175	175	175	82.3	72.9	85.1	83.1
6	92	92	119	84.8	73.3	84.8[b]	83.3[k]
7	223	220	220	74.4	70.7	87.3	85.1
8	149	149	149	71.8	63.3	81.2	77.6
9	141	141	141	77.3	74.0	80.1	68.1
10	1,102	1,106	1,119	69.1	75.9	77.3	79.3
Total exon	2,328	2,344	2,387				
Intron							
1	318 (-)[c]	306 (-)	329 (-)	55.9		64.2	
2	484 (0)	417 (0)	452 (0)	56.4[d]		68.6	
3	137 (I)	146 (I)	157 (I)	66.2		62.4	
4	626 (I)	603 (I)	329 (I)	57.8[e,f]		65.3[f]	
5	396 (II)	193 (II)	187 (II)	66.3[g]		71.7	
6	143 (I)	157 (I)	161 (I)	63.1		49.4	
7	220 (II)	221 (II)	225 (II)	63.3		71.1	
8	574 (I)	666 (I)	644 (I)	58.8		63.4	
9	306 (I)	346 (I)	326 (I)	59.4		65.0	
10	1,178 (0)	989 (0)	655 (0)	57.8[h,i]		71.2[i]	
Total intron	4,382	4,044	3,465				
Total[j]	6,710	6,388	5,852				

[a]Exon is entirely noncoding.

[b]Calculated omitting the 27-nucleotide/9 amino acid segment unique to porcine exon 6.

[c]Roman numerals in parentheses indicate intron placement; -, introns occurring within noncoding sequence; 0, between codons; I, between the first and second nucleotides of a codon; II, between the second and third nucleotides of a codon.

[d]Calculated omitting nucleotides 801–858 of the mouse gene that contain the repeat $(AG)_{29}$.

[e]Calculated omitting nucleotides 1,428–1,745 of the mouse gene that contain a B2 family repeat and the repeat $(AC)_{21}$.

[f]Calculated omitting nucleotides 1,429–1,736 of the human gene that contain an Alu family repeat.

[g]Calculated omitting nucleotides 2,075–2,281 of the mouse gene that contain a B2 family repeat.

[h]Calculated omitting nucleotides 4,686–5,223 of the mouse gene that contain a B1 family repeat and the NE sequence.

[i]Calculated omitting nucleotides 4,853–5,159 of the human gene that contain an Alu family repeat.

[j]Total size of gene from transcription initiation site to polyadenylation site.

Adapted from Frizner Degen et al., 1987.

TABLE 8.2. uPA and tPA antigen in serum-free media conditioned for 24 hours by various human endothelial cell types.

Human endothelial cell type	Antigen in conditioned media (ng/10⁵)[a]	
	uPA	tPA
Renal microvascular	60.48	0.96
Renal artery	50.42	5.27
Omental microvascular	<1.50[b]	8.80
Umbilical Vein	<1.50[b]	2.17

[a]Values represent mean of three experiments, each done in triplicate.
[b]Below limit of detection.
Adapted from Wojta et al., 1989.

Other researchers demonstrated production of a single-chain uPA by non-renal endothelial cells under certain conditions. In characterizing the single-chain uPA produced by subcultured human umbilical vein endothelial cells, Booyse, Lin, Traylor, & Bruce (1988) noted that the uPA produced by these subcultured cells was similar to that isolated in urine.

The ability of tPA, urinary two-chain uPA, and single-chain uPA derived from human umbilical vein endothelial cells to bind to fibrin clots was evaluated in vitro (Booyse et al., 1988). Only a low level of binding (5% to 20%) was observed with either form of uPA. In contrast, a high level of binding (>80%) was evident with tPA. Thus, it appears that endothelial cell fibrinolysis is triggered primarily by tPA (Figure 8.4). The role of uPA in endothelial cell function has not yet been elucidated, although it may play a primary role in the initiation and modulation of biological processes requiring extracellular proteolysis, such as maintenance of ad luminal antithrombogenicity.

In addition to expressing plasminogen activators, endothelial cells also express a plasminogen activator inhibitor (PAI). Although at least three distinct forms of these inhibitors are known, endothelial cells express primarily one version—PAI-1. PAI-1 inhibits both tPA and uPA and is the predominant PAI of unstimulated endothelial cells. In one series of experiments, unstimulated, cultured human umbilical vein endothelial cells were shown to contain approximately 670 PAI-1 mRNA molecules/cell whereas another plasminogen activator inhibitor, PAI-2, was not detectable (Scarpati & Sadler, 1989). Coordinated regulation of the various PAI proteins may promote the fibrin deposition that accompanies inflammation (Scarpati & Sadler, 1989).

Urokinase was shown to be chemotactic for polymorphonuclear leukocytes in the concentration range of 2×10^{-13} to 2×10^{-15} mol/L when injected into the air sac on the backs of mice (Boyle, Chiodo, Lawman, Gee, & Young, 1987). Interestingly, higher concentrations of urokinase did not induce a chemotactic response. The chemotactic effect of urokinase is in part dependent upon its serine protease activity.

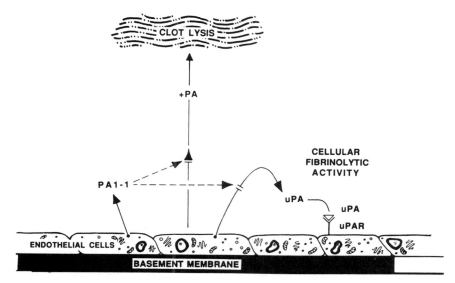

FIGURE 8.4. Currently, tPA is thought to be involved in the clot lysis in the fluid phase, and uPA, through binding to a cellular receptor for uPA, is thought to mediate cell-associated clot lysis. uPAR, uPA receptor.

Postsurgical Cells

Macrophages are the most common cell in the exudative fluid following peritoneal insult and in critical components of the tissue repair process (see Chapter 6). The ability of macrophages to secrete plasminogen activator is well recognized (e.g., Unkeless, Dano, Kellerman, & Reich, 1974; Furman & Schnyder, 1984). Interestingly, macrophages secrete protease inhibitors, such as alpha$_2$-macroglobulin (e.g., Klimetsek & Sorg, 1979; Wohlwend, Belin, & Vassalli, 1987). Fukasawa and colleagues (1989) evaluated the synthesis and secretion of plasminogen activator and protease inhibitors by macrophages harvested at various times following ileal resection and reanastomosis in the rabbit. Intracellular plasminogen activator activity of postsurgical macrophages on days 1 to 3 was significantly less than that of resident (i.e., nonsurgical) macrophages (Figure 8.5). By day 7, PAA of postsurgical macrophages had returned to resident levels. The PAA of the macrophages was shown via electrophoretic analysis to be of the urokinase type. Media conditioned from postsurgical macrophages inhibited uPA; this inhibition was most potent from conditioned media derived from macrophages on postsurgical days 1 to 3 (Figure 8.6). This same pattern of results, namely diminished PAA initially after peritoneal insult with a gradual return to nonsurgical cell levels by day 7, was also described for macrophages obtained from rabbits following bowel resection and reanastomosis (Orita, Campeau, Gale, Nakamura, & diZerega, 1986). Through their ability to both inhibit and

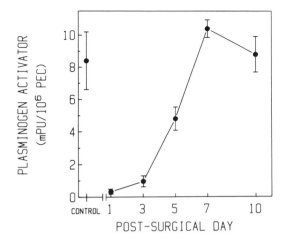

FIGURE 8.5. Plasminogen activator (PA) activity is cytosol of postsurgical macrophages recovered from the peritoneum of rabbits at various days after surgery. PA activity of supernatant was determined in sonicates after centrifugation. On days 1 to 3 after surgery, the plasminogen activator activity of postsurgical macrophages was significantly less than that of nonsurgical macrophages. Each data point represents the mean ± SEM of 8 to 12 samples. PEC, peritoneal exudate cells. (From Fukasawa et al., 1989. Reproduced by permission of Academic Press.)

stimulate plasmin formation and activity, macrophages directly modulate fibrinolytic activity during peritoneal re-epithelialization following tissue insult or trauma.

Summary

The fibrinolytic system includes several components. Plasminogen is activated via PA to plasmin. uPA and tPA are the products of two genes and are secreted by a variety of cell types including postsurgical peritoneal macrophages. Peritoneal trauma can diminish PA activity and this depression may, in turn, contribute to intraperitoneal thrombogenic events including fibrin deposition and adhesion formation.

Inhibitors of Fibrinolysis

The fibrinolytic balance is regulated at many stages including inhibition of both PA and plasmin by specific and nonspecific protease inhibitors. Blood contains at least three kinds of plasmin inhibitors. Alpha$_2$-macroglobulin is a nonspecific proteinase inhibitor that can rapidly inhibit plasmin along with other proteases and growth factors. Another inhibitor of plasmin is slow reacting alpha$_1$-antitrypsin. However, alpha$_2$-antiplas-

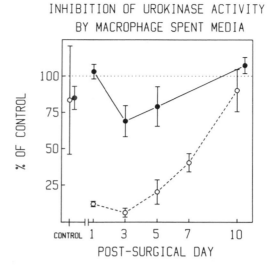

FIGURE 8.6. Plasminogen activator inhibitor activity in macrophage-conditioned media. Standard urokinase (UK; 12.5 mPU/ml final concentration) was incubated with the macrophage-conditioned media and the remaining UK activity was determined (○, without acid treatment, ●, after acid treatment). Data are expressed as percentage activity of control. Each point represents the mean ± SEM. (From Fukasawa et al., 1989. Reproduced by permission of Academic Press.)

min, which is a specific inhibitor of plasmin, is probably the most important inhibitor of plasmin activity in vivo.

Inhibitors of PA are released by a variety of cells including platelets (PAI-1), macrophages (PAI-2), and endothelial cells (PAI-1) (Dosne, Dupuy, & Bodevin, 1978; Esnard, Dupuy, Dosne, & Bodevin, 1982; Emeis, Van Hinsbergh, Verheijen, & Wijngaards, 1983; Levin, 1983; Loskutoff, Van Movrik, Erickson, & Lawrence, 1983; Erickson, Ginsberg, & Loskutoff, 1984; Philips, Juul, & Thorsen, 1984; Sprengers, Verheijen, Van Hinsbergh, & Emeis, 1984; Booth, Anderson & Bennett, 1985; Laug, 1985; Ny, Bjersing, Hsuek, & Loskutoff, 1985). PAI-1 is synthesized in an active form but is rapidly inactivated in vitro through alterations in folding of the protein. PAI-2 was originally isolated from human placenta, but was subsequently found to be produced by macrophages that are present in the placenta. PAI-2 is an inhibitor of both high and low molecular weight uPA, and tPA, especially two-chain tPA. Protease nexin I is an inhibitor with broad specificity that includes uPA, tPA and plasmin. This protein was originally identified as a substance that produces a link between thrombin or plasminogen activator and normal human fibroblasts, hence the term *nexin* (from the Latin *nexes,* meaning a tying or binding together) (Baker, Low, Simmer, & Cunningham, 1980). It is produced by a variety of anchorage-dependent cells including fibroblasts, heart, muscle, and kidney epithelium.

The secretion of inhibitors is also highly regulated. PA-inhibitory activity rapidly increases after surgery. This increase is also observed following exposure of endothelial cells in culture to these stimulants. In addition, when human peritoneum was harvested at the time of surgery, PAI-1 was not detectable in control peritoneum, but was present in inflamed tissue (Vipond et al., 1990). Long-term administration of synthetic anabolic steroids can modulate basal, but not postsurgical levels of PA-inhibitory activity in blood.

Regulation of Secretion by Growth Factors and Interleukins

Urokinese PA production is influenced by numerous agents including growth factors (e.g., Lee & Weinstein, 1978; Grimaldi et al., 1986), intracellular cyclic adenosine monophosphate (cAMP) (Degen, Estensen, Nagamine, & Reich, 1985) and oncogene products (e.g., Unkeless et al., 1974). In several systems, changes in uPA gene transcription leads to changes in uPA synthesis. Grimaldi and colleagues (1986) demonstrated that the expression of uPA in normal murine cells is modulated by factors that influence cell growth. In particular, these researchers demonstrated an early and transient rise in uPA mRNA levels in quiescent fibroblasts following stimulation with fetal calf serum. This rise preceded by several hours the onset of DNA synthesis. The profile of induction of uPA mRNA during the cellular transition from quiescent to proliferative states coincided with the elevation in c-*myc*. The increased expression of uPA mRNA was related to an augmented transcriptional activity of the gene.

Levin and Santell (1988) demonstrated that the kinetics of the enhanced tPA release in epithelial cells after phorbol esters and histamine were similar: a 4-hour lag followed by a period of rapid release and then a decline toward pretreatment values. After the stimulation of tPA secretion, cells became refractile to additional stimulation by the homologous agent. The changes in tPA antigen secretion appear to be directly related to changing levels of tPA mRNA since the characteristics of the response of tPA mRNA to phorbol esters mimics and precedes those of tPA antigen (Levin, Marotti, & Santell, 1989). Activation of protein kinase C appears to mediate enhanced tPA secretion as evidenced by findings that inhibitors of protein kinases, H-7 and staurosporine inhibited phorbol ester– and cAMP-induced elevations in tPA mRNA levels or antigen secretion (Levin et al., 1989). These researchers speculated that the mechanisms underlying the stimulation of tPA secretion by phorbol esters are the same as those responsible for the response of tPA to thrombin and other physiologic agonists.

Urokinase PA synthesis in porcine kidney cell cultures is inducible by phorbol esters and cAMP; the induction was related to increased uPA mRNA levels (Degen et al., 1985). Enhanced uPA synthesis with both of these agents was rapid in onset (changes in transcription rate were detectable within 10 to 20 minutes) and neither inducer agent required protein synthesis to stimulate uPA transcription. These researchers reported that the main difference between the uPA response to phorbol esters and to cAMP is in the time course of the response. The uPA response to phorbol esters was transient, whereas the response to cAMP was more prolonged.

Stimulation of both uPA and tPA synthesis was induced in cultured bovine capillary endothelial cells by basic fibroblast growth factor (FGF; Saksela, Moscatelli, & Rifkin, 1987). These same researchers reported an opposite effect on PA synthesis in these cells with the addition of transforming growth factor-β (TGF-β). The stimulatory effects of FGF could not be completely suppressed by the addition of TGF-β nor could the inhibitory effects of TGF-β be abolished by the addition of FGF, suggesting that the effects of the two growth factors on PAA are mediated by separate receptors. This hypothesis was supported by the finding that TGF-β did not compete with FGF receptor binding in hamster kidney cells (Saksela et al., 1987). Contributing to the inhibitory effect of TGF-β on PAA was its ability to dramatically increase production of an endothelial-type PAI. The effects of TGF-β on PA and PAI activities appear to be transient; after prolonged incubation of cell cultures treated simultaneously with FGF and TGF-β, the effects of FGF on PA synthesis predominated (Saksela et al., 1987). These researchers concluded that the interaction of these two growth factors—particularly with respect to their influence on PAA—may be important in the regulation of several endothelial functions involving hemostasis and wound healing.

Interleukin-1 also supports a balance between procoagulant and anticoagulant activities in the resolution of injury or inflammation. tPA synthesis was shown to be reduced and PAI activity enhanced after incubation of human umbilical vein endothelial cells with human interleukin-1 (Bevilacqua, Schleef, Gimbrone, & Loskutoff, 1986). Maximal effects (i.e., approximate 50% reduction in tPA antigen and 400 to 800% increase in PAI antigen) were observed following 24-hour incubation with 2.5 to 5 U/mL interleukin-1. These changes persisted for more than 48 hours. Interleukin-1 also has a procoagulant effect as it induces a rapid (maximal effect after 6 hours) and transient (no longer apparent by 24 hours) expression of tissue factor procoagulant activity in cultured endothelial monolayers (Bevilacqua et al., 1986). These research findings suggest that interleukin-1 may contribute to the generation and maintenance of fibrin in pathophysiologic conditions.

Of particular interest, postsurgical peritoneal macrophages secrete interleukin-1 with a peak effect observed on postsurgical day 14 (Abe, Rodgers, Ellefson, & diZerega, 1991). The occurrence of relatively high levels of interleukin-1 during the latter stage of wound repair may indicate that this endogenous secretory product is involved in facilitating the remodeling of healing tissue under normal conditions.

Summary

The release of tPA from human endothelial cells is influenced in a dose- and time-dependent manner by a variety of agents, including interleukin-1, growth factors, tumor-promoting phorbol esters, histamine, and cAMP (Table 8.3). Human interleukin-1 and transforming growth factor-β (Bevilacqua et al., 1986; Saksela et al., 1987) inhibit tPA secretion, whereas fibroblast growth factor, tumor-promoting phorbol esters, histamine, and cAMP stimulate tPA secretion (Saksela et al., 1987; Levin & Santell, 1988; Santell & Levin, 1988).

Plasminogen Activator Receptors

A specific cell-surface receptor for uPA was identified on human peripheral blood monocytes and normal fibroblasts (e.g., Bajpai & Baker, 1985; Nielsen et al., 1988). The receptor-binding domain is located in the 15,000 amino-terminal fragment of the uPA molecule (Appella et al., 1987). uPA has a high affinity for this receptor ($K_d = 0.1$ nM) and the rates of dissociation and exchange of bound uPA are low; furthermore, bound uPA is not internalized (Stoppelli et al., 1985; Vassalli, Baccino, & Belin, 1985). Nielsen and colleagues (1988) isolated the uPA receptor in four tumor cell lines and characterized it as a Mr 55,000 to 60,000 protein that was specifically cross-linked to uPA and proenzyme uPA but not to tPA or unrelated proteins.

Data from Barnathan and co-researchers (1988) indicate that tPA and PAI-1 are expressed on the surface of cultured human umbilical vein endothelial cells. Their studies demonstrated that recombinant tPA binds to at least two sites on the surface of these cells. Recombinant tPA bound with high affinity to a limited number of surface sites through the catalytic portion of the molecule; this binding appeared to be mediated by PAI-1 expressed on the cell surface. Lower affinity binding of tPA to a second class of surface binding sites on endothelial cells was also found; this site did not appear to involve the catalytic site of the tPA molecule. Binding to this low affinity site was rapidly reversible and the bound tPA fully retained its PAA. The results of these experiments suggest that endothelial cells may help to regulate fibrinolysis through differential expression of the high affinity PAI-1 and low affinity tPA binding sites on the cell surface.

Peritoneum

Several studies examined the level of fibrinolytic activity present in peritoneum. Using a fibrin slide technique, Porter, Ball, and Silver (1971)

TABLE 8.3. Modulation of protease and protease inhibitor secretion by various molecules.

Cell type	IL-1	TNF	PDGF	IL-6	TGF-β	LPS	PMA	FGF	m-CSF
Endothelial tPA	↓	↓			↓		↑	↑	
Cells PAI-1	↑	↑			↑		↑	↑	
Chondrocytes PA	↑					↑			
Collagenase		↑	↓				↑		
Synoviocytes PA	↑	±↑	—	—					
Fibroblast tPA	↑								
uPA	—								
PAI-1	↑								
PAI-2	—								
Collagenase	↑		↑		↑		↑		
Collagenase	↑								
Inhibitor									
Peritoneal									
Macrophage PA	↑								
Macrophage PAI	↑								
Macrophages PA						↑	↑		
PAI						↑	↑		↑

IL-1, interleukin-1; TNF, tumor necrosis factor; PDGF, platelet-derived growth factor; IL-6, interleukin-6; TGF-β, transforming growth factor-β; LPS, lipopolysaccharides; PMA, phorbol myristate acetate; FGF, fibroblast growth factor; m-CSF, macrophage colony stimulating factor; PA, plasminogen activator; PAI, plasminogen activator inhibitor; tPA, tissue plasminogen activator; uPA, urokinase plasminogen activator; ↑, increased; ↓, decreased; ± equivocal results.

showed that mesothelial tissue contains large amounts of PA activity. A further study examining a single layer of mesothelial cells from human peritoneum showed fibrinolytic activity in all areas of peritoneal serosa, but there were differences between areas. For example, the fibrinolytic activity of the serosa obtained from different areas of the sigmoid colon contained different amounts of PA activity (see Chapter 7). Species differences in the level of fibrinolytic activity in the peritoneal mesothelium were observed. The mesothelium of rats and guinea pigs contains relatively more fibrinolytic activity than rabbits (Myhre-Jensen, Larsen, & Astrup, 1969).

Peritoneal surgical injury results in a depression of the fibrinolytic activity (Raftery, 1981). Surgical trauma that reduced peritoneal fibrinolytic activity also increases adhesion formation, suggesting that depressed fibrinolytic activity contributes to adhesion formation. Vipond et al. (1990) found that tPA is the principal PA in human peritoneal tissue. In addition, the PA activity of the inflamed peritoneum in humans is much lower than control tissue. This reduction was shown to be due to an increase in PAI-1 production rather than a decrease in tPA antigen (see Chapter 7).

A recent study examined the nature of human omental mesothelial cells and characterized the production of PAs and PA inhibitory activity by these cells (van Hinsbergh, Kooistra, Scheffer, van Bockel, & van Muijen, 1990). This study showed that human peritoneal mesothelial cells produce tPA along with PAI-1 and PAI-2. PAI-1 antigen was present in the culture medium of the mesothelial cells, whereas PAI-2 antigen remained cell-associated. Upon exposure of the mesothelial cultures to TNF, the level of tPA antigen was reduced (Figure 8.7) whereas levels of both PAI-1 and PAI-2 antigens were elevated (Figure 8.8). Therefore, inflammatory cytokines, such as TNF, effectively modulated the fibrinolytic activity of human mesothelial cells.

Bleeding can be associated with increased fibrinolysis. Hyperfibrinolysis may be due to surgical stress, perhaps mediated through catecholamines (Britton, Giddings, Brooks, & Bloom, 1977). In patients who do not develop thrombosis, PA activity does not decrease but inhibitor activity increases, lasting 7 to 10 days. Some investigators reported that stress and anesthesia can activate the fibrinolytic system (Engqvist & Winther, 1972; Pike, Turner, Manohitharajah, & Deverall, 1975). In addition, there is a normal diurnal alteration in fibrinolytic activity in the blood (Korsan-Bengtsen, Wilhelmsen, & Tibblin, 1973).

Thrombosis and adhesion formation are complications that are due to a relative reduction in fibrinolytic activity after surgery. Tolmetin, a nonsteroidal anti-inflammatory drug that prevents adhesion formation, elevates the fibrinolytic activity of the peritoneum of traumatized animals and reduces PA-inhibitory activity in early postsurgical peritoneal fluid (see Chapter 10). The level of PA inhibitory activity was reduced through

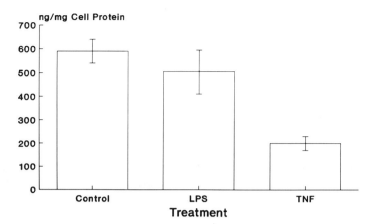

FIGURE 8.7. The effect of TNF and LPS on tPA antigen of human omental cells. TNF significantly reduced the secretion of tPA antigen from these cells. (Adapted from van Hinsbergh et al., 1990, reproduced with the permission of W.B. Saunders Co.)

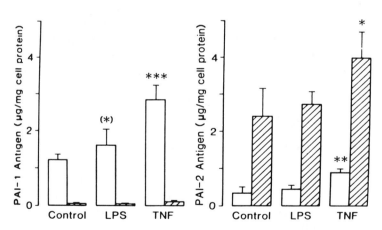

FIGURE 8.8. Effect of TNF and LPS on the production of PAI-1 and PAI-2 antigen by human omental cell. Confluent cells were incubated for 24 hours in M199 medium supplemented with 20% human serum, 150 μg/mL ECGF, and 5 U/mL heparin without (control) or with the addition of 10 μg/mL LPS or 500 U/mL TNF. Open bars represent the amount of PAI antigen in the condition medium (mean ± SD, five experiments); hatched bars represent the amount of PAI in the cell extracts after the incubation period (two to three experiments). Significance from the t-test for paired data: (*) $p = .05$; *$p < .02$; **$p < .01$; ***$p < .001$. (From van Hinsbergh et al., 1990, reproduced with the permission of W.B. Saunders Co.)

in vitro exposure of postsurgical macrophages to tolmetin (Figure 8.9; Rodgers, 1990; Rodgers, Ellefson, Girgis, & diZerega, in press). These latter data were confirmed by addition of tolmetin to postsurgical peritoneal lavage fluid (Figure 8.10). This inhibition of PA inhibitor activity may allow increased PA activity and hence increased fibrinolysis. In vivo administration of tolmetin to rats after surgical trauma increased the level of fibrinolytic activity of the injured peritoneum in an in vitro assay. These data suggest that tolmetin can alter the protease–protease inhibitor balance such that increased fibrinolysis is possible at early postsurgical time points.

Summary

The fibrinolytic system involves the interaction of many enzymes and inhibitors and is regulated at many levels. This is due to a need to balance coagulation and fibrinolysis to restore and maintain physiologic homeostasis. Fibrin deposition is required for hemostasis and tissue repair, yet fibrin resolution is necessary for the return of normal conditions. Bleeding can be a complication of increased fibrinolysis. However, reduction of fibrinolysis can result in adhesion formation and thrombosis. The level of fibrinolytic activity can be reduced by inflammatory cytokines (which may contribute to adhesion formation, see Chapter 3) or elevated by anti-inflammatory drugs.

Collagenase

Interstitial collagens types I, II, and III are the major structural proteins of the extracellular matrix (see Chapter 5). Their triple helical structure makes them resistant to proteolytic degradation except by the neutral protease collagenase. Thus, collagenase is crucial to the process of collagen turnover and in connective tissue remodeling associated with healing. Elevated collagenase activity occurs in disorders such as rheumatoid arthritis and periodontal disease, which may be responsible for the excessive tissue destruction found in these diseases.

Collagenase was isolated from a number of connective tissue and inflammatory cells, including macrophages and monocytes (e.g., Harris & Krane, 1974; Dayer, Beutler, & Cerami, 1985; Welgus, Campbell, Bar-Shavit, Senior, & Teitelbaum, 1985; Wahl & Lampel, 1987). Collagenases were also isolated from microvascular endothelial cells, although these cells (both human and rabbit) secrete substantially less collagenase in response to an inducing agent than do synovial fibroblasts (Banda, Herron, Murphy, & Werb, 1986). Collagenase is secreted from cells as an inactive proenzyme that can be activated by other proteinases found in the extracellular matrix. In rabbits, the metalloproteinase activator that

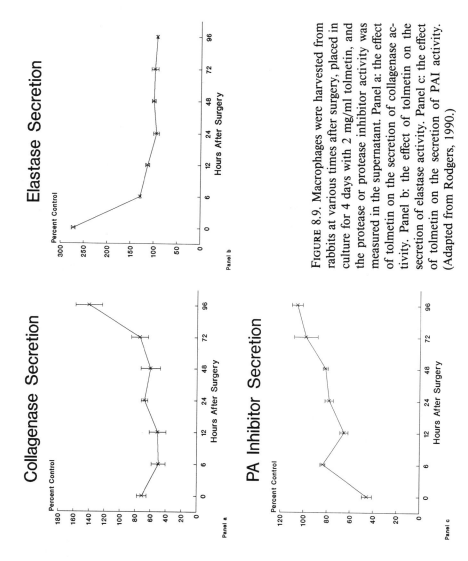

FIGURE 8.9. Macrophages were harvested from rabbits at various times after surgery, placed in culture for 4 days with 2 mg/ml tolmetin, and the protease or protease inhibitor activity was measured in the supernatant. Panel a: the effect of tolmetin on the secretion of collagenase activity. Panel b: the effect of tolmetin on the secretion of elastase activity. Panel c: the effect of tolmetin on the secretion of PAI activity. (Adapted from Rodgers, 1990.)

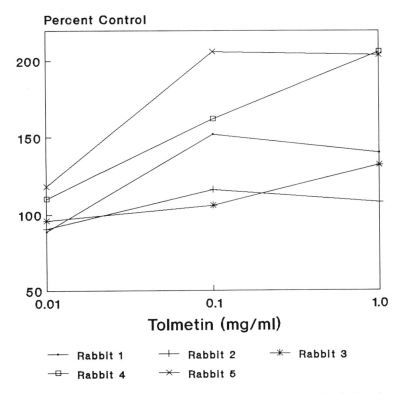

FIGURE 8.10. The effect of tolmetin in the assay on the level of plasminogen activator activity observed in peritoneal lavage fluid after peritoneal surgery, as a function of tolmetin concentrations and postsurgical time.

converts collagenase proenzyme to the active moiety is stromelysin. Stromelysin is a metalloproteinase that both activates the proenzyme of collagenase and degrades noncollagenous matrix (e.g., Chin, Murphy, & Werb, 1985).

The gene structure for a collagenase mRNA produced by rabbit synovial cells was mapped and determined to be 9.1 kilobases with 10 exons and 9 introns (Fini, Plucinska, Mayer, Gross, & Brinckerhoff, 1987). Since the interstitial collagenase isolated from skin fibroblasts and macrophages has similar properties to that isolated from synovial cells, these researchers hypothesized that all three are products of the same gene. Sequence analysis of rabbit synovial cell collagenase and human skin and synovial cell collagenase indicates that they contain approximately 86% homology (Fini et al., 1987).

The collagenase produced by fibroblasts, macrophages and monocytes is specific for interstitial collagen types I to III and is not effective in cleaving basement membrane collagen types IV and V. Table 8.4 shows

TABLE 8.4. Comparison of collagen type specificity of human monocyte, macrophage and fibroblast collagenases.

Enzyme source	Collagen type	K_m (μmol/L)	K_{cat} (h^{-1})
Monocyte	I	1.1	21.5
	II	ND[a]	ND[a]
	III	2.2	347
Macrophage[b]	I	0.8	28.4
	II	1.7	1.0
	III	1.9	598
Skin fibroblast[b]	I	0.9	22.5
	II	2.1	1.0
	III	1.4	565

[a]Catalytic activity of available enzyme was too low to accurately quantify.
[b]Relative rates of cleaving with the rate against type II collagen arbitrarily defined as 1.0.
Adapted from Campbell et al., 1987.

the comparative specificity of human peripheral blood monocytes, human alveolar macrophages, and human skin fibroblasts for types I to III collagen. Seltzer and colleagues (1989) presented data indicating that the collagenase produced by human skin fibroblasts could also degrade the type VII collagen helix, a major structural protein of anchoring fibrils.

Regulation of Secretion

Growth factors, such as interleukin-1, TGF-β, and epidermal growth factor (EGF), enhance collagenase secretion from different cells, including human skin fibroblasts and inflammatory synovial cells (Postlethwaite, Lachman, Mainardi, & Kang, 1983; Chua, Geiman, Keller, & Ladda, 1985; Kumkumian et al., 1989). The activation of cells to produce collagenase appears to occur via a prostaglandin-dependent pathway. Agents that inhibit prostaglandin E_2 synthesis, including the nonsteroidal anti-inflammatory agent indomethacin and the glucocorticoid dexamethasone, prevent enhanced collagenase secretion by macrophages and monocytes in response to lipopolysaccharide (LPS) or concanavalin A (Con-A) (Werb, 1978; Wahl & Winter, 1984; Wahl & Wahl, 1985; Wahl & Lampel, 1987). Further supportive evidence for the involvement of prostaglandins comes from experimental findings that indicate that PGE_2 or phospholipase A_2 can restore collagenase secretion from cells exposed to indomethacin or dexamethasone (Wahl & Winter, 1984; Wahl & Lampel, 1987). The mechanism by which PGE_2 can regulate collagenase production appears to involve elevation of cAMP. In macrophages or peripheral blood monocytes treated with indomethacin or dexamethasone, di-butyryl-cAMP also restored collagenase secretion (Wahl & Winter, 1984; Wahl & Lampel, 1987). Thus, the pathway leading to the activation of macrophages and monocytes to produce collagenase likely requires a primary stimulus, such as lipopolysaccharide followed by increased production of PGE_2 which, through stimulation of adenylate cyclase, elevates intracellular cAMP levels. Increased collagenase secretion in response to a stimulus is dependent upon synthesis of the proenzyme molecule by the cells and not simply the release of preformed molecules, since treatment with cycloheximide abolishes the effect (e.g., Wahl & Winter, 1984).

The enhancement of collagenase secretion from fibroblasts and synovial cells by interleukin-1 also appears to follow the same prostaglandin-mediated pathway, since this cytokine increases PGE_2 production (Kumkumian et al., 1989). Interleukin-1, but not platelet-derived growth factor (PDGF), increases transcription of collagenase by synovial cells (Kumkumian et al., 1989); PDGF inhibited the effect of interleukin-1 on collagenase transcription in these cells. The effects of PDGF on collagenase gene expression in synovial cells differs from its effects in dermal fibroblasts; in this latter cell type, collagenase secretion and gene expression were augmented by PDGF (Chua et al., 1985).

Collagenase Inhibitor

An endogenous inhibitor of collagenase was identified for fibroblasts (Stricklin & Welgus, 1983; Welgus & Stricklin, 1983), macrophages (Welgus et al., 1985) and monocytes (Campbell, Davis Cury, Lazarus, & Welgus, 1987). This glycoprotein, which appears to be immunologically and functionally identical in all three cell types (Campbell et al., 1987), is termed tissue inhibitor of metalloproteinases (TIMP). In unstimulated alveolar macrophages, the amount of TIMP released is about $100 \text{ ng}/10^6$ cells per 24 hours, which can be markedly enhanced by LPS or phorbol myristate acetate (PMA) (Welgus et al., 1985). Campbell et al. (1987) reported that the collagenase and collagenase inhibitor molecules produced by human peripheral blood monocytes are similar to those produced by human alveolar macrophages, although there are some qualitative and quantitative differences. In particular, monocytes normally secrete high levels of TIMP and virtually no procollagenase; conversely, macrophages secrete comparatively higher levels of procollagenase. Thus, under normal conditions, monocytes favor collagenase inhibition, whereas macrophages favor collagenolytic activity. Monocyte production of TIMP and procollagenase is largely unaffected by stimulatory agents, whereas macrophage TIMP production can be augmented by LPS and PMA. Macrophage procollagenase activity could also be stimulated by LPS.

Summary

Collagenase is produced by a number of cell types in a proenzyme form and cleaves a variety of collagen types. Growth factors can enhance collagenase production by a prostaglandin-dependent pathway. A collagenase inhibitor, TIMP, was also identified and isolated.

Elastase

Elastase is a specific proteolytic enzyme that degrades elastin, a fibrous and insoluble protein of the extracellular matrix. Neutrophils, alveolar macrophages (Chapman & Stone, 1984) and peritoneal macrophages (Werb, 1978) secrete elastase (Scheele, Bartelt, & Bieger, 1981). Three elastase isoenzymes, elastase I, II, III, were isolated from the human pancreas (Largman, Brodrick, & Geokas, 1976; Tani, Ohsumi, Mita, & Takiguchi, 1988). Chapman and Stone (1984) reported marked differences between the elastolytic activity of human alveolar macrophages and neutrophils. Neutrophils inherently possess greater elastinolytic potential than do alveolar macrophages; however, in the presence of proteinase inhibitors, macrophages have the ability to degrade substantially more elastin than do neutrophils. Macrophage elastase activity is primarily expressed at the cell surface or in the immediate microenvironment, and thus reflects a rather close association of intact cells with the substrate. The elastase activity of neutrophils, in contrast, appears to involve less intimate contact with the substrate. Such a difference between the two cell types could explain the differential effect of proteinase inhibitors on the elastase activity of macrophages and neutrophils.

Peritoneal surgery modulates the secretion of elastase by macrophages (Figure 8.11). Early after surgery (day 1), there was a decrease in elastase secretion. However, by days 3 to 5, the elastase levels were comparable to nonsurgical controls. On days 7 to 14, the secretion of elastase by macrophages from postsurgical rabbits was elevated. These data indicate that the secretion of elastase is modulated such that it is elevated during the remodeling phase of wound repair.

Glucocorticoids (dexamethasone and cortisol) suppress, in a dose- and time-dependent manner, elastase secretion by both resident- and thioglycolate-elicited mouse peritoneal macrophages and rabbit alveolar macrophages (Werb, 1978). Progesterone and the steroids, estradiol and dihydrotestosterone, did not effect secretion of these proteinases. The inhibition of elastase secretion by dexamethasone was less than that for plasminogen activator secretion (97% to 100%) (Figure 8.12). Such inhibition was reversible in that secretion of elastase was restored to at least 80% of control values within 24 hours after treatment with dexamethasone. Reversal of the inhibitory effects of this glucocorticoid on plasminogen activator secretion was quicker than that for elastase; some attenuation occurred within 2 hours.

Alpha$_1$-proteinase is a relatively specific inhibitor of neutrophil elastase. An elastase inhibitor has also been identified in equine leukocyte cytosol

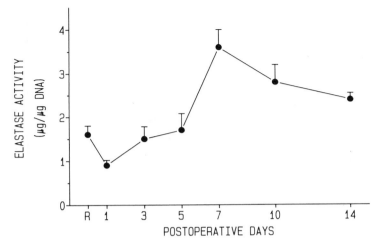

FIGURE 8.11. Elastase activity in the spent media of nonsurgical and postsurgical peritoneal macrophages. The secretion of elastase is modulated as a function of postsurgical time. Each point represents the mean ± SEM of four or five experiments performed in rabbits (Kuraoka et al., 1992).

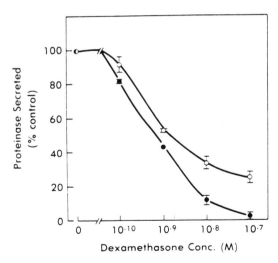

FIGURE 8.12. Comparison of effects of dexamethasone on elastase and plasminogen activator secretion by thioglycolate-elicited mouse macrophages. Dexamethasone inhibits the secretion of both plasminogen activator and elastase by macrophages. Values represent the mean ± SD ($n = 3$); elastase (○); plasminogen activator (●). (From Werb, 1978. Reproduced by permission of Rockefeller University Press.)

that reacts with porcine pancreatic elastase as well as human and equine elastase (Dubin, Potempa, & Silberring, 1985; Dubin, Potempa, & Turynea, 1986; Potempa, Dubin, Watorek, & Travis, 1988). Of particular note, this leukocyte elastase inhibitor belongs to the intracellular protein pool.

Kornecki, Ehrlich, De Mars, and Lenox (1986) demonstrated that even low concentrations of porcine elastase can result in an irreversible exposure of fibrinogen-binding sites on the surface of human platelets. Aggregation of platelets induced by fibrinogen is possible even in the absence of the normal triggering stimulus, i.e., a rise in intracellular cAMP levels. Such findings suggest that deleterious hemostatic changes may be a consequence of elevated levels of circulating elastase.

Miscellaneous Proteases

Protein C System

Coagulation is also regulated by serine proteases. One of these, protein C, functions as an anticoagulant and circulates as an inactive zymogen. It is activated by a complex of thrombin and its endothelial cell receptor thrombomodulin. Activation involves proteolytic removal of a 12-residue activation peptide from the NH_2 terminus of the protein C heavy chain (Ehrlich, Jaskunas, Grinnell, Yan, & Bang, 1989). It appears that the binding of thrombomodulin with thrombin induces a conformational change in the latter's substrate binding such that it will bind effectively with protein C and hence change from inducing procoagulant to anticoagulant activities (Esmon, Galvin, Johnson, DeBault, & Esmon, 1987).

Activated protein C proteolytically degrades coagulation cofactors VIIIa and Va and therefore acts as an anticoagulant (Marlar, Kleiss, & Griffin, 1982). Both phospholipids and calcium are necessary cofactors for the anticoagulant effects of protein C (Marlar et al., 1982). Esmon et al. (1987) hypothesized that calcium induced a conformational change in protein C such that the molecule binds effectively to the thrombin-thrombomodulin complex. An additional cofactor also appears crucial to the ability of protein C to degrade coagulation factor Va; this is the vitamin K–dependent plasma protein, protein S. Protein S forms a 1:1 complex with activated protein C and thus confers an increased activity of the latter for the membrane surface (Harris & Esmon, 1985). Deficiencies in either protein C or protein S are associated with recurrent thrombotic disease (e.g., Griffin, Evatt, Zimmerman, Kleiss, & Wideman, 1981; Comp, Nixon, Cooper, & Esmon, 1984).

Harris and Esmon (1985) demonstrated that protein S accelerated the rate of factor Va inactivation by protein C at the platelet surface by about ten-fold. Their experiments further suggest that platelets contain protein

S, which is made available as a cofactor for protein C upon stimulation with thrombin and that the presence of proteins permits specific, saturable binding of activated protein C to the platelet surface. No specific binding was observed in vitro in the absence of protein S.

Multicatalytic Proteinase

A high molecular weight proteinase (Mr of 700,000) was isolated from a variety of mammalian tissues. This molecule, generally referred to as multicatalytic proteinase, can cleave bonds on the carboxyl side of 1, basic; 2, hydrophobic; and 3, acidic amino acid residues (Rivett, 1989). These activities are called 1, trypsin-like; 2, chymotrypsin-like; and 3, peptidyl-glutamyl-peptide bond hydrolyzing activities, respectively. Rivett (1989) demonstrated that the multicatalytic proteinase isolated from rat liver has at least two distinct catalytic sites. All proteolytic activity is lost after dissociation by urea or acid treatment.

Proteinase Inhibitors

Proteinase inhibitors make up approximately 10% of the protein in plasma (Travis & Salvesen, 1983) and are one of the largest functional groups of protein. These proteins control a variety of events associated with peritoneal and connective tissue turnover, fibrinolysis, coagulation, inflammatory reactions, and complement activation. Although most of the proteinase inhibitors can react with a number of proteinases, only their ability to inactivate a particular proteinase is usually of physiological relevance. The one exception is alpha$_2$-macroglobulin. This inhibitor has the ability to interact with members of each proteinase class, i.e., serine, aspartate, cysteine, or metalloproteinases.

The role of proteinase inhibitors is to regulate proteolytic activity. Proteinase inhibitors act competitively by allowing their target enzyme to bind directly to a substrate-like region on the inhibitor molecule. In general, proteinase–proteinase inhibitor complexes are equimolar with respect to reactive sites and the reaction between enzyme and proteinase inhibitor is typically second-order.

Derangements in the normal proteolytic response are believed to underlie the physiological sequelae associated with numerous diseases, including emphysema, thrombotic disorders, rheumatoid arthritis, and postsurgical peritoneal adhesion formation. Adhesion formation results from a reduction in the normal proteolytic activity that accompanies peritoneal healing and tissue remodeling. Such a reduction could be the consequence of increased proteinase inhibitor activity. Similarly, endothelial cell growth and maintenance are, in part, dependent upon proteinase inhibitor activity. For example, cell retention on endothelium-lined prosthetic vascular grafts was improved following stimulation of serine proteinase inhibitors (Ashworth et al., 1987). The following sections summarize information regarding specific proteinase inhibitors (Table 8.5).

Alpha₁-Proteinase Inhibitor

Human alpha₁-proteinase inhibitor is a glycoprotein of approximately Mr 53,000. It exists as a single polypeptide chain with no internal disulfide bonds and only a single cysteinyl residue. Although human alpha₁-proteinase inhibitor is capable of inactivating virtually all serine proteinases, its primary role is to inactivate neutrophil elastase. The rate of inactivation (k_{ass}) for this proteinase is approximately tenfold higher than that of other proteinases and is only 12-fold lower than diffusion-controlled limits (Travis & Salvesen, 1983).

Human alpha₁-proteinase inhibitor is predominantly derived from the liver; however it is also expressed at extrahepatic sites by monocytes and macrophages. Although the alpha₁-proteinase inhibitor molecules synthesized and secreted from both hepatic and extrahepatic sources are identical, there are some interesting distinctions. For example, transcription of the alpha₁-proteinase inhibitor gene in macrophages is initiated at a promoter located about 2 kilobases upstream from that which initiates transcription in hepatocytes. Furthermore, expression of alpha₁-proteinase inhibitor from monocytes and macrophages is subject to regulation by elastase and bacterial LPS. Both mediate increased expression of the inhibitor in an additive fashion (Perlmutter & Punsal, 1988). Distinct pretranslational and translational mechanisms of action for elastase and LPS, respectively, account for the additive effect of the two on human alpha₁-proteinase inhibitor expression.

A molecular change occurs when alpha₁-proteinase inhibitor inhibits a serine proteinase. The proteinase splits a 6,000 to 8,000 Mr peptide from the alpha₁-proteinase inhibitor molecule, which then undergoes rearrangement and covalent acyl bond formation with the hydroxyl group of the serine in the proteinase's reactive site (Heimburger, 1974). Methionine is present in the active site of alpha₁-proteinase inhibitor and its oxidation apparently destroys the ability of the molecule to inhibit proteinases.

Harada and colleagues (1987) demonstrated that extravascular levels of serum alpha₁-proteinase inhibitor within inflammatory tissue differ during the wound healing process. In culture fluids of dermal sulfur mustard lesions in rabbits, alpha₁-proteinase inhibitor levels were elevated approximately nine-fold on the first day after lesion formation relative to normal skin. During the healing process, levels declined and by day 6 were only about three-fold greater than those observed in normal skin. Approximately two-thirds of the alpha₁-proteinase inhibitor found in the

TABLE 8.5. Characteristics of select proteinase inhibitors.

Proteinase inhibitor	Mr	Normal concentration in plasma	Primary target	Rate of inactivation (k_{ass} in $M^{-1}\ sec^{-1}$)
Alpha$_1$-proteinase inhibitor	53,000	15–130 mg/100 mL	Neutrophil elastase	6.5×10^7
Antithrombin III	58,000	2.9 mg/100 mL	Thrombin	1×10^3
Alpha$_2$-antiplasmin	65,000–75,000	6 mg/100 mL	Plasmin	$1.8–3.8 \times 10^7$
PAI-1	53,000	N/A	uPA, tPA	10^6 to 10^7
PAI-2	47,000	N/A	uPA	N/A
Alpha$_2$-macro-globulin	725,000	250 mg/100 mL	All proteinase classes	Differs depending upon specific proteinase

Adapted from Travis & Salvesen, 1983.

culture fluids existed as a complex with a proteinase. A similar pattern of results was observed with alpha$_1$-macroglobulin, the rabbit equivalent of human alpha$_2$-macroglobulin.

Antithrombin III

Human antithrombin III has a major role in controlling serine proteinases involved in the coagulation process. As reviewed by Travis and Salvesen (1983), the purified protein is a single-chain molecule of Mr 58,000 with six disulfide bonds and four apparent glycosylation sites. Significant homology exists between the amino acid sequence of human antithrombin III and human alpha$_1$-proteinase inhibitor. Although human antithrombin III inactivates a variety of proteinases, the only reaction of any discernible physiological importance is its ability to inhibit the activity of thrombin. The effect of antithrombin III on thrombin is significantly accelerated by the presence of heparin. Heparin is an allosteric activator in which binding at one site of the human antithrombin III protein effected a conformational change that facilitates the inhibition of thrombin and other serine proteinases. Since thrombin also binds heparin, Travis and Salvesen (1983) speculated that heparin could also induce a conformational change in thrombin which accelerates its binding by antithrombin III. The inhibition of thrombin by human antithrombin III apparently occurs by the same mechanism as that described for human alpha$_1$-proteinase inhibitor, namely formation of a covalently bound, stable, equimolar complex between the inhibitor and the proteinase.

Alpha$_2$-Antiplasmin

In the mid-1970s, a single-chain glycoprotein of Mr 65,000 to 70,000 that markedly and rapidly inhibits plasmin was purified from human plasma; this glycoprotein was subsequently termed alpha$_2$-antiplasmin. The interaction of alpha$_2$-antiplasmin with plasmin is very rapid. Like other proteinase inhibitors, alpha$_2$-antiplasmin interacts with a variety of proteinases but none of the interactions appears to be physiologically relevant except for that with plasmin and trypsin.

The process by which alpha$_2$-antiplasmin inhibits plasmin is similar to that of antithrombin III and alpha$_1$-proteinase inhibitor, e.g., formation of equimolar, covalently bound inhibitor-proteinase complex. The ability of alpha$_2$-antiplasmin to rapidly inhibit plasmin may depend upon the existence of unoccupied lysine binding sites on the plasmin A-chain since the rate of inhibition is approximately 10 times slower in the presence of a lysine analogue than in its absence. Wiman and Collen (1979) demonstrated that inactivation of plasmin by alpha$_2$-antiplasmin proceeds much slower when the plasmin molecule is bound to fibrin than when it is free in circulation. The interaction of plasmin with fibrin also involves lysine binding sites on the plasmin molecule. Travis and Salvesen (1983) postulated that alpha$_2$-antiplasmin evolved sites on its surface that enable it to distinguish plasmin molecules that are actively involved in clot lysis from those molecules that are unbound.

Alpha$_2$-antiplasmin may play a prominent role in fibrinolytic states and in the control of clot lysis. The concentration of alpha$_2$-antiplasmin in the plasma of patients with disseminated intravascular coagulation and fibrinolysis was significantly reduced relative to healthy adults; in contrast, plasma concentrations of the proteinase inhibitors, alpha$_2$-macroglobulin and alpha$_1$-antitrypsin, were unchanged in this patient group (Aoki, Moroi, Matsuda, & Tachiya, 1977). A role for alpha$_2$-antiplasmin in postsurgical adhesion formation has also been implicated. Dhabuwala, Dawe, Mammem, and Silva (personal communication) reported that the concentrations of alpha$_2$-antiplasmin in peritoneal exudate obtained 2, 4, and 6 hours after abrasion of rabbit cecum was significantly greater than those observed in plasma obtained immediately prior to injury. Of primary interest, this difference was only apparent in animals that developed adhesions. The concentration of alpha$_2$-antiplasmin in peritoneal exudate was also greater than that in peritoneal fluid obtained prior to surgery, and this difference was also more apparent in animals with adhesions.

Alpha-Macroglobulins

Alpha-macroglobulins are large glycoproteins found in both vertebrates and invertebrates that appear to function as sophisticated binding proteins for proteinases. They belong to a family of high molecular weight molecules that also include the complement components C3 and C4. Most alpha-macroglobulins are tetramers and differences in quaternary structure give rise to alpha-macroglobulins with distinct proteinase binding properties. One human alpha-macroglobulin, alpha$_2$-macroglobulin, shares significant nucleotide sequence similarity with the complement proteins C3 and C4. Alpha-macroglobulins recognize proteinases by presenting a specific exposed peptide stretch that has been termed the bait region. The sequences of bait regions differ among species. Alpha-macroglobulins undergo extensive conformational changes following cleavage in the bait region by a particular proteinase. As a result of this cleavage, the reactivity of internal thiol esters is enhanced. In their short-lived nascent state, the activated thiol esters provide the potential for covalent binding of activated proteinases to alpha-macroglobulins. Bait region cleavage also results in the exposure of previously concealed sites that are recognized by high affinity receptors on several cell types. Thus, by binding to alpha-macroglobulins, proteinases trigger conformational changes in the alpha-macroglobulins that not only effectively "trap" the proteinase but also make the alpha-macroglobulin–proteinase complex destined for clearance by cells such as hepatocytes.

Circulating levels of alpha-macroglobulin–proteinase complexes are very low, with a half-life of 2 to 5 minutes. The complexes bind with high affinity to hepatocytes as well as fibroblast-like cells and monocytes/macrophages. The nature of the complexed proteinase does not appear to significantly alter the degree or rate of receptor binding to these cells. Receptor binding of the alpha-macroglobulin–proteinase complex is Ca^{2+}-dependent. Following binding, the alpha-macroglobulin–proteinase complex is internalized and degraded. The existence of specific proteinase inhibitors coupled with the relative nonspecificity of alpha-macroglobulins led Sottrup-Jensen (1989) to propose that alpha-macroglobulins may function as backup inhibitors of proteinase under conditions where the specific primary inhibitors become depleted, such as clotting.

Plasminogen Activator Inhibitors, Types 1 and 2

Three immunologically distinct classes of plasminogen activator inhibitors are known: the endothelial cell type PA inhibitor or PAI-1, the placental type PA inhibitor or PAI-2, and the fibroblast type plasminogen activator inhibitor or protease nexin (Sprengers & Kluft, 1987). The latter form has a higher second-order rate constant with thrombin and trypsin than with either uPA or tPA and thus cannot be considered a true, specific plasminogen activator inhibitor (Sprengers & Kluft, 1987). Thus, the remainder of this section focuses on PAI-1 and PAI-2.

PAI-1 is synthesized from endothelial, cells although other cells, including cultured hepatocytes (Sprengers, Pincen, Kooistra, & Van Hinsbergh, 1985), some hepatoma cell lines (Coleman, Batouski, & Gelehrter, 1982; Sprengers et al., 1985), and the MJZJ human melanoma cell line (Wagener & Binder, 1986), are capable of synthesizing PAI-1. PAI-1 interacts with both uPA and tPA with a second-order constant above 10^6 to 10^7 mol/L^{-1} sec^{-1} (Sprengers & Kluft, 1987). The reaction of PAI-1 with either PA results in the formation of a covalently bound, stable complex between the two molecules.

Both an active form and an inactive form of PAI-1 were isolated from endothelial cell–conditioned medium and blood platelets. The latter form does not inhibit PA nor does it form complexes with either uPA or tPA. The inactive form of PAI-1 can be activated following incubation with protein denaturing agents, such as sodium dodecyl sulfate (SDS), urea, and guanidine, and the inhibitory activity of this "activated" latent form is identical to that of the active form (Hekman & Loskutoff, 1985). Kooistra, Springers, and Van Hinsbergh (1986) demonstrated that at least part of the inactive PAI-1 found in the endothelial cell–culture medium is derived from the rapid inactivation of newly synthesized PAI-1 upon release from the cell. The calculated half-life for the inactivation of active

PAI-1 is 0.29 hours. A slower inactivation process was also identified in vitro, which occurred with a half-life of 2 to 4 hours (Kooistra et al., 1986). Accumulation of the inactive form was more rapid under standard culture conditions than that of the active form, with estimates of 40- to 80-fold excess accumulation of the inactive form reported in 24-hour conditioned medium (Hekman & Lostutoff, 1985; Levin 1986). Although the molecular mechanism(s) involved in inactivation of the PAI-1 molecule are unknown, it may involve oxidation of at least one critical methionine residue. Lawrence and Loskutoff (1986) demonstrated that PAI-1 is unusually sensitive to oxidative inactivation, being at least one order of magnitude more sensitive to chloramine-T than alpha$_1$-proteinase inhibitor, with great sensitivity to oxidants. Data from these researchers suggest that, as with alpha$_1$-proteinase inhibitor, the conversion of a critical methionine residue into methionine sulfoxide may be responsible for the inactivation of PAI-1.

PAI-2, isolated from human placenta, may be of macrophage origin (Chapman & Stone, 1985). PAI-2 inhibits uPA, two-chain tPA, and, to a lesser extent, single-chain tPA (Sprengers & Kluft, 1987). PAI-2 is not found in normal human plasma (Sprengers & Kluft, 1987). Like PAI-1, PAI-2 forms stable, covalently bound equimolar complexes with plasminogen activator. Wun and Reich (1987) reported that the rate of inactivation with PAI-2 was much faster for uPA than for tPA.

PA inhibitor activity in plasma increases rapidly in response to insults such as major surgery, severe trauma, or myocardial infarction. Since PAI-2 or protease nexin are undetectable in normal human plasma, the increase in PA inhibitor activity is due to elevations in PAI-1. PAI-1 in plasma behaves as an acute-phase reactant protein in that the levels of PAI-1 return toward normal very shortly after the occurrence of the insult. For example, Kluft and colleagues (1985) found increased PAI-1 activity on the first day following surgery. Although the amount of tPA antigen was also elevated after surgery, the overall PA activity was diminished (Figures 8.13 and 8.14). PA inhibitor activity can also be enhanced by interleukin-1 and bacterial LPS (Colucci, Paramo, & Collen, 1985; Emeis & Kooistra, 1986; Michel & Quertermous, 1989). The increased activity observed in response to these agents was maximal 4 hours after administration and was no longer apparent by 24 hours (Emeis & Kooistra, 1986).

PA inhibitor activity is very quickly cleared from circulation; half-lives of 3.5 and 7 minutes are reported in the rat and rabbit, respectively (Colucci et al., 1985; Emeis, 1985). Clearance apparently takes place in the liver. PA inhibitor activity in endothelial cell–conditioned medium can be inactivated by thrombin and activated protein C (Sprengers & Kluft, 1987). The latter molecule can form 1:1 complexes with PAI (Sakata, Griffin, & Loskutoff, 1985).

Certain disease states are associated with changes in PA inhibitor ac-

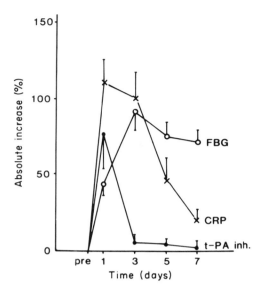

FIGURE 8.13. Plasminogen activator inhibitory activity after surgery. tPA inhibitory activity has kinetics of secretion similar to the acute phase proteins fibrinogen (FBG) and C reactive protein (CRP). (From Kluft et al., 1985. Reproduced by permission of Blackwell Scientific.)

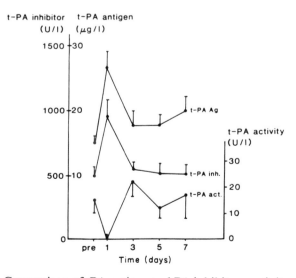

FIGURE 8.14. Comparison of tPA antigen and PA inhibitory activity after surgery. Although the amount of tPA antigen is elevated after surgery, the levels of tPA activity are reduced. This may be due to an elevation in tPA inhibitor activity. (From Kluft et al., 1985. Reproduced by permission of Blackwell Scientific.)

tivity. For example, elevated PA inhibitor levels are frequently observed in patients with deep venous thrombosis (Paramo, DeBoer, Colucci, Jonker, & Collen, 1985; Wiman et al., 1985). Since increased PA inhibitor levels were observed in a variety of other conditions (e.g., hyperlipoproteinemia, pancreatitis, myocardial infarction), Sprengers and Kluft (1987) proposed that an increase in the level of this proteinase inhibitor is indicative of acute illness per se and is not specific for any particular disease.

PA inhibitor activity plays a pivotal role in the coagulation process. In normal human plasma two distinct pools of PA inhibitor activity are known. One is a platelet-poor pool that has a very rapid turnover and for which there is large interindividual variation (ranging from 0.0 to 1.3 nmol/L). The other is a platelet pool that has a turnover time approximating that of platelets themselves and for which a mean normal value of 6.7×10^{-14} mol/platelet (standard deviation $= 3.0 \times 10^{-14}$; Sprengers, Akkerman & Jansen, 1986). The PA inhibitor activity in platelets is about four times higher than that in plasma for a given volume of blood (Sprengers & Kluft, 1987). During coagulation, PA inhibitor derived from platelets may play an important role in protecting the blood clot against premature lysis. Inactivation of PA inhibitor by thrombin and protein C may result in the gradual elimination of the inhibitor from the clot, thus permitting PA and the resultant plasmin to lysis the clot.

Metalloproteinase Inhibitors

A role for one catalytic class of proteinases, the metalloproteinases, in a variety of intracellular membrane fusion events was suggested (e.g., Baxter, Johnston, & Strittmatter, 1983; Couch & Strittmatter, 1983). Fusion of membrane vesicles is implicated in the intracellular processes underlying the transport of proteins destined for secretion or storage. Strous, van Kerkhof, Dekker, and Schwartz (1988) (1988) demonstrated that the transport and secretion of newly synthesized proteins as well as receptor-mediated endocytosis and receptor recycling were inhibited in hepatoma cells by inhibitors of metalloproteinases. The inhibition was rapid, reversible, and specific.

Summary

Proteinase inhibitors are ubiquitous proteins that are instrumental in the regulation of activity. Alpha$_1$-proteinase inhibitor is capable of inhibiting nearly all serine proteinases, but its primary role is inhibition of elastase. Antithrombin III plays a major role in the regulation of coagulation processes. The physiologic role of alpha$_2$-antiplasmin appears to be in the inhibition of plasmin and trypsin. Alpha$_2$ macroglobulin is a nonspecific proteinase inhibitor that seems to act as a backup to specific proteinase inhibitors. Lastly, PAI-1, PAI-2, and protease nexin inhibit the activity of a major regulatory protein, the plasminogen activator.

Conclusions

Proteinases and proteinase inhibitors are crucial in the regulation of wound healing and tissue remodeling. The activity of proteases, including plasminogen activator, plasmin, collagenase, and elastase, is highly regulated by protease inhibitors. These proteases are involved in tissue remodeling, inflammation, coagulation, and fibrinolysis. Protease inhibitors such as, alpha$_2$-macroglobulin, PAI-1, PAI-2, alpha$_1$-antiprotease, alpha$_2$-antiplasmin, and antithrombin III tightly regulate the activity of these proteases. The level of protease activity is also regulated at the level of protease secretion. The secretion of proteases and protease inhibitors is regulated by surgical trauma, inflammation, and inflammatory mediators. Several studies showed that circulating levels of PA, plasmin, and protease inhibitors are rapidly increased by these stimuli. The increase in the secretion of proteases induced by surgical trauma is further modulated by exposure to tolmetin, an NSAID. The proper balance between protease and protease inhibitor activities is necessary to prevent excessive bleeding on one hand and excess fibrin deposition on the other hand. A reduction in fibrinolysis has been linked to increased intraperitoneal adhesion formation by many authors.

References

Abe H, Rodgers KE, Ellefson D, diZerega GS. (1991). Kinetics of interleukin-1 and tumor necrosis factor secretion by rabbit macrophages recovered from the peritoneal cavity after surgery. *J Invest Surg.* 4:141–151.

Albrechtsen OK. (1956). The fibrinolytic activity of the human endometrium. *Acta Endocrinol.* 23:207–218.

Albrechtsen OK. (1957a). The fibrinolytic activity of human tissues. *Br J Haematol.* 3:284–291.

Albrechtsen OK. (1957b). The fibrinolytic activity of animal tissues. *Acta Physiol Scand.* 39:284–290.

Andersson L, Nilsson IM, Olow B. (1962). Fibrinolytic activity in man during surgery. *Thromb Diath Haemorrh.* 7:392–403.

Andersson L. (1964). Antifibrinolytic treatment with epsilon-amino-caproic acid in connection with prostatectomy. *Acta Chir Scand.* 127:552–557.

Aoki N, Moroi M, Matsuda M, Tachiya K. (1977). The behavior of alpha$_2$-plasmin inhibitor in fibrinolytic states. *J Clin Invest.* 60:361–369.

Appella E, Robinson EA, Ullrich SJ, Stoppelli MP, Corti A, Cassani G, Blasi F. (1987). The receptor binding sequence of urokinase. A biological function for growth factor module of proteases. *J Biol Chem.* 262:4437–4440.

Ashworth EM, Herring MB, Hoagland WP, Arnold M, Glover JL, Darsing MC.

(1987). Endothelial linings: the effect of serine protease inhibition. *J Surg Res.* 43:10–13.

Astrup T, Albrechtsen OK. (1957). Estimation of the plasminogen activator and the trypsin inhibitor in animal and human tissues. *Scand J Clin Lab Invest.* 9:233–243.

Astrup T, Claassen M. (1957). Fibrinolytic activity of peritoneum. Trans. 6th Congr. European Soc Haematol, Copenhagen, Basel: Karger; 455–459.

Astrup T, Albrechtsen OK, Claassen M, Rasmussen J. (1959). Thromboplastic and fibrinolytic activity of human aorta. *Circ Res.* 7:969–974.

Bajpai A, Baker JB. (1985). Cryptic urokinase binding sites on human foreskin fibroblasts. *Biochem Biophys Res Commun.* 133:475–482.

Baker JB, Low DA, Simmer RL, Cunningham DD. (1980). Protease nexin: a cellular component that links thrombin and plasminogen activator and mediated their binding to cells. *Cell.* 21:37–45.

Banda MJ, Herron GS, Murphy G, Werb Z. (1986). Regulation of metalloproteinase activity by microvascular endothelial cells. In: Rifkin DB, Klagsburn M, eds. *Current Communcations in Molecular Biology-Angiogenesis Mechanisms and Pathology.* Cold Spring Harbor: 101–109.

Barnathan ES, Kuo A, Van der Keyl H, McCral KR, Larsen GR, Cines DB. (1988). Tissue-type plasminogen activator binding to human endothelial cells. *J Biol Chem.* 263:7792–7799.

Baxter DA, Johnston D, Strittmatter WJ. (1983). Protease inhibitors implicate metalloendoprotease in synaptic transmission at the mammalian neuromuscular junction. *Proc Natl Acad Sci USA.* 80:4174–4178.

Bevilacqua MP, Schleef RR, Gimbrone MA, Loskutoff DJ. (1986). Regulation of the fibrinolytic system of cultured human vascular endothelium by interleukin-1. *J Clin Invest.* 78:587–591.

Booth NA, Anderson JA, Bennett B. (1985). Platelet release protein which inhibits plasminogen activators. *J Clin Pathol.* 38:825–830.

Booyse FM, Lin PH, Traylor M, Bruce R. (1988). Purification and properties of a single-chain urokinase-type plasminogen activator form produced by subcultured human umbilical vein endothelial cells. *J Biol Chem.* 263:15139–15145.

Boyle MDP, Chiodo VA, Lawman JP, Gee AP, Young M. (1987). Urokinase: a chemotactic factor for polymorphonuclear leukocytes in vivo. *J Immunol.* 139:169–174.

Britton BJ, Giddings JC, Brooks L, Bloom AL. (1977). Fibrinolytic, factor VIII and pulse rate responses to repeated adrenaline infusion followed by haemorrhagia. *Thromb Haemost.* 37:527–534.

Campbell EJ, Davis Cury J, Lazarus CJ, Welgus HG. (1987). Monocyte procollagenase and tissue inhibitor of metalloproteinases. *J Biol Chem.* 263:15862–15868.

Chakrabarti R, Hocking ED, Fearnley GR. (1969). Reaction pattern to three stresses—electroplexy, surgery and myocardial infarction—of fibrinolysis and plasma fibrinogen. *J Clin Pathol.* 22:659–662.

Chapman HA, Stone OL. (1984). Comparison of live human neutrophil and alveolar macrophage elastolytic activity in vitro. *J Clin Invest.* 74:1693–1700.

Chapman HA Jr, Stone OL, Vavrin Z. (1984). Degradation of fibrin and elastin by intact human alveolar macrophages in vitro. Characterization of a plasminogen activator and its role in matrix degradation. *J Clin Invest.* 73:806–815.

Chapman HA, Stone OL. (1985). Characterization of a macrophage-derived plasminogen-activator inhibitor. Similarities with placenta urokinase inhibitor. *Biochem J.* 230:109–114.

Chin JR, Murphy G, Werb Z. (1985). Stromelysin: a connective tissue degrading metalloendopeptidase secreted by stimulated rabbit synovial fibroblasts in parallel with collagenase biosynthesis, isolation, characterization and substrates. *J Biol Chem.* 260:12367–12376.

Chua CC, Geiman DE, Keller GH, Ladda RL. (1985). Induction of collagenase secretion in human fibroblast cultures by growth promoting factors. *J Biol Chem.* 260:5213–5216.

Coccheri S, Astrup T. (1961). Thromboplastic and fibrinolytic activities of large human vessels. *Proc Soc Exp Biol Med.* 108:369–372.

Coleman PI, Batouski PA, Gelehrter TD. (1982). The dexamethasone-induced inhibitor of fibrinolytic activity in hepatoma cells. A cellular product which specifically inhibits plasminogen activation. *J Biol Chem.* 257:4260–4263.

Colucci M, Paramo JA, Collen D. (1985). Generation in plasma of a fast-acting inhibitor of plasminogen activator in response to endotoxin stimulation. *J Clin Invest.* 75:818–824.

Comp PC, Nixon RR, Cooper MR, Esmon CT. (1984). Familial proteins deficiency is associated with recurrent thrombosis. *J Clin Invest.* 74:2082–2088.

Couch CB, Strittmatter WJ. (1983). Rat myoblast fusion requires metalloendoprotease activity. *Cell.* 32:257–265.

Dastre A. (1893). Fibrinolyse dans le sang. *Arch Physiol Norm Pathol.* 5:661–663.

Dayer J-M, Beutler B, Cerami A. (1985). Cachectin/tumor necrosis factor stimulates collagenase and prostaglandin E_2 production by human synovial cells and dermal fibroblasts. *J Exp Med.* 162:2163–2168.

Degen JL, Estensen RD, Nagamine Y, Reich E. (1985). Induction and desensitization of plasminogen activator gene expression by tumor promoters. *J Biol Chem.* 260:12426–12433.

Deutsch DG, Mertz ET. (1970). Plasminogen purification from human plasma by affinity chromatography. *Science* 170:1095–1096.

Doody KJ, Dunn RC, Buttram VC. (1989). Recombinant tissue plasminogen activator reduces adhesion formation in a rabbit uterine horn model. *Fertil Steril.* 51:509–512.

Dosne AM, Dupuy E, Bodevin E. (1978). Production of a fibrinolytic inhibitor by cultured endothelial cells derived from human umbilical vein. *Thromb Res.* 12:377–387.

Dubin A, Potempa J, Silberring J. (1985). Horse leucocyte proteinase inhibitor system. Kinetic parameters of the inhibiton reaction. *Int J Biochem.* 17:509–513.

Dubin A, Potempa J, Turynea B. (1986). The interaction between some serine proteinases and horse leukocyte inhibitor. *Folia Histochem Cytobiol.* 24:163–168.

Ehrlich HJ, Jaskunas RJ, Grinnell BW, Yan SB, Bang NU. (1989). Direct expression of recombinant activated human protein C, a serine protease. *J Biol Chem.* 264:14298–14304.

Ellis H, Harrison W, Hugh TB. (1965). The healing of peritoneum under normal and pathologic conditions. *Br J Surg.* 52:471–476.

Emeis JJ, Van Hinsbergh VWM, Verheijen JH, Wijngaards G. (1983). Inhibition of tissue-type plasminogen activator by conditioned medium from cultured human and porcine vascular endothelial cells. *Biochem Biophys Res Commun.* 110:392–398.

Emeis JJ. (1985). Fast hepatic clearance of plasminogen activator inhibitor. *Thromb Haemost.* 54:230.

Emeis JJ, Kooistra T. (1986). Interleukin-1 and lipopolysaccharide induces a fast-acting inhibitor of tissue-type plasminogen activator in vivo and in cultured endothelial cells. *J Exp Med.* 163:1260–1272.

Ende N, Auditore J. (1961). Fibrinolytic activity of human tissues and dog mast cell tumors. *Am J Clin Pathol.* 36:16–24.

Engqvist A, Winther O. (1972). Variations of plasma cortisol and blood fibrinolytic activity during anaesthetic and surgical stress. *Br J Anaesth.* 44:1291–1297.

Erickson LA, Ginsberg MH, Loskutoff DJ. (1984). Detection and partial characterization of an inhibitor of plasminogen activator in human platelets. *J Clin Invest.* 74:1465–1472.

Esmon CT, Galvin JB, Johnson AE, DeBault LE, Esmon NL. (1987). Thrombomodulin: an example of cell surface regulation of protease function. *Perspect Inflamm Neoplasia Vascular Cell Biol.* 263:213–221.

Esnard F, Dupuy E, Dosne AM, Bodevin E. (1982). Partial characterization of a fibrinolytic inhibitor produced by cultured endothelial cells derived from human umbilical vein. *Thromb Haemost.* 47:128–131.

Fini ME, Plucinska IM, Mayer AS, Gross RH, Brinckerhoff GF. (1987). A gene for rabbit synovial cell collagenase: member of a family of metalloproteinases that degrade the connective tissue matrix. *Biochemistry.* 26:6156–6165.

Friezner Degen SJ, Heckel JL, Reich E, Degen JL. (1987). The murine urokinase-type plasminogen activator gene. *Biochemistry.* 26:8270–8279.

Fukasawa M, Campeau JD, Girgis W, Bryant SM, Rodgers KE, diZerega GS. (1989). Production of protease inhibitors by postsurgical macrophages. *J Surg Res.* 46:256–261.

Furman W, Schnyder M. (1984). Alveolar macrophage plasminogen activator. *Exp Lung Res.* 6:159–169.

Griffin JH, Evatt B, Zimmerman TS, Kleiss AJ, Wideman C. (1981). Deficiency in protein C in congenital thrombotic disease. *J Clin Invest.* 68:1370–1373.

Grimaldi G, DiFiore P, Kajtaniak Locatelli E, Falco J, Blasi F. (1986). Modulation of urokinase plasminogen activator gene expression during the transition from quiescent to proliferative state in normal mouse cells. *EMBO J.* 5:855–861.

Grossbard EB. (1987). Recombinant tissue plasminogen activator: a brief review. *Pharmacol Res.* 4:375–378.

Hamilton JA, Slywka J. (1981). Stimulation of human synovial fibroblast plasminogen activator production by mononuclear cell supernatants. *J Immunol.* 126:851–855.

Harada S, Dannenberg AM, Vogt RF, Myrick JE, Tanaka F, Redding LC, Merkhofer RM, Pula PJ, Scott AL. (1987). Inflammatory mediators and modulators released in organ culture from rabbit skin lesions produce *in vivo* by sulfur mustard. *Am J Pathol.* 126:148–162.

Harris ED, Krane SM. (1974). Collagenases. *N Engl J Med.* 291:557–563, 605–609, 652–661.

Harris KW, Esmon CT. (1985). Protein S is required for bovine platelets to support activated protein C binding and activity. *J Biol Chem.* 260:2007–2010.

Hau T, Payne D, Simmons RL. (1979). Fibrinolytic activity of the peritoneum during experimental peritonitis. *Surg Gynecol Obstet.* 148:415–418.

Hedlund PO. (1969). Antifibrinolytic therapy with cyklokapron in connection with prostatectomy. *Scand J Urol Nephrol.* 3:177–182.

Heimburger N. (1974). Biochemistry of proteinase inhibitors from human plasma: a review of recent development. Bayer Symposium. In: Fritz H, Tschesche H, Greene LJ, Truscheit E, eds. *Proteinase Inhibitors.* New York: Springer-Verlag; 14–22.

Hekman CM, Loskutoff DJ. (1985). Endothelial cells produce a latent inhibitor of plasminogen activators that can be activated by denaturants. *J Biol Chem.* 260:11581–11585.

Innes D, Sevitt S. (1974). Coagulation and fibrinolysis in injured patients. *J Clin Pathol.* 17:1–13.

Jespersen J, Astrup TA. (1983). Study of the fibrin plate assay of fibrinolytic agents. *Haemostasis.* 13:301–315.

Klimetsek V, Sorg C. (1979). The production of fibrinolysis inhibitors as a parameter of the activation state in murine macrophages. *Eur J Immunol.* 9:613–619.

Kluft C, Verheijen JH, Jie AFH, Rijken DC, Preston FE, Sue-Ling HM, Jespersen J, Aasen AO. (1985). The postoperative fibrinolytic shutdown: a rapidly reverting acute phase pattern for the fast-acting inhibitor of tissue-type plasminogen activator after trauma. *Scand J Clin Lab Invest.* 45:466–471.

Kooistra T, Sprengers ED, Van Hinsbergh VWM. (1986). Rapid inactivation of the plasminogen-activator inhibitor upon secretion from cultured human endothelial cells. *Biochem J.* 239:497–503.

Kornecki E, Ehrlich YH, De Mars DD, Lenox RH. (1986). Exposure of fibrinogen receptors in human platelets by surface proteolysis with elastase. *J Clin Invest.* 77:750–756.

Korsan-Bengtsen K, Wilhelmsen L, Tibblin G. (1973). Blood coagulation and fibrinolysis in relation to degree of physical activity during work and leisure time. *Acta Med Scand.* 193:73–77.

Kruithof EKO, Tran-Thang C, Ransijn A, Backmann F. (1984). Demonstration of a fast-acting inhibitor of plasminogen activators in human plasma. *Blood.* 64:907–913.

Kumkumian GK, Lafyatis R, Remmers EF, Case JP, Kimsj W, Ider RL. (1989). Platelet-derived growth factor and IL-1 interactions in rheumatoid arthritis. *J Immunol.* 143:833–837.

Kuraoka S, Campeau JD, Rodgers KE, Nakamura RM, diZerega GS. (1992). Effects of interleukin-1 (IL-1) on postsurgical macrophage secretion of protease and protease inhibitor activities. *J Surg Res.* 52:71–78.

Largman C, Brodrick JW, Geokas MC. (1976). Purification and characterization of two human pancreatic elastases. *Biochemistry.* 15:2491–2500.

Laug WE. (1985). Vascular smooth muscle cells inhibit plasminogen activator secreted by endothelial cells. *Thromb Haemost.* 20:165–172.

Lawrence DA, Loskutoff DJ. (1986). Inactivation of plasminogen activator inhibitor by oxidants. *Biochemistry.* 25:6351–6355.

Lee LS, Weinstein IB. (1978). Epidermal growth factor, like phorbol esters induces plasminogen activator in HeLa cells. *Nature.* 274:696–697.

Leizer T, Hamilton JA. (1989). Plasminogen activator and prostaglandin E2 levels in human synovial fibroblasts. Differential stimulation by synovial activator and other cytokines. *J Immunol.* 143:971–978.

Levin EG. (1983). Latent tissue plasminogen activator produced by human endothelial cells in culture: evidence for an enzyme-inhibitor complex. *Proc Natl Acad Sci USA.* 80:6804–6808.

Levin EG. (1986). Quantitation and properties of the active and latent plasminogen activator inhibitors in cultures of human endothelial cells. *Blood.* 67:1309–1317.

Levin EG, Santell L. (1988). Stimulation and desensitization of tissue plasminogen activator release from human endothelial cells. *J Biol Chem.* 263:9360–9365.

Levin EG, Marotti KR, Santell L. (1989). Protein kinase C and the stimulation of tissue plasminogen activator release from human endothelial cells. *J Biol Chem.* 264:16030–16036.

Loskutoff DJ, Van Mourik JA, Erickson LA, Lawrence D. (1983). Detection of an unusually stable fibrinolytic inhibitor produced by bovine endothelial cells. *Proc Natl Acad Sci USA.* 80:2956–2961.

Macfarlane RG. (1937). Fibrinolysis following operation. *Lancet.* 1:10.

Markwardt F, Klocking HP. (1977). Heparin-induced release of plasminogen activator. *Haemostasis.* 6:370–374.

Marlar RA, Kleiss AJ, Griffin JH. (1982). Mechanism of action of human activated protein C, a thrombin-dependent anticoagulant enzyme. *Blood.* 59:1067–1072.

Mayer M, Yedgar S, Hurwitz A, Palti Z, Finzi Z, Milwidsky A. (1988). Effect of viscous macromolecules on peritoneal plasminogen activator activity: a potential mechanism for their ability to reduce postoperative adhesion formation. *Am J Obstet Gynecol.* 159:957–963.

Medcalf RL, Hamilton JA. (1986). Human synovial fibroblasts produce urokinase-type plasminogen activator. *Arthritis Rheum.* 29:1397–1402.

Menzies D, Ellis H. (1989). Intra-abdominal adhesions and their prevention by topical tissue plasminogen activator. *J R Soc Med.* 82:534–535.

Merlo G, Fausone G, Barbero C, Castagna B. (1980). Fibrinolytic activity of the human peritoneum. *Eur Surg Res.* 12:433–438.

Michel JB, Quertermous T. (1989). Modulation of mRNA levels for urinary- and tissue-type plasminogen activator and plasminogen activators inhibitors 1 and 2 in human fibroblasts by interleukin-1. *J Immunol.* 143:890–895.

Mochan E, Uhl J. (1984). Elevations in synovial fluid plasminogen activator in patients with rheumatoid arthritis. *J Rheumatol.* 11:123–131.

Moroz LA, Gilmore NJ. (1976). Fibrinolysis in normal plasma and blood: evidence for significant mechanisms independent of the plasminogen-plasmin system. *Blood.* 48:531–545.

Myhre-Jensen O, Larsen SB, Astrup T. (1969). Fibrinolytic activity in serosal and synovial membranes. *Arch Pathol.* 88:623–625.

Nagamine Y, Pearson D, Altus MS, Reich E. (1984). cDNA and gene nucleotide sequence of porcine plasminogen activator. *Nucleic Acids Res.* 12:9525–9541.

Nielsen LS, Kellerman GM, Behrendt N, Picone R, Dano K, Blasi F. (1988). A 55,000–60,000 Mr receptor protein for urokinase-type plasminogen activator. *J Biol Chem.* 263:2358–2363.

Nilsson IM, Pandolfi M. (1970). Fibrinolytic response of the vascular wall. *Thromb Diath Haemorrh Suppl.* 40:231–242.

Ny T, Bjersing L, Hsuek AJW, Loskutoff DJ. (1985). Cultured granulosa cells produce two plasminogen activators and an antiactivator, each regulated differently by gonadotropins. *Endocrinology.* 116:1666–1668.

Orita H, Campeau JD, Gale JA, Nakamura RM, diZerega G. (1986). Differential secretion of plasminogen activator activity by postsurgical activated macrophages. *J Surg Res.* 41:569–573.

Orita H, Girgis W, diZerega GS. (1991). Inhibition of postsurgical adhesions in a standardized rabbit model: intraperitoneal administration of tissue plasminogen activator. *Int J Fertil.* 36:172–177.

Paramo JA, De Boer A, Colucci M, Jonker JJC, Collen D. (1985). Plasminogen activator inhibitor (PA-inhibitor) activity in the blood of patients with deep vein thrombosis. *Thromb Haemost.* 54:725–729.

Perlmutter DH, Punsal PI. (1988). Distinct and additive effects of elastase and endotoxin on expression of alpha$_1$-proteinase inhibitor in mononuclear phagocytes. *J Biol Chem.* 263:16499–16503.

Philips M, Juul AG, Thorsen S. (1984). Human endothelial cells produce a plasminogen activator inhibitor and a tissue-type plasminogen activator-inhibitor complex. *Biochim Biophys Acta.* 802:99–110.

Pike GJ, Turner RL, Manohitharajah SM, Deverall PB. (1975). Fibrinolysis in cyanotic and acyanotic children before and after open intracardiac operations with the Bentley temptrol oxygenator. *J Thorac Cardiovasc Surg.* 69:922–926.

Porter JM, Ball AP, Silver D. (1971). Mesothelial fibrinolysis. *J Thorac Cardiovasc Surg.* 62:725–730.

Postlethwaite AE, Lachman LB, Mainardi CL, Kang AH. (1983). Interleukin 1 stimulation of collagenase production by cultured fibroblasts. *J Exp Med.* 157:801–806.

Potempa J, Dubin A, Watorek W, Travis J. (1988). An elastase inhibitor from equine leukocyte cytosol belongs to the serpin superfamily. Further characterization and amino acid sequence of the reaction center. *J Biol Chem.* 263:7364–7369.

Raftery AT. (1979). Regeneration of peritoneum: a fibrinolytic study. *J Anat.* 129:659–664.

Raftery AT. (1981). Effect of peritoneal trauma on peritoneal fibrinolytic activity and intraperitoneal adhesion formation. *Eur Surg Res.* 13:397–401.

Ratnoff OD. (1953). Studies on a proteolytic enzyme in human plasma. IX. Fibrinogen and fibrin as substrated for the proteolytic enzyme of plasma. *J Clin Invest.* 32:473–479.

Rennie JAN, Bennett B, Ogston D. (1977). Effect of local exercise and vessel occlusion on fibrinolytic activity. *J Clin Pathol.* 30:350–352.

Riccio A, Grimaldi G, Verde P. (1985). The human urokinase plasminogen activator gene and its promoter. *Nucleic Acids Res.* 13:2759–2771.

Rivett AJ. (1989). The multicatalytic proteinase. Multiple proteolytic activities. *J Biol Chem.* 264:12215–12219.

Rodgers KE. (1990). Nonsteroidal anti-inflammatory drugs (NSAIDs) in the treatment of postsurgical adhesions. In: diZerega GS, Malinak LR, Diamond MD, Linsky C, eds. *Treatment of Postsurgical Adhesions.* (Progress in Clinical Biology Research). New York: Wiley Liss Press; 358:119–130.

Rodgers K, Ellefson D, Girgis W, diZerega GS. (in press). Protease and protease inhibitor secretion following in vitro exposure to tolmetin. *Agents Actions.*

Sakata Y, Griffin JH, Loskutoff DJ. (1985). Role of protein C in fibrinolysis. *Thromb Haemost.* 54:118–123.

Saksela O, Moscatelli D, Rifkin DB. (1987). The opposing effects of basic fibroblast growth factor and transforming growth factor beta on the regulation of plasminogen activator activity in capillary endothelial cells. *J Cell Biol.* 105:957–963.

Santell L, Levin EG. (1988). Cyclic AMP potentiates phorbol ester stimulation of tissue plasminogen activator release and inhibits secretion of plasminogen activator inhibitor-1 from human endothelial cells. *J Biol Chem.* 263:16802–16808.

Scarpati EM, Sadler JE. (1989). Regulation of endothelial cell coagulant properties. *J Biol Chem.* 264:20705–20713.

Scheele G, Bartelt D, Bieger W. (1981). Characteristization of human exocrine pancreatic proteins by two dimensional isoelectric focusing dodeceyl sodium sulfate gel electrophoresis. *Gastroenterology.* 80:461–473.

Seltzer JL, Eisen AZ, Bauer EA, Morris NP, Glanville RW, Burgeson RE. (1989). Cleavage of type VII collagen by interstitial collagenase and type IV collagenase (gelatinase) derived from human skin. *J Biol Chem.* 264:3822–3826.

Sottrup-Jensen L. (1989). Alpha-macroglobulins: structure, shape and mechanism of proteinase complex formation. *J Biol Chem.* 264:11539–11542.

Sprengers ED, Verheijen JH, Van Hinsbergh VWM, Emeis JJ. (1984). Evidence for the presence of two different fibrinolytic inhibitors in human endothelial cell conditioned medium. *Biochim Biophys Acta.* 801:163–170.

Sprengers ED, Pincen HMG, Kooistra T, Van Hinsbergh VWM. (1985). Inhibition of plasminogen activators by conditioned medium of human hepatocytes and hepatoma cell line Hep G2. *J Lab Clin Med.* 105:751–759.

Sprengers ED, Akkerman JWN, Jansen BG. (1986). Blood platelet plasminogen activator inhibitor: two different pools of endothelial cell type plasminogen activator inhibitor in human blood. *Thromb Haemost.* 55:325–329.

Sprengers ED, Kluft C. (1987). Plasminogen activator inhibitors. *Blood.* 69:381–387.

Stoppelli MP, Corti A, Soffientini A, Cassani G, Blasi F, Assoian RK. (1985). Differentiation-enhanced binding of the amino terminal fragment of human urokinase plasminogen activator to aspecific receptor on U937 monocytes. *Proc Natl Acad Sci USA.* 82:4939–4943.

Stricklin GP, Welgus GP. (1983). Human skin fibroblast collagenase inhibitor: purification and biochemical characterization. *J Biol Chem.* 258:12252–12258.

Strous GJ, van Kerkhof P, Dekker J, Schwartz AL. (1988). Metalloendoprotease inhibitors block protein synthesis, intracellular transport, and endocytosis in hepatoma cells. *J Biol Chem.* 263:18197–18204.

Tani T, Ohsumi J, Mita K, Takiguchi Y. (1988). Identification of a novel class of elastase isozyme, human pancreatic elastase III, by cDNA and genomic gene cloning. *J Biol Chem.* 263:1231–1239.

Thompson JN, Paterson-Brown S, Harbourne T, Whawell SA, Kalodiki E, Dudley HA. (1989). Reduced human peritoneal plasminogen activating activity: possible mechanism of adhesion formation. *Br J Surg.* 76:382–384.

Thorsen S, Philips M. (1984). Isolation of tissue-type plasminogen activator-inhibitor complexes from human plasma. Evidence for a rapid plasminogen activator inhibitor. *Biochim Biophys Acta.* 802:111–118.

Travis J, Salvesen GS. (1983). Human plasma proteinase inhibitors. *Annu Rev Biochem.* 52:655–709.

Unkeless JC, Dano K, Kellerman GM, Reich E. (1974). Fibrinolysis associated with oncogenic transformation. Partial purification and characterization of the cell factor, a plasminogen activator. *J Biol Chem.* 249:4295–4305.

van Hinsbergh VWM, Kooistra T, Scheffer MA, van Bockel JH, van Muijen GNP. (1990). Characterization and fibrinolytic properties of human omental tissue mesothelial cells. Comparison with endothelial cells. *Blood.* 75:1490–1497.

Vassalli JD, Baccino D, Belin D. (1985). A cellular binding site for the Mr 55,000 form of the human plasminogen activator, urokinase. *J Cell Biol.* 100:86–92.

Vipond MN, Whawell SA, Thompson JN, Dudley HAF. (1990). Peritoneal fibrinolytic activity and intra-abdominal adhesions. *Lancet.* 335:1120–1122.

Wagner OF, Binder BR. (1986). Purification of an active plasminogen activator inhibitor immunologically related to the endothelial type plasminogen activator inhibitor from the conditioned media of a human melanoma cell line. *J Biol Chem.* 261:14474–14481.

Wahl LM, Winter CC. (1984). Regulation of guinea pig macrophage collagenase production by dexamethasone and colchicine. *Arch Biochem Biophys.* 230:661–667.

Wahl SM, Wahl LM. (1985). Regulation of macrophage collagenase, prostaglandin, and fibroblast-activating-factor production by anti-inflammatory agents: different regulatory mechanisms for tissue injury and repair. *Cell Immunol.* 92:302–312.

Wahl LM, Lampel L. (1987). Regulation of human peripheral blood monocyte collagenase by prostaglandins and anti-inflammatory drugs. *Cell Immunol.* 105:411–422.

Wallenbeck IAM, Tangen O. (1975). On the lysis of fibrin formed in the presence of dextran and other macromolecules. *Thromb Res.* 6:75–86.

Welgus HG, Stricklin GP. (1983). Human skin fibroblast collagenase inhibitor: comparative studies in human connective tissues, serum, and amniotic fluid. *J Biol Chem.* 258:12259–12264.

Welgus HG, Campbell EJ, Bar-Shavit Z, Senior RM, Teitelbaum SL. (1985). Human alveolar macrophages produce a fibroblast-like collagenase and collagenase inhibitor. *J Clin Invest.* 76:219–224.

Werb Z. (1978). Biochemical actions of glucocorticoids on macrophages in culture. *J Exp Med.* 147:1695–1711.

Whitaker D, Papadimitriou JM, Walters N-I. (1982). The mesothelium: its fibrinolytic properties. *J Pathol.* 136:295–299.

Wiman B, Collen D. (1979). Fibrinolysis inhibitors. In: Collen D, Winman B, Verstraete M, eds. *Physiological Inhibitors of Blood Coagulation and Fibrinolysis.* Amsterdam: Elsevier; 247–254.

Wiman B, Ljungberg B, Chmielewska J, Urden G, Blombaeck M, Johnsson H. (1985). The role of the fibrinolytic system in deep vein thrombosis. *J Lab Clin Med.* 105:265–270.

Wohlwend A, Belin D, Vassalli JD. (1987). Plasminogen activator-specific inhibitors in mouse macrophages: in vivo and in vitro modulation of their synthesis and secretion. *J Immunol.* 139:1278–1284.

Wojta J, Hoover RL, Daniel TO. (1989). Vascular origin determines plasminogen activator expression in human endothelial cells. *J Biol Chem.* 264:2846–2852.

Wun TC, Reich E. (1987). An inhibitor of plasminogen activation from human placenta. *J Biol Chem.* 262:3646–3653.

9

Intraperitoneal Adhesions

A MAJOR CLINICAL PROBLEM RELATING TO PERITONEAL REPAIR IS THE formation of intra-abdominal and pelvic adhesions. Although the term *adhesions* is used in reference to ophthalmic, orthopedic, central nervous system, cardivascular, and intrauterine repair processes, the formation of peritoneal adhesions is unique and specific to the peritoneal response to injury.

Incidence

The most common cause of peritoneal adhesions is prior surgery (Weibel & Majno, 1973). Perry, Smith, and Yonehiro (1955) found that 79% of the 388 patients they surveyed with abdominal adhesions had a history of surgery, 18% had a history of inflammatory disease, and 11% had congenital adhesions. In a further analysis of patients with adhesions related to inflammatory disease, Perry et al. reported that 42% had acute appendicitis, 14.5% had diverticulitis, and the remaining patients had pelvic inflammatory disease, cholecystitis, and Crohn's disease. Raf (1969) reported that 86% of patients with adhesions had a history of peritoneal surgery. In a survey of 142 patients with obstruction of the small intestine due to adhesions, Nemir (1952) reported that 73% had prior surgery, 20% had inflammatory disease, and 6% had congenital adhesions. In a prospective analysis of 210 patients undergoing laparotomy who previously underwent one or more abdominal operations, 93% had intra-abdominal adhesions. This contrasted with 115 first-time laparotomies in which only 10% of patients had adhesions (Menzies & Ellis, 1990). Bowel obstruction from adhesion is most prevalent in the pediatric age group where 8% of neonates undergoing abdominal surgery will require a future laparotomy for this complication (Wilkins & Spitz, 1986).

Adhesions occur in 55% to 100% of fertility-enhancing procedures as determined by second-look laparoscopy performed in a number of large, multicenter studies (Table 9.1; Adhesion Study Group, 1983; Interceed

TABLE 9.1. Pelvic adhesions noted at second-look laparoscopy.

	Time from initial procedure	Total no. of patients	Total no. with adhesions	% with adhesions
Diamond et al. (1987)	1 wk–12 wk	106	91	86
Decherney & Mezer (1984)	4 wk–16 wk	20	15	75
	1 yr–3 yr	41	31	76
Surrey & Friedman (1982)	6 wk–8 wk	31	22	71
	≥6 mo	6	5	83
Pittaway et al. (1985)	4 wk–6 wk	23	23	100
Trimbos-Kemper et al. (1985)	8 days	188	104	55
Daniell and Pittaway (1983)	4 wk–6 wk	25	24	96

From Diamond, 1988.

(TC7) Adhesion Barrier Study Group, 1989). Diamond et al. (1987) used second-look laparoscopy to evaluate the location of adhesions in 161 infertility patients after reproductive pelvic surgery. Fifty percent of the pelvic sites that did not contain adhesions at the time of the initial procedure developed adhesions following this procedure. In a prospective study of 955 patients undergoing laparoscopic sterilization, Szigetvari, Feinman, Barad, Bartfai, and Kaali (1989) confirmed that significant adhesions were more frequent among patients with prior pelvic or abdominal surgery (28% versus 2% in the no-prior-surgery group). DeCherney and Mezer (1984) found that 75% of the 61 infertile females they evaluated after salpingostomy contained adhesions upon follow-up laparoscopy. Appendectomy and gynecologic surgery are the most frequent surgical procedures implicated in the formation of clinically significant adhesions (Raf, 1969).

Predisposing Factors

Age

In two large surveys postsurgical adhesion formation did not appear to be age-dependent (Perry et al., 1955; Weibel & Majno, 1973); however, no prospective evaluation of the effect of age on adhesion formation is available. Weibel and Majno (1973) reported a slightly higher frequency of "spontaneous" adhesions (i.e., those adhesions that form without any apparent cause) after age 60.

Sex

There does not appear to be a sex bias in the development of postoperative adhesions. Weibel and Majno (1973) reported a slightly higher frequency of adhesions among male patients. After excluding adhesions resulting from gynecologic procedures, Raf (1969) reported that the incidence of intraperitoneal adhesions was 47% in male patients and 53% in female patients.

Anatomical Site

The omentum is particularly susceptible to adhesion formation. In Weibel and Majno's studies (1973), the omentum was involved in 92% of postoperative adhesions. The omentum was also the predominant organ involved in "spontaneous" adhesions (i.e., those with no prior history of surgery); 100% of the 126 spontaneous adhesions examined by Weibel and Majno involved the omentum. These reports raise the question of omentectomy during pelvic surgery where postoperative adhesion formation is likely to occur. With the exception of the omentum, the internal organs involved in postoperative adhesions may vary as a function of the surgical procedure. The small intestine was involved in 21% of the adhesions present after appendectomy but in only 6% of those formed following gynecologic laparotomy; 47% and 19% of adhesions that form after appendectomy and gynecologic laparotomy, respectively, involve the colon (Turunen, 1933). The ovary is the most common site for adhesions to form after reconstructive surgery of the female pelvis (Adhesion Study Group, 1983; Diamond et al., 1987; Interceed (TC7) Adhesion Barrier Study Group, 1989). Ovarian adhesions were found at second-look laparoscopy in over 90% of cases after ovarian surgery (Pittaway, Daniell, & Maxson, 1985).

Blood

The role of blood in the peritoneal cavity in the formation of adhesions is controversial. Hertzler (1919) reported that large volumes of clotted blood could be completely absorbed by normal peritoneum within 48 hours. Jackson (1958) found that 100 ml of free blood and a well-formed clot were absorbed from the peritoneal cavity within 8 days. Nisell and Larsson (1978) suggested that trauma to the serosa rather than blood was the instigator of adhesion formation. Bronson and Wallach (1977), on the other hand, finding no etiological factor in 46% of their infertile patients with pelvic adhesions, suggested that ovarian bleeding associated with follicle rupture at the time of ovulation may produce significant adhesions.

Ryan, Grobety, and Majno (1971) showed that blood may play an important part in the pathogenesis of adhesions. Addition of fresh blood to an otherwise uninjured peritoneal cavity resulted in omental adhesions, whereas preformed clots produced widespread adhesions even without peritoneal injury. When 0.2 to 2 ml of fresh blood was dripped onto a dried peritoneal surface and allowed to clot, adhesions formed at the site of injury. If peritoneum was excised, the degree to which clot induced adhesion formation was markedly enhanced. When addition of fresh blood was delayed, adhesions formed if blood was added to the injured site. The addition of blood alone without cecal drying led to more limited adhesion formation. Serosal damage, no matter how mild, may lead to adhesions in the presence of blood. Clotted blood may constitute a fibrinous network upon which fibroblasts may proliferate, resulting in adhesions (Pfeffer, 1980). Golan and Winston (1989) confirmed the findings of Ryan et al. (1971), reporting that blood in conjunction with trauma to the serosa is more important in adhesion formation than either trauma alone or trauma and serum.

Laparoscopic Surgery

Although there are obvious advantages to laparoscopy relative to laparotomy with respect to the duration of hospitalization and recovery time, no clinical studies adequately compare the occurrence of adhesions following the two groups of procedures (see Chapter 10). Luciano, Maier, Koch, Nielsen, and Whitman (1989) found greater postoperative adhesion formation after laparotomy compared to laparoscopy in a rabbit model. In addition, less adhesion reformation was noted after salpingo-ovariolysis by laparoscopy than by laparotomy. In contrast, the mean area of uterine adhesions was similar between rats after uterine injury by microsurgery involving laparoscopy or laparotomy (Filmar, Jetha, McComb, & Gomel, 1989a, 1989b). Mecke, Semm, Freys, Argirious, and Gent (1989) reported a 52% incidence in pelvic adhesions in 33 patients who previously underwent adhesiolysis during removal of ectopic pregnancy by laparoscopy. Although intraoperative bleeding can usually be controlled during laparoscopic surgery, rigorous removal of clot and complete postoperative hemostasis may be more problematic.

Previous laparotomy is sometimes considered a relative contraindication for laparoscopy because of the potential for adhesion formation following the initial procedure. In a prospective study of 955 patients undergoing laparoscopic sterilization, Szigetvari et al. (1989) reported that the risk of major complications arising from the laparoscopic procedure was not increased in patients with previous laparotomies, suggesting that the risk of adhesion formation from prior surgical procedures does not necessarily preclude laparoscopic procedures.

Peritoneal Closure

Adhesions, delayed healing, and wound breakdown are often attributed to failure of peritoneal suturing or the presence of deperitonealized areas within the abdomen. To reconstruct the pelvis after removal of viscera and peritoneum seems a logical procedure for good surgical practice. However, examination of the data indicates that approximation of peritoneum by sutures to cover vascularized areas denuded by the previous dissection may not facilitate peritoneal repair. After resection of peritoneal tissue, natural healing is associated with less adhesion formation than after reapproximation with staples or sutures (McDonald et al., 1988). There is no difference in adhesions to the previous laparotomy incisions after closure with or without peritoneal suturing (Tulandi, Hum, & Gelfand, 1988).

Animal Studies

Milewczyk (1989) evaluated adhesion formation to anterior peritoneum in rabbits after laparotomy with and without peritoneal closure. Following laparotomy in 50 rabbits (two incisions in each), the wound was closed in 25 rabbits without suturing the parietal peritoneum whereas in the remaining 25 rabbits the parietal peritoneum was sutured closed. On the 1st, 3rd, 7th, 14th, and 21st days following the procedure, five rabbits from each group were sacrificed. It was found that in the nonsutured group adhesions appeared in only 3 out of 50 incisions, whereas in the sutured group 17 adhesions formed out of 50 wounds. This significant difference indicates that parietal peritoneum that has not been sutured heals better and with a smaller number of adhesions than sutured parietal peritoneum. Similar results were reported by McDonald et al. (1988). Resection of peritoneal tissue followed by natural healing is preferable to reapproximation of free peritoneal edges with either staples or sutures.

The effect of peritoneal closure after reproductive surgery through Pfannenstiel incisions was studied by second-look laparoscopy (Table 9.2; Tulandi et al., 1988). No difference was found in the length of hospital stay, the incidence of wound complications, or other postoperative complications after abdominal closure with or without peritoneal suturing. There is no difference in postoperative complications, wound healing, and adhesions to previous laparotomy incisions after laparotomy closure with or without peritoneal suturing.

The effects of suturing and stapling peritoneal edges or excising, cauterizing, and abrading areas of peritoneum on adhesion formation were evaluated by McDonald et al. (1988) in rabbits. Two weeks after peritoneal injury, the amount of adhesion formation was noted. Resection of peritoneal tissue with natural healing was preferable to reapproximation of free peritoneal edges with either staples or sutures. Ling, Sto-

TABLE 9.2. Postoperative complications after reproductive operations in which the abdomen was closed with or without peritoneal suturing.

Postoperative complications	Peritoneal closure ($n = 168$) (%)	No peritoneal closure ($n = 165$) (%)
Wound infection	6 (3.6)	4 (2.4)
Pneumonia	1 (0.6)	1 (0.6)
Urinary tract infection	1 (0.6)	2 (1.2)
Leak of dextran	1 (0.6)	4 (2.4)

From Tulandi et al., 1988.

vall, Meyer, Elkins, and Muram (1989) assessed adhesion formation after peritoneal closure with absorbable staples. Absorbable staples were associated with increased adhesion formation when compared to the other methods of injury. The amount of adhesion formation correlates with the presence and quantity of suture material (Luciano, Hauser, & Benda, 1983). Sutured peritoneum is twice as likely to be associated with adhesion formation that is associated with postoperative bowel obstruction (Conolly & Stephens, 1968).

Peritoneal Closure: Horse

Similar conclusions were reached by Swanwick, Stockdale and Milne (1973) in a study of parietal peritoneum after abdominal surgery using horses with and without intraperitoneal infection. Adhesions to the peritoneum occurred in 50% of the peritoneal closures contrasted to 27% of the incisions where peritoneum was not closed. Reapproximated peritoneal defects contained adhesions in 53% of the sites, in contrast to 17% of the cases where peritoneal defects were left unopposed. In ponies with iatrogenic peritonitis, adhesions occurred in 9 of the 12 ponies with peritoneal closure, and 3 of the 12 without. Overall well being of the infected ponies was similar between the two groups. The unsutured midline peritoneal incision appeared to be spontaneously closed by the sixth to eighth postoperative day. In contrast the sutured peritoneum contained evidence of trauma or tears from the tension of the suture lines. Sutured peritoneum of midline incisions appeared healed 2 days after surgery whereas the unsutured peritoneal incisions required 6 to 8 days for closure. Some of the infected unsutured defects in the ponies were not healed after 8 days. In ponies with fecal contamination, adhesions were present in 75% of the sutured and 25% of the unsutured incisions. Thus the combination of suture material and infection is particularly prone to adhesion formation.

Clinical Studies

Clinical reports after cancer surgery demonstrate normal healing of unsutured peritoneum (Robbins, Brunschwig, & Foote, 1949; Williams,

1955; Hubbard, Khan, Carag, Albites, & Hricko, 1967). No instance of bowel obstruction occurred and at later reoperation the surgical sites were covered by a smooth, glistening peritoneal surface. Trimpi and Bacon (1952) reported 49 cases of abdominoperineal resection of the rectum. In 18 patients the peritoneal floor was closed and there were four instances of intestinal obstruction. In 28 patients no reperitonealization was performed and there were no instances of obstruction. Ulfelder and Quinby (1951) found that, after combined abdominoperineal resection, 50% of postoperative intestinal obstructions were due to incarceration of small bowel between sutures of the newly constructed peritoneal floor. All experimental evidence indicates that areas denuded of peritoneum will heal satisfactorily (Singleton, Rowe, & Moore, 1952; Rhoades & Schwegman, 1965; Glucksman & Warren, 1966; Hubbard et al., 1967) and that the suturing of peritoneum actually increases the incidence of adhesions (Chester, Zimmer, & Hoffman, 1948; Thomas & Rhoads, 1950; Singleton et al., 1952; Trimpi & Bacon, 1952; Brunschwig & Robbins, 1954; Williams, 1955; Ellis, Harrison, & Hugh, 1965; Hubbard et al., 1967).

The value of peritoneal closure at the time of Cesarean birth was evaluated prospectively. Hull and Varner (1991) as well as Pietrantoni et al. (1991) compared the clinical outcome of post–Cesarean section patients who did ($n = 59, 121$) or did not ($n = 54, 127$) undergo peritoneal closure. Closure of the peritoneum extended the duration of the surgical procedure by 5 minutes. There were no differences between the groups in the postoperative incidence of wound infection, dehiscence, endometritis, ileus, or length of hospital stay. Nonclosure of the visceral and parietal peritoneum after low transverse Cesarean section had no adverse effects on recovery and decreased the operating time. Thus, leaving the parietal peritoneum unsutured is an acceptable way to manage patients at Cesarean delivery.

Morphogenesis of Adhesion Formation

The initiation of adhesion formation begins with a fibrin matrix that typically occurs during coagulation (Figure 9.1). This matrix is gradually replaced by vascular granulation tissue containing macrophages, fibroblasts, and giant cells. The clots are slow to achieve complete organization. In the process, they consist of erythrocytes separated by strands or condensed masses of fibrin that are covered with two or three layers of flattened cells and contain a patchy infiltrate of mononuclear cells (Figure 9.2). Eventually the adhesion matures into a fibrous band, often containing small nodules of calcification. The adhesions are often covered by mesothelium and contain blood vessels and connective tissue fibers, including elastin. Even at 6 months, collections of hemosiderin-filled macrophages are present in many adhesions.

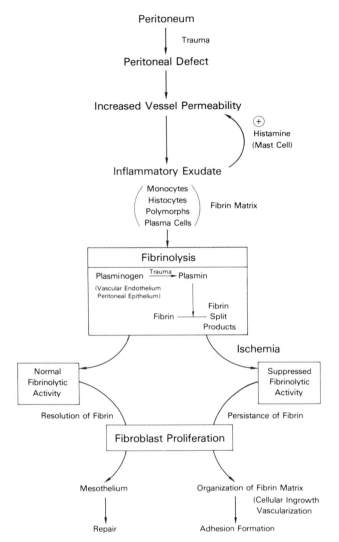

FIGURE 9.1. Summary of normal tissue repair and adhesion formation following surgical trauma. After trauma to the peritoneum, there is increased vascular permeability, mediated by histamine, which produces an inflammatory exudate and formation of fibrin matrix. As with other parts of the body, this fibrin matrix is normally removed by fibrinolysis. Under normal conditions, where fibrinolytic activity is allowed to occur, fibroblast proliferation results in remesothelialization. However, under the ischemic conditions present in surgical trauma, fibrinolytic activity is suppressed and fibrin is allowed to persist. Once the fibrin bands are infiltrated with fibroblasts, they become organized into adhesions. (From Montz et al., 1987. Reproduced by permission of Year Book Medical Publishers.)

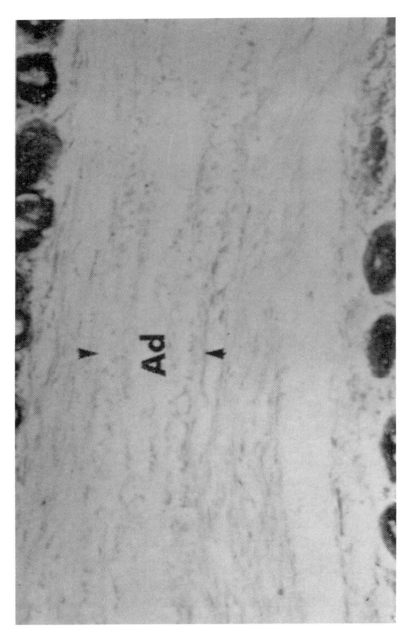

FIGURE 9.2. Adhesion of colon to cecum at 1 day. There is a complete absence of mast cells within the adhesion (Ad). Light photomicrograph; toluidine blue. (×381). (From Milligan & Raftery, 1974. Reproduced by permission of Butterworth.)

Milligan and Raftery (1974) described the histological and morphological features of postsurgical adhesion formation in rats using light and electron microscopic techniques. They compared adhesions arising from the liver, cecum, and ileal-cecal junction using both peritoneal abrasion and stripping techniques to create petechial bleeding or a clear, well demarcated peritoneal defect. Rats were sacrificed 7 or 14 days as well as 1 or 2 months after the initial trauma.

At day 1 to 3 the adhesion was characterized by the variety of cellular elements encased in fibrin matrix (Figure 9.3). The cells were primarily polymorphonuclear leukocytes (PMNs) but also included macrophages, eosinophils, red blood cells (RBC), and tissue debris, as well as necrotic cells presumably desquamated from the peritoneal injury (Figure 9.4). By 4 days macrophages were the predominant leukocyte in the fibrin mesh, which primarily contained large strands of fibrin associated with a few fibroblasts. A few mast cells were seen at day 5 and unorganized fibrin was not apparent. In contrast, many fibroblasts were lying together assuming the formation of a syncytium together with macrophages. Distinct bundles of collagen were evident as were scattered foreign body granulomas. At 7 days collagen and fibroblasts were the predominant components of the adhesion. However, small vascular channels containing endothelial cells were present. The number of mast cells slightly increased between 2 weeks and 2 months. During this interval the cellularity of the adhesion was replaced almost entirely by collagen fibrils associated with macrophages (Figure 9.5). Occasional macrophages and lymphocytes persisted for ~2 weeks.

Electron Microscopy

A wide heterogeneity exists among adhesions when examined by electron microscopy (Milligan & Raftery, 1974). Two days after injury fibrin appears as fibrils. The number of macrophages exceeds the number of PMNs, whereas a scattering of eosinophils is present throughout the damaged peritoneum. Fibroblasts and collagen are found; however, fibroblasts appear in areas not associated with eosinophils. Early on there is no evidence of mesothelial cell attachment to the surface of the adhesion. By 4 days most of the fibrin is gone and larger numbers of fibroblasts and collagen are present. Through days 5 to 10, fibroblasts become aligned while collagen deposition and organization advance (Figure 9.6). The other cells involved at this time include macrophages and eosinophils. Similar studies performed by Abe and diZerega also identified the presence of eosinophils in the peritoneal cavity of rabbits after surgical injury (unpublished observation). At 2 weeks the relatively few cells present are predominantly fibroblasts. At 1 to 2 month after injury the collagen fibrils are organized into discrete bundles interposed by spindle-shaped fibroblasts and a rare macrophage.

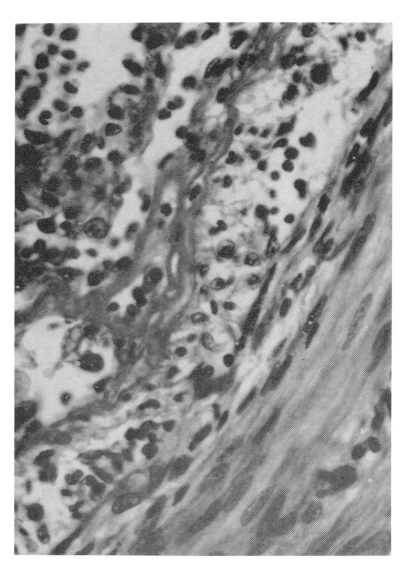

FIGURE 9.3. Adhesion of peritesticular fat pad to cecum at 3 days. Interspersed among the fibrin strands are numerous mononuclear cells, mainly monocytes and macrophages, with a few PMNs and fibroblasts. Light photomicrograph; HE. (×454). (From Milligan & Raftery, 1974. Reproduced by permission of Butterworth.)

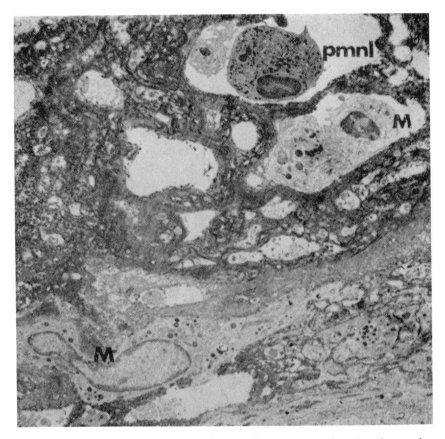

FIGURE 9.4. Adhesion of ileum to parietal peritoneum at 1 day. A polymorpho-nuclear leukocyte (pmnl) and two macrophages (M) are embedded in a network of fibrin. Electron photomicrograph; uranyl acetate (UA) + lead citrate (LC) (×3700). (From Milligan & Raftery, 1974. Reproduced by permission of Butterworth.)

Animal Models: Adhesion Induction

To obtain peritoneal adhesions in animals, it is necessary to inflict severe damage usually involving two adjacent surfaces or to use artificial methods (see reviews: Richardson, 1911; Boys, 1942; Connolly & Smith, 1960). The following are descriptions of injuries used to induce adhesion formation in standard animal models.

1. Mechanical injury: crushing the bowel, (Thomas, & Rhoads, 1950; Spagna, & Peskin, 1961; Choate, Just-Viera, & Yaeger, 1964; Grosz,

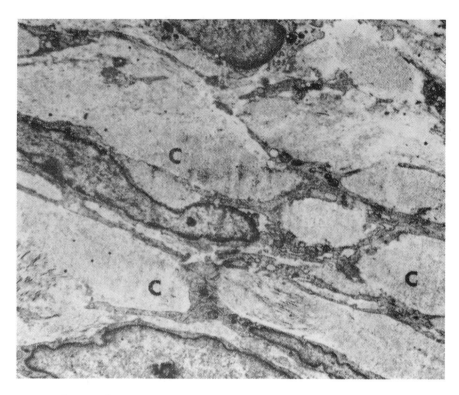

FIGURE 9.5. Typical adhesion at 2 months. Fibroblasts form an interlacing network around dense bundles of collagen (C). Electron micrograph. (From Milligan & Raftery, 1974. Reproduced by permission of Butterworth.)

Aka, Zimmer, & Alterwein, 1966; Perriard, & Mirkovitch, 1966; Swolin, 1966; Goldman & Rosemond, 1967); stripping or scrubbing away the outer layers from long segments of bowel wall (Pope, 1914; Warren, 1928; Lacey, 1930; Trusler, 1931; Thomas & Rhoads, 1950; Hubay, Weckesser, & Holden, 1953; de Sanctis, Schatten, & Weckesser, 1955; Gustavsson, Blombäck, Blombäck, & Wallen, 1955).

2. Ischemia: dividing major vessels to loops of intestine, (Ellis, 1963; James, Ellis, & Hugh, 1965).

3. Introduction of foreign material: talcum (German, 1943; Seelig, Verda, & Kidd, 1943; Zachariae, 1954; Luttwak, Behar, & Saltz, 1957; Myllärniemi, Frilander, Turumen, & Saxén, 1966; Myllärniemi, 1967, 1973); colloidal silica, (Schade & Williamson, 1968; Green, French, & Fingerhut, 1970); gauze sponges (Adams, 1913; Donaldson, 1938; Lehman & Boys, 1940); toxic chemicals (Warren, 1928; Lacey, 1930; Heinz, 1900; Chandy, 1950); bacteria (Adams, 1913; Mion & Boen, 1965); feces (Jackson, 1958).

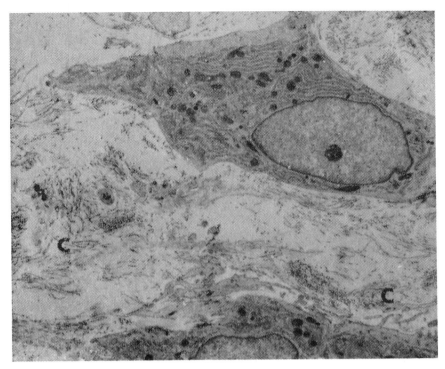

FIGURE 9.6. Adhesion of cecum to cecum at 5 days. Two fibroblasts and numerous small bundles of collagen (C) are seen. (×2700). (From Milligan & Raftery, 1974. Reproduced by permission of Butterworth.)

Mast Cells and Adhesion

Bridges, Johnson, and Whitting (1965) found a species difference in adhesion formation between rats and rabbits after implantation of polyethylene sheets into the peritoneal cavity. Adhesions formed readily in the rat, whereas they did not in the rabbit. Rat peritoneum is densely populated with mast cells, whereas that of the rabbit is not. Injury to the rat peritoneum was followed by a disappearance of mast cells from in and around the wound, which reappear in large numbers 3 to 4 days after surgery at the sites of adhesion formation and in the adjacent wound.

Fibrin

Fibrinous exudate is a necessary precursor for fibrous adhesions. Highly mobile intraperitoneal structures will not permanently adhere to each other unless held in continuous, close apposition until fibroblast invasion leads to collagen deposition beginning on the third postoperative day. Thus, the crucial consideration is the factor that determines whether the fibrinous band is absorbed, or persists and is organized into an adhesion (Ellis, 1971, 1983).

Further evidence for the role of fibrin in the formation of adhesions comes from the observation that use of defibrinated blood or blood products is less frequently associated with adhesion formation. Serosal injury, though relatively innocuous per se, readily leads to adhesions if combined with blood products. Injury only requires removal of the mesothelial surface: not only drying but even prolonged moistening is sufficient to denude the surface of peritoneal mesothelium. Plasma alone on dried areas creates fibrinous attachments, most of which disappear within a few days. Fibrin provides the initial bridge between two surfaces; when the bridge is made of fibrin only, it is amenable to lysis by fibrinolytic mechanisms; but when it contains cellular elements (erythrocytes, leukocytes, platelets, etc.) within the fibrin it will likely undergo organization into an adhesion. Under these experimental conditions (1) desquamation of mesothelial cells appears to be the critical event in adhesion formation and (2) adhesions apparently develop when two denuded surfaces are involved.

Foreign Body

Schade and Williamson (1968) evaluated the temporal course of adhesion formation in rats after the addition of foreign body (colloidal silica oxide) into the peritoneal cavity. Three phases were discernible in foreign body–induced adhesion formation. The first phase (0 time to 6 hours) involved degeneration and desquamation of mesothelial cells. In the second phase (7 hours to 10 days) fibrin deposition on exposed basement membranes led to formation of fibrinous adhesions. This transformation of fibrinous exudate into fibrous adhesions occurred over an extended period of time (10 days to 1 month). The sequence of events which leads to adhesion formation in response to foreign body injury is similar to that which follows surgical trauma; however, the time course is significantly prolonged.

Radiation

The pathogenesis of radiation-induced adhesions is complex. Practically all of the tissue layers of the gut can be involved as well as the surrounding connective tissues that form gut-associated adhesions (Chu & Smathers, 1974). Several mechanisms can give rise to enteropathy; which one predominates will depend upon the radiation dose, treatment site, volume

TABLE 9.3. The incidence of adhesions following total abdominal radiation as a function of radiation dose and time.

Dose of radiation	Incidence of adhesions (%) on day of sacrifice[a]		
	28–84 days	112–140 days	168–224 days
13.5 Gy	0% ($n = 80$)	1.25% ($n = 80$)	0% ($n = 50$)
13.6–15.5 Gy	0% ($n = 18$)	8.3% ($n = 36$)	14.3% ($n = 84$)
15.6–16.5 Gy	16.7% ($n = 24$)	24.3% ($n = 37$)	26.2% ($n = 42$)
16.6–17.5 Gy	nd	60% ($n = 5$)	16.7% ($n = 6$)

Note: Animals were sacrificed on 28, 56, 84, 112, 126, 140, 168, 182, 210, and 224 days after total abdominal radiation. Groups were combined as shown to increase the significance of the data points to mirror the three phases found from mortality data.
[a]Mice with adhesions as a percent of survivors.
From McBride et al., 1989b.

irradiated, time to development of symptoms, and the end point chosen as well as nonradiation-associated variables including species, bacteriological status, diet, and ongoing inflammation.

Adhesions formation as a function of time and radiation dose was evaluated in a murine model (McBride, Mason, Davis, & Withers, 1989a,b). Up to 14% of mice receiving 13.5 to 14.5 Gy total abdominal radiation (TAI) developed adhesions within 224 days. This increased by 12% when the radiation dose was increased 16 Gy TAI. Adhesion formation after radiation injury is time-dependent (Table 9.3). No adhesions were found before day 56 after total abdominal radiation; most adhesions were present by 140 days with little further increase in incidence thereafter. A total dose of 19 Gy in two fractions produced fewer adhesions and fewer deaths than a single dose of 16 Gy. In contrast, 20.5 Gy in two fractions yielded higher incidences of both sequelae (Table 9.4). From these data it is possible to estimate that 19.9 Gy total abdominal radiation split dose would give the same effect as 16 Gy total abdominal radiation single dose for adhesion formation after 140 days. Interestingly, a very similar split dose figure of 19.8 Gy total abdominal radiation can be estimated for mortality equivalent to a single dose of 16 Gy total abdominal radiation.

TABLE 9.4. The effect of splitting the radiation dose into two fractions within a 24-hour interval upon the incidence of adhesions and mortality following total abdominal radiation.

Dose of radiation	Incidence of Adhesions %	Deaths %
16 Gy	35.0 ($n = 20$)	36.7 ($n = 30$)
9.5 Gy ×2	11.5 ($n = 26$)	13.3 ($n = 30$)
10.25 Gy ×2	57.1 ($n = 14$)	60.0 ($n = 30$)

From McBride et al., 1989b.

After total abdominal radiation, the serosal surface of the bowel desquamates with underlying serosa undergoing varying degrees of disintegration (McBride et al., 1989a). These changes were more evident in large gut and in mice with adhesions than in mice that did not form adhesions. In addition, total abdominal radiation induces the development of prominent highly reactive lymphoid follicles in the colon and adjoining lymph nodes in the connective tissue. This site preference for adhesion formation in rodents after radiation exposure is different from humans where the ileocecal region appears to be the main site of obstruction (Withers & Mason, 1974; Withers et al., 1974, 1981; McLaren, 1977; Withers & Romsdahl, 1977; Localio, Pachter, & Gouge, 1979; Kinsella & Bloomer, 1980). The difference may stem from gut fixation, which is a more important risk factor in clinical situations.

Oxygen Free Radicals

Oxygen-derived free radicals induced by ischemia may be important for peritoneal adhesion formation (Korthuis, Granger, Townsley, & Taylor, 1985; McCord, 1985; Tsimoyiannis et al., 1988). Tsimoyiannis et al. (1989) developed an ischemic bowel model to evaluate the role of these radicals in adhesion formation. They induced ileal ischemia in rats, which was followed by reperfusion. This procedure resulted in an 80% incidence of adhesion formation. Xanthine oxidase is the principal source of oxygen radicals after 30 minutes of complete ischemia. Administration of superoxide dismutase (a superoxide anion scavenger), catalase (a hydrogen peroxide scavenger), dimethyl sulfoxide (a hydroxyl radical scavenger), and allopurinol (a xanthine oxidase inhibitor) significantly reduced the intestinal injury and consequently the incidence and severity of peritoneal adhesion formation in a rat bowel ischemia/reperfusion model.

Further support for the concept that oxygen-derived free radicals mediate ischemia/reperfusion damage in the intestinal wall was provided by the observation that allopurinol (the first identified source of superoxide anion) was as effective as free radical scavengers. Xanthine oxidase is formed by conversion of xanthine dehydrogenase, an enzyme widely distributed thoughout the body and with particularly high concentrations in intestine, liver, and lungs. In ischemic tissue rapid conversion of xanthine dehydrogenase to xanthine oxidase occurs (Parks, Bulkley, Granger, Hamilton, & McCord, 1982). This finding suggests that xanthine oxidase is the principal source of oxygen radicals in the intestinal wall subjected to 30 minutes of complete ischemia followed by reperfusion.

During ischemia of an ileal segment, much of the cellular adenosine triphosphate pool is converted to hypoxanthine. The final substrate necessary to produce superoxide anion is molecular oxygen, which is supplied during reperfusion of the tissues with oxygenate blood, and with which the enzyme xanthine oxidase can produce anion, hydrogen peroxide, and hydroxyl radical (Tsimoyiannis et al., 1988). Thus hydroxyl radicals may induce injury on the outer muscular layer of the intestinal wall.

Complications Arising from Intraperitoneal Adhesions

Intestinal Obstruction

The most serious complication of intraperitoneal adhesions is intestinal obstruction. It was estimated that one-third of all intestinal obstructions are caused by adhesions (Table 9.5). Intestinal obstruction can be fatal and often requires immediate surgical correction. In Nemir's (1952) survey of 129 patients presenting with intestinal obstruction due to adhesion formation, the mortality rate was 6%. Perry et al. (1955) and Raf (1969) reported overall mortality rates of 6% and 8%, respectively, among their patients with intestinal obstruction from intraperitoneal adhesions. Among patients with intestinal obstruction due to adhesions, many present with strangulated or gangrenous obstructions (15% in Nemir's survey and 25% in Perry et al.'s survey). The mortality rate among patients with strangulated obstructions may be higher than that for all patients with intestinal obstruction (Table 9.6); Leffall and Syphax (1970) reported that 30% of the 74 patients with strangulated intestinal obstructions died.

Menzies and Ellis (1990) reviewed hospital records over a 25-year period; 261 of 28,297 adult general surgical admissions were for intestinal obstruction from adhesions (0.9%). Of 4,502 laparotomies, 148 were for adhesion-related obstruction (3.3%). Over a 13-year period all laparotomies were followed up for an average of 14.5 months (range 0 to 91

TABLE 9.5. Adhesions as causes of bowel obstruction.

Author	Year	Place	Total adhesion		Notes
			No.	(%)	
Nemir (1952)	1952	Philadelphia	430	33	
Perry et al. (1955)	1955	Minneapolis	1252	31	
Raf (1969)	1969	Stockholm	2295	64	Small intestine only and excludes hernias, neoplasms and Crohn's disease
Playforth et al. (1970)	1970	Lexington	111	54	Small intestine only
Stewardson et al. (1978)	1978	Chicago	238	64	Small intestine only
Ellis (1982)	1982	London	253	26	Adults only

From Ellis, 1982.

TABLE 9.6. Etiology and mortality in small bowel obstruction.

Etiology	No. of patients	Deaths
Adhesions	152 (64%)	4 (3%)
Hernia	57 (24%)	1 (1.8%)
Malignancy	17 (7%)	7 (41.2%)
Volvulus	6 (3%)	1 (16.7%)
Intussusception	3 (1%)	0
Regional enteritis	3 (1%)	0
Total	238	13 (5.5%)

From Stewardson et al. 1978.

months). From these 2,708 patients, 26 developed intestinal obstruction due to postoperative adhesions within 1 year after surgery (1%). The majority of the operations producing intestinal obstruction were lower abdominal, usually involving the colon.

Paralytic ileus and intestinal adhesions are common events following intra-abdominal surgery (Glucksman, 1966). The hypothesis that "stimulation of the postoperative bowel will reduce intestinal adhesions" was tested in a rat model of intestinal adhesions in which postoperative bowel motility was pharmacologically manipulated (Sparnon & Spitz, 1989). Immediate postoperative stimulation of gastrointestinal motility by the prokinetic agent cisapride, resulted in a significant reduction in both the number and extent of adhesions (Verlinden et al., 1985). Inhibition of postoperative intestinal motility with the anticholinergic agent atropine resulted in a greater number of more dense adhesions involving an increased length of bowel (Table 9.7).

TABLE 9.7. Effect of medication on the number of adhesions.

Medication	Number of adhesions			
	At 7 days		At 35 days	
	Mean	SEM	Mean	SEM
Cisapride	1.4	0.30	2.6	0.27
Saline	2.2	0.13	4.4	0.64
Atropine	3.6	0.34	4.7	0.34

(Rats (n = 10) treated with the three medications at both 7 and 35 days; p <.05 when comparing saline with cisapride (an agent that reduces bowel motility) and atropine (an agent that increases bowel motility) at 7 days and when comparing saline with cisapride at 35 days.
From Sparnon and Spitz, 1989.

Equine Model

Lundin et al. (1989) established an equine model to evaluate the formation of bowel adhesion. Twenty-two foals were divided into groups of intestinal distention and intestinal ischemia as methods to induce peritoneal adhesions. In the first group, the lumen of a segment of distal small intestine was occluded without extramural vascular compromise and distended with lactated Ringer's solution. The ischemic group underwent 70 minutes of total vascular occlusion of identical bowel segments. Serosal biopsies were obtained before and after each experimental procedure and after 60 minutes of reperfusion. The foals were sacrificed 10 days after surgery and tissues were collected for histological and ultrastructural evaluation.

Serosal edema and cellular infiltration were observed following reperfusion of the ischemic segments and were present after 2 hours of distention. Experimental and control mesothelial surfaces were denuded immediately after experimental occlusions. All foals developed bowel-to-bowel and bowel-to-mesentery adhesions of the experimental segments. Control foals younger than 30 days exhibited mesenteric contraction and thickening of the isolated segment, whereas those older than 30 days had little or no mesenteric contraction. Fibrous tissue formed on the outer boundary of the original serosa, and new mesothelial-like cells were present on the surface of fibrous tissue in some area. Some serosal fibrosis was also seen in most of the control segments.

Canine Model

Booth, Zimny, Kaufman, and Cohn (1973) characterized the development of small bowel obstruction in dogs. Strangulation of the bowel induces an early loss of serosal integrity, which is accompanied by gross bloody congestion of the bowel wall. Using the scanning electron microscope, a variety of topographic changes followed strangulation and obstruction. Control specimens revealed broad, tongue-shaped villi on the mucosal surface. Morphologic changes after only 3 hours of strangulation-obstruction were obscured by extravasated erythrocytes and cellular debris that covered the normal mucosal surface. Loss of serosal mesothelium began at 1 hour after strangulation-obstruction and was nearly complete after 6 hours (Figure 9.7). Only intermediate sized pits were observed in the subserosal layer after 1 hour, but clefts up to 60 μm in diameter appeared by 3 hours. These serosal defects filled with erythrocytes at six hours, and the bowel wall became covered with a coagulum by 9 hours.

By 3 hours, progressive congestion produced shreading of the smooth muscle and connective tissue, which at this time made up the outer layer of the bowel wall. Defects in the wall filled with blood and proteinaceous

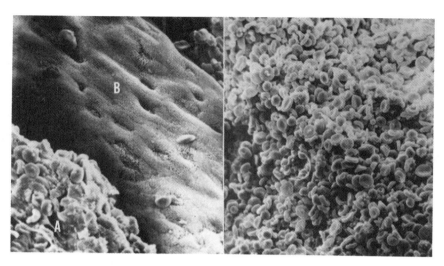

FIGURE 9.7. Strangulated dog ileum at 1 hour, mucosal surface (OM ×2,000). Extravasated erythrocyte and cellular debris (A) are interspersed with areas of normal-appearing mucosa (B) on which microvilli are clearly seen (left panel). Strangulated dog ileum at 6 hours, mucosal surface (OM ×2,000, right panel). The usual mucosal surface is obscured by erythrocytes and other cellular debris (Booth, et al., 1973. Reproduced by permission of Reed Publishing.)

debris produced a coagulum that persisted up to 24 hours. It is likely that within 24 to 36 hours the coagulum began to lose integrity because of lytic enzymes present both intramurally and intraluminally, and the highly toxic fluid contained within the strangulated loop began to filter through the microscopic crevices that appear in the bowel wall as early as 3 hours after injury. Thus, nonreversible injury to bowel occurs soon after strangulation and leads to multiple gross and microscopic changes that result in obstruction.

Clinical Considerations

Patients with acute intestinal obstruction secondary to postoperative adhesions typically present with colicky abdominal pain, vomiting, abdominal distention, and abdominal tenderness. Many of these patients have a history of previous, short-duration episodes of subacute intestinal obstruction with colicky pain, mild distention, vomiting, and constipation that were either relieved spontaneously or with purgatives (Ellis, 1983). Miller and Winfield (1959) reported that of the 63 patients they followed, 94% presented with abdominal pain, 90% presented with vomiting, 76% had some degree of abdominal distention, and 75% had abdominal tenderness. The severity of pain was rated as intense by significantly more patients with strangulation than in those with simple obstruction; however, these clinicians reported no discernible difference in the degree of abdominal distention or vomiting between patients with simple or strangulated obstructions (Miller & Winfield, 1959). In addition to other symptoms such as abdominal pain and vomiting, Leffall and Syphax (1970) reported that tachycardia (>100 bpm), leukocytosis (>10,000 mm³), and fever (>100 °F) were present in 70%, 64%, and 50%, respectively, of the patients with strangulated obstructions.

In the majority of patients with intestinal obstruction secondary to postoperative adhesion formation, the presenting symptoms occur long after surgery; however, in a minority of patients, acute obstruction is observed in the immediate postoperative period (Table 9.8). Menzies and Ellis (1990) prospectively evaluated 2,708 laparotomies for an average of 14 months (range 0 to 91 months); 1% of patients developed intestinal obstruction within 1 year of surgery. Among the 63 patients with intestinal obstruction secondary to postoperative adhesions, obstruction was observed within an average of 1 week in 14 (22%) patients (Miller & Winfield, 1959). Sannella (1975) also reported that 37% of his 35 patients developed an obstruction of the small bowel within 30 days of abdominal surgery; in his patients, the cause of the obstruction was not limited to adhesion formation. In the largest survey published to date, Raf (1969) reported that the interval between the initial laparotomy and surgery for obstruction due to adhesion formation was less than 1 year in only 16% of the 1,477 patients evaluated. In 17% of the patients in this survey, the interval was greater than 20 years.

Chronic Pelvic Pain

Peritoneal adhesions are one of the major causes of chronic or recurrent pelvic pain. In three surveys, adhesions were identified as the primary cause of chronic pelvic pain in 13% to 26% of females (Lundberg, Wall, & Mathers, 1973; Goldstein, deCholnoky, Emans, & Leventhal, 1980;

TABLE 9.8. Time to obstruction from postoperative adhesions.

Time from surgery	No. (%)
<1 month	17 (21.25%)
1 month–1 year	14 (17.5%)
1–5 years	17 (21.25%)
5–10 years	5 (6.25%)
>10 years	17 (21.25%)
Unknown	10 (12.5%)
Total	80

From Menzies & Ellis, 1990.

Malinak, 1980; Renaer, 1981; Rapkin, 1986). Removal of adhesions in women with pelvic pain often leads to relief of symptoms (Malinak, 1980; Renaer, 1981). It was suggested that chronic pain arises as a result of the restriction of pelvic organ mobility imposed by adhesions (Kresch, Seifer, Sachs, & Barrese, 1984). Since both sensory and vasomotor nerves supply the peritoneum, most of the parietal peritoneum is sensitive to pain. Painful stimuli to the anterior and lateral regions are localized to the point of stimulation (see Chapter 1). Pain fibers have not been clearly demonstrated for visceral peritoneum. Rather visceral pain is perceived via the viscus itself or stretch or spasm of smooth muscles within the viscus.

From a clinical point of view, the relationship between pelvic pain and adhesions is unclear. Rapkin (1986) reported that of 88 infertility patients undergoing laparotomy, 39% had adhesions; however, only 12% of these patients presented with pelvic pain. Stovall, Elder, and Ling (1989) found that the incidence of adhesions in their patients with chronic pelvic pain (48%) was not significantly different from the overall incidence of adhesion (34%) in their study population. The only significant predictor of adhesions was prior pelvic surgery, whereas the significant physical findings that predicted adhesions were an adnexal mass and decrease in uterine mobility. In this study approximately 25% of all patients with intraperitoneal adhesions had no pelvic pain and a normal physical examination.

Stout, Steege, Dodson, and Hughes (1991) compared laparoscopic findings to the patient's self-report of pelvic pain. Patients with laparoscopically diagnosed pathological conditions reported higher pain levels and greater interference with their lives than the group who reported pain and had negative laparoscopic results. Kresch et al. (1984) discovered endometriosis or adhesions in 29% of asymptomatic women during laparoscopic surgery for tubal ligation. Rapkin (1986) found laparoscopically diagnosed evidence of pelvic adhesions in 26% of patients with chronic pain and 39% of infertility patients; however, only a small portion of the infertility patients with pelvic adhesions complained of pelvic pain. In clinical practice, many gynecologists observe patients with a few small implants of endometriosis or adhesions who report significant pain, whereas other patients who are found to have significant disease may not describe pain symptoms. Stout et al. found that the majority of women reporting pelvic pain may be expected to have some type of physical abnormality, primarily endometriosis or adhesions. The location of the pain usually corresponded with the location of the abnormality.

Stout et al. (1991) reported partial (35%) and complete (35%) resolution of pelvic pain in women with chronic pain following laparoscopic lysis of adhesions. Prognosis was not related to the extent of adhesions that were lysed. About 25% of their patients returned with pain within 3 to 5 months. Others found that lysis of adhesions may benefit up to 85%

of patients with pelvic pain (Figure 9.8 and 9.9; Chan & Wood, 1985; Daniell, 1989; Sutton & MacDonald, 1990).

Individual differences exist in how persons experience or interpret physical sensory input from the pelvis. Within a group of women who reported pelvic pain, a significant portion (21% in this sample) showed no evidence of physical disease at laparoscopy (Stout et al., 1991). A few women in this sample who underwent laparoscopic surgery for reasons other than investigation of pain had comparable physical findings that were not associated with pain symptoms. These general findings were confirmed and extended by Peters et al. (1991) who found that both organic and other causative factors usually constitute the etiology(s) of pelvic pain. As a result, consideration of psychosocial factors in conjunction with traditional laparoscopy are more likely to result in reduction of pelvic pain.

Secondary Sterility in Females

Adhesion formation is well-recognized as a major cause of infertility in females. Drake and Grunert (1980) reported that of 38 infertile females with otherwise normal outpatient evaluations, 32% had adhesions upon diagnostic laparoscopy. DeCherney and Mezer (1984) found that approximately 75% of the 61 infertile females they evaluated who had undergone prior salpingostomy had adhesions upon follow-up laparoscopy. Trimbos-Kemper, Trimbos, and van Hall (1985) observed a similar

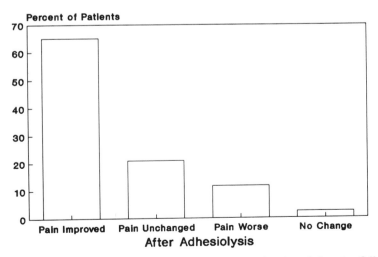

FIGURE 9.8. Pelvic pain improves after lysis of adhesion involving the fallopian tubes and/or ovaries in the majority of patients (Chan & Wood, 1985. Reproduced with the permission of the Royal Australian College of Obstetricians and Gynaecologists.)

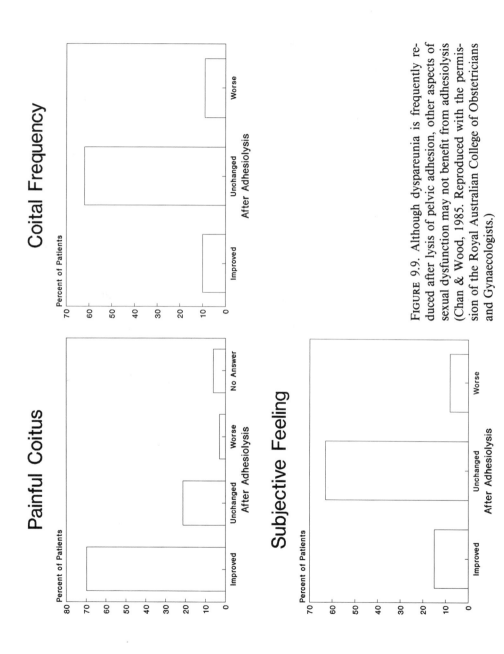

FIGURE 9.9. Although dyspareunia is frequently reduced after lysis of pelvic adhesion, other aspects of sexual dysfunction may not benefit from adhesiolysis (Chan & Wood, 1985. Reproduced with the permission of the Royal Australian College of Obstetricians and Gynaecologists.)

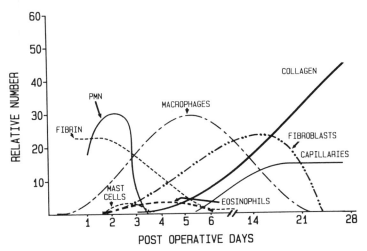

FIGURE 9.10. Immediately after peritoneal injury, polymorphonuclear (PMN) cells appear in large numbers throughout the surgical site and fibrin matrix forms. Their number rapidly increases, then falls in the absence of infection. In the presence of infection, however, the PMN count continues to increase. Rapid increase in the number of PMNs and amount of fibrin underscores the importance of preventing adhesions as quickly as possible after surgery. The principal cellular elements in control of peritoneal healing are macrophages, which appear in large numbers 1 to 2 days after surgery. The macrophage is involved in regulating fibroblast and mesothelial cell functions. About postsurgical day 2, mesothelial cells appear in large numbers over the damaged peritoneal surface. By day 6 or 7 after surgical injury, virtually all of the peritoneal injury will be covered by at least one layer of mesothelial cells. Thus, adhesion formation is initiated by surgical trauma, and any methods employed to prevent adhesion formation should begin during the surgical procedure and persist for at least 3 to 4 days.

incidence of periadnexal adhesions among the 188 infertile patients they studied.

Ovarian Surgery

Surgical procedures are often used in attempts to restore fertility although postoperative adhesions can contribute to infertility. For example, wedge resection of the ovaries is used in the treatment of polycystic ovarian disease and temporarily restores the menstrual cycle (Kistner, 1969; Buttram & Vaquero, 1975; Toaff, Toaff, & Peyser, 1976). Nevertheless, adhesion formation usually follows wedge resection and thereby impairs fertility. McLaughlin (1984) observed adhesions in 18 of 49 ovaries (37%) from 25 patients following ovarian wedge resection by microlaser. Weinstein and Polishuk (1975) did not find a greater incidence of adhesions resulting in infertility following ovarian wedge resection relative to other pelvic surgical procedures. In their study of 57 patients after ovarian wedge resection, adhesions resulted in infertility in 14%. Because of the risk of infertility arising from peritubal and periovarian adhesions after ovarian wedge resection, numerous clinicians utilize medical protocols including clomiphene citrate, hCG, human menopausal gonadotropin, and gonadotropin releasing hormone (Gn-RH) analogues to manage patients with polycystic ovarian disease in an effort to avoid surgery (Toaff et al., 1976; Aboulghar, Mansour, & Serour, 1989).

Conclusion

Adhesions form as a result of residual fibrin matrix deposited between tissue surfaces in apposition (Figure 9.10). In the presence of active fibrinolysis, the fibrin deposits are removed. In a hypoxic environment fibrinolysis is suppressed and fibrin persists, undergoes organization, and forms adhesions. Previous surgery is the most common cause of adhesions followed by infection. Clinical problems caused by adhesions include (1) pelvic pain, (2) infertility, and (3) bowel obstruction.

References

Aboulghar MA, Mansour RT, Serour GI. (1989). Ovarian superstimulation in the treatment of infertility due to peritubal and periovarian adhesions. *Fertil Steril.* 51:834–837.

Adams JE. (1913). Peritoneal adhesions (an experimental study). *Lancet.* 1:663–668.

Adhesion Study Group. (1983). Reduction of postoperative pelvic adhesions with intraperitoneal 32% dextran 70: a prospective, randomized clinical trial. *Fertil Steril.* 40:612–619.

Bloom W, Fawcett DW. (1975). *A Textbook of Histology.* 9th ed. Philadelphia: W.B. Saunders, 186–188.

Booth WV, Zimny M, Kaufman HJ, Cohn I Jr. (1973). Scanning electron microscopy of small bowel strangulation obstruction. *Am J Surg.* 125:129–133.

Boys F. (1942). The prophylaxis of peritoneal adhesions: a review of the literature. *Surgery.* 11:118–168.

Bridges JB, Johnson FR, Whitting HW. (1965). Peritoneal adhesion formation. *Acta Anat (Basel).* 61:203–212.

Bronson RA, Wallach EE. (1977). Lysis of periadnexal adhesions for correction of infertility. *Fertil Steril.* 28:613–619.

Brunschwig A, Robbins GF. (1954). Regeneration of peritoneum: experimental observations and clinical experience in radical resections of intra-abdominal cancer. In: *XV. Congr. Soc. Internat. Chir., Lisbonne 1953.* Bruxelles: Henri de Smedt: 756–765.

Buttram VC, Vaquero C. (1975). Post-ovarian wedge resection adhesive disease. *Fertil Steril.* 26:874–876.

Chan CLK, Wood C. (1985). Pelvic adhesiolysis—the assessment of symptom relief by 100 patients. *Aust N Z J Obstet Gynaecol.* 25:295–298.

Chandy J. (1950). Use of heparin in the prevention of peritoneal adhesions. *Arch Surg.* 60:1151–1153.

Chester J, Zimmer CH, Hoffman LD. (1948). The use of free peritoneal grafts in intestinal anastomosis. *Surg Gynecol Obstet.* 89:605–608.

Choate WH, Just-Viera JO, Yaeger GH. (1964). Prevention of experimental peritoneal adhesions by dextran. *Arch Surg.* 88:249–254.

Connolly JE, Smith JW. (1960). The prevention and treatment of intestinal adhesions. *Int Abstr Surg.* 110:417–431.

Conolly WB, Stephens FO. (1968). Factors influencing the incidence of intraperitoneal adhesions: An experimental study. *Surgery.* 63:976–979.

Daniell JF, Pittaway DE. (1983). Short interval second-look laparoscopy after infertility surgery: a preliminary report. *J Reprod Med.* 28:281–283.

Daniell JF. (1989). Laparoscopic enterolysis of chronic abdominal pain. *J Gynecol Surg.* 5:61–66.

DeCherney AH, Mezer HC. (1984). The nature of posttuboplasty pelvic adhesions as determined by early and late laparoscopy. *Fertil Steril.* 41:643–646.

de Sanctis AL, Schatten WE, Weckesser EC. (1955). Effect of hydrocortisone in the prevention of intraperitoneal adhesions. *Arch Surg.* 71:523–530.

Diamond MP, Daniell JF, Feste J, Surrey MW, McLaughlin DS, Friedman S, Vaughn WK, Martin DC. (1987). Adhesion formation and de novo adhesion formation after reproductive pelvic surgery. *Fertil Steril.* 47:864–866.

Diamond MP. (1988). Surgical aspects of infertility. In: Sciarra JW, ed. *Gynecology and Obstetrics,* Chapter 61. Philadelphia: Harper & Row; 5:5.

Donaldson JK. (1938). Abdominal adhesions and the use of papain: a discussion and an experimental study. *Arch Surg.* 36:20–27.

Drake TS, Grunert GM. (1980). The unsuspected pelvic factor in the infertility investigation. *Fertil Steril.* 34:27–31.

Ellis H. (1963). The aetiology of post-operative abdominal adhesions: an experimental study. *Br J Surg.* 50:10–16.

Ellis H, Harrison W, Hugh TB. (1965). The healing of peritoneum under normal and pathological conditions. *Br J Surg.* 52:471–476.

Ellis H. (1971). The cause and prevention of postoperative intraperitoneal adhesions. *Surg Gynecol Obstet.* 133:497–511.

Ellis H. (1982). *Intestinal Obstruction.* New York: Appleton-Century-Crofts.

Ellis H. (1983). Prevention and treatment of adhesions. *Infect Surg.* 803–818.

Filmar S, Jetha N, McComb P, Gomel V. (1989a). A comparative histologic study on the healing process after tissue transection. I. Carbon dioxide laser and electromicrosurgery. *Am J Obstet Gynecol.* 160:1062–1067.

Filmar S, Jetha N, McComb P, Gomel V. (1989b). A comparative histologic study on the healing process after tissue transection. II. Carbon dioxide laser and surgical microscissors. *Am J Obstet Gynecol.* 160:1068–1072.

German WMCK. (1943). Dusting powder granulomas following surgery. *Surg Gynecol Obstet.* 76:501–507.

Glucksman D. (1966). Serosal integrity and intestinal adhesions. *Surgery.* 60:1009–1011.

Glucksman DL, Warren WD. (1966). The effect of topically applied corticosteroids in the prevention of peritoneal adhesions: An experimental approach with a review of the literature. *Surgery.* 60:352–360.

Golan A, Winston RML. (1989). Blood and intraperitoneal adhesion formation in the rat. *J Obstet Gynaecol.* 9:248–252.

Goldman LI, Rosemond GP. (1967). 5-Fluorouracil inhibition of experimental peritoneal adhesions. *Am J Surg.* 113:491–493.

Goldstein DP, deCholnoky C, Emans SJ, Leventhal JM. (1980). Laparoscopy in the diagnosis and management of pelvic pain in adolescents. *J Reprod Med.* 24:251–256.

Green N, French S, Fingerhut A. (1970). Radiation inhibition of peritoneal adhesions: an experimental study. *Proc Soc Exp Biol Med.* 133:544–550.

Grosz C, Aka E, Zimmer J, Alterwein R. (1966). The effect of intraperitoneal fluids on the prevention of experimental adhesions. *Surgery.* 60:1232–1234.

Gustavsson E, Blombäck B, Blombäck M, Wallen P. (1955). Plasmin in the prevention of adhesions: preliminary report. *Acta Chir Scand.* 109:327–333.

Heinz. (1900). Ueber die Herkunft des. Fibrins und die Enstehung von Verwachsuger bie acutes ad häsiver Entzündung seröser Haute. *Virchows Arch [A].* 160:365–377.

Hertzler AE. (1919). *The Peritoneum.* St. Louis: CV Mosby; 20–69.

Hubay CA, Weckesser EC, Holden WD. (1953). The effect of cortisone on the prevention of peritoneal adhesions. *Surg Gynecol Obstet.* 96:65–70.

Hubbard TB, Khan MZ, Carag VR, Albites VE, Hricko GM. (1967). The pathology of peritoneal repair: its relation to the formation of adhesions. *Ann Surg.* 165:908–916.

Hull DB, Varner MW. (1991). A randomized study of closure of the peritoneum at Cesarean delivery. *Obstet Gynecol.* 77:818–821.

Interceed. (TC7). Adhesion Barrier Study Group. (1989). Prevention of postsurgical adhesions by Interceed (TC7), an absorbable adhesion barrier: a prospective, randomized multicenter clinical study. *Fertil Steril.* 51:933–938.

Jackson BB. (1958). Observations on intraperitoneal adhesions, an experimental study. *Surgery* 44:507–518.

James DCO, Ellis H, Hugh TB. (1965). The effect of streptokinase on experimental intraperitoneal adhesion formation. *J Pathol Bact.* 90:279–287.

Kinsella TJ, Bloomer WD. (1980). Tolerance of the intestine to radiation therapy. *Surg Gynecol Obstet.* 151:273–284.

Kistner RW. (1969). Peri-tubal and peri-ovarian adhesions subsequent to wedge resection of the ovaries. *Fertil Steril.* 20:35–42.

Korthuis RJ, Granger DN, Townsley MI, Taylor AE. (1985). The role of oxygen-derived free radicals in ischaemia induced increases in canine skeletal muscle vascular permeability. *Circ Res.* 57:599–609.

Kresch AJ, Seifer DB, Sachs LB, Barrese I. (1984). Laparoscopy in 100 women with chronic pelvic pain. *Obstet Gynecol.* 64:672–674.

Lacey JT. (1930). The prevention of peritoneal adhesions by amniotic fluid. *Ann Surg.* 92:281–293.

Leffall LD, Syphax B. (1970). Clinical aids in strangulation intestinal obstruction. *Am J Surg.* 120:756–759.

Lehman EP, Boys F. (1940). The prevention of peritoneal adhesions with heparin: an experimental study. *Ann Surg.* 111:427–435.

Ling FW, Stovall TG, Meyer NL, Elkins TE, Muram D. (1989). Adhesion formation associated with the use of absorbable staples in comparison to other types of peritoneal injury. *Int J Gynaecol Obstet.* 30:361–366.

Localio SA, Pachter HL, Gouge TH. (1979). The radiation induced bowel. *Surg Ann.* 11:185–205.

Luciano AA, Hauser KS, Benda J. (1983). Evaluation of commonly used adjuvants in the prevention of postoperative adhesion. *Am J Obstet Gynecol.* 146:88–92.

Luciano AA, Maier DB, Koch EI, Nielsen JC, Whitman GF. (1989). A comparative study of postoperative adhesions following laser surgery by laparoscopy versus laparotomy in the rabbit model. *Obstet Gynecol.* 74:220–224.

Lundberg WI, Wall JE, Mathers JE. (1973). Laparoscopy in evaluation of pelvic pain. *Obstet Gynecol.* 42:872–876.

Lundin C, Sullins KE, White NA, Clem MC, Debowes RM, Pfeiffer CA. (1989). Induction of peritoneal adhesions with small intestinal ischemia and distention in the foal. *Equine Vet J.* 21:451–458.

Luttwak EM, Behar AJ, Saltz NJ. (1957). Effect of fibrinolytic agents and corticosteroid hormones on peritoneal adhesions: a comparative experimental study. *Arch Surg.* 75:96–101.

Malinak LR. (1980). Operative management of pelvic pain. *Clin Obstet Gynecol.* 23:191–200.

McBride WH, Mason KA, Davis C, Withers HRW. (1989a). The effect of interleukin-1, inflammation and surgery on the incidence of adhesion formation and death after abdominal surgery. *Cancer Res.* 49:169–173.

McBride WH, Mason KA, Davis C, Withers HR, Smathers JB. (1989b). Adhesion formation in experimental chronic radiation enteropathy. *Int J Radiat Oncol Biol Phys.* 16:737–743.

McCord JM. (1985). Oxygen-derived free radicals in postischemic tissue injury. *N Engl J Med.* 312:159–163.

McDonald MN, Elkins TE, Wortham GF, Stovall TG, Ling FW, McNeely SG. (1988). Adhesion formation and prevention after peritoneal injury and repair in the rabbit. *J Reprod Med.* 33:436–439.

McLaren JR. (1977). Sequelae of abdominal radiation and their medical management. *Compr Ther.* 3:25–33.

McLaughlin DS. (1984). Evaluation of adhesion reformation by early second-look laparoscopy following microlaser ovarian wedge resection. *Fertil Steril.* 42:531–537.

Mecke H, Semm K, Freys I, Argirious C, Gent HJ. (1989). Incidence of adhesions in the true pelvis after pelviscopic operative treatment of tubal pregnancy. *Obstet Invest.* 28:202–204.

Menzies D, Ellis H. (1990). Intestinal obstruction form adhesions—how big is the problem? *Ann R Coll Surg Engl.* 72:60–63.

Milewczyk M. (1989). [Experimental studies on the development of peritoneal adhesions in cases of suturing and non-suturing of the parietal peritoneum in rabbits]. *Ginekol Pol.* 60:1–6.

Miller EM, Winfield JM. (1959). Acute intestinal obstruction secondary to postoperative adhesions. *Arch Surg.* 78:148–153.

Milligan DW, Raftery AT. (1974). Observations on the pathogenesis of peritoneal adhesions: a light and electron microscopical study. *Br J Surg.* 61:274–280.

Mion CM, Boen ST. (1965). Analysis of factors responsible for the formation of adhesions during chronic peritoneal dialysis. *Am J Med Sci.* 250:675–679.

Montz FJ, Shimanuki T, diZerega GS. (1987). Postsurgical mesothelial re-epithelialization. In: DeCherney AH, Polan ML, eds. *Reproductive Surgery*. Chicago: Year Book Medical Publishers; 31–47.

Myllärniemi H, Frilander M, Turunen M, Saxén L. (1966). The effect of glove powders and their constituents on adhesion and granuloma formation in the abdominal cavity of the rabbit. *Acta Chir Scand*. 131:312–318.

Myllärniemi H. (1967). Foreign material adhesion formation after abdominal surgery: a clinical and experimental study. *Acta Chir Scand*. 377:1–48.

Myllärniemi H. (1973). Healing and adhesion formation of peritoneal wounds. *Acta Chir Scand*. 139:258–263.

Nemir P Jr. (1952). Intestinal obstruction: ten year survey at the Hospital of the University of Pennsylvania. *Ann Surg*. 135:367–375.

Nisell H, Larsson B. (1978). Role of blood and fibrinogen in development of intraperitoneal adhesions in rats. *Fertil Steril*. 30:470–473.

Parks DA, Bulkley GB, Granger DN, Hamilton SR, McCord JM. (1982). Ischemic injury in the cat small intestine: role of superoxide radicals. *Gastroenterology*. 82:9–15.

Perriard M, Mirkovitch V. (1966). L'effet du diméthyloplysiloxane surla prévention d'adhérences abdominals chez le rat. *Helv Chir Acta*. 33:536–540.

Perry JF Jr, Smith GA, Yonehiro EG. (1955). Intestinal obstruction caused by adhesions. A review of 388 cases. *Ann Surg*. 142:810–816.

Peters AAW, van Dorst E, Jellis B, van Zuuren E, Hermans J, Trimbos JB. (1991). A randomized clinical trial to compare two different approaches in women with chronic pelvic pain. *Obstet Gynecol*. 77:740–744.

Pfeffer WH. (1980). Adjuvants in tubal surgery. *Fertil Steril*. 33:245–255.

Pietrantoni M, Parsons MT, O'Brien WF, Collins E, Knuppel RA, Spellacy WN. (1991). Peritoneal closure or non-closure at Cesarean. *Obstet Gynecol*. 77:293–296.

Pittaway DE, Daniell JF, Maxson WS. (1985). Ovarian surgery in an infertility patient as an indication for a short-interval second-look laparoscopy: a preliminary study. *Fertil Steril*. 44:611–614.

Playforth RH, Holloway BJ, Griffen WO. (1970). Mechanical small bowel obstruction: a plea for earlier surgical intervention. *Ann Surg*. 171:783–788.

Pope S. (1914). The use of citrate solutions in the prevention of peritoneal adhesions. *Ann Surg*. 59:101–106.

Raf LE. (1969). Causes of abdominal adhesions in cases of intestinal obstruction. *Acta Chir Scand*. 135:73–76.

Rapkin AJ. (1986). Adhesions and pelvic pain: a retrospective study. *Obstet Gynecol*. 68:13–15.

Renaer M. (1981). *Chronic Pelvic Pain in Women*. New York: Springer-Verlag; 78–92.

Rhoades JE, Schwegman CW. (1965). One-stage combined abdominoperineal resection of the rectum (Miles) performed by two surgical teams. *Surgery*. 58:600–606.

Richardson EH. (1911). Studies on peritoneal adhesions: with a contribution to the treatment of denuded surfaces. *Am Surg*. 54:758–797.

Robbins GF, Brunschwig A, Foote FW. (1949). Deperitonealization: clinical and experimental observations. *Am Surg*. 130:466–479.

Ryan GB, Grobety Y, Majno G. (1971). Postoperative peritoneal adhesions. *Am J Pathol*. 65:117–148.

Sannella NA. (1975). Early and late obstruction of the small bowel after abdominoperineal resection. *Am J Surg.* 130:270–272.

Schade DS, Williamson JR. (1968). The pathogenesis of peritoneal adhesions: an ultrastructural study. *Ann Surg.* 167:500–510.

Seelig MG, Verda DJ, Kidd FH. (1943). The talcum powder problem in surgery and its solution. *JAMA.* 23:950–954.

Singleton AO Jr, Rowe EB, Moore RM. (1952). Failure of reperitonealization to prevent abdominal adhesions in the dog. *Am J Surg.* 18:789.

Spagna PM, Peskin GW. (1961). An experimental study of fibrinolysis in the prophylaxis of peritoneal adhesions. *Surg Gynec Obstet.* 113:547–550.

Sparnon AL, Spitz L. (1989). Pharmacological manipulation of postoperative intestinal adhesions. *Aust N Z J Surg.* 59:725–730.

Stewardson RH, Bombeck T, Nyhus LM. (1978). Critical operative management of small bowel obstruction. *Ann Surg.* 187:189–193.

Stout AL, Steege JF, Dodson WC, Hughes CL. (1991). Relationship of laparoscopic findings to self-report of pelvic pain. *Am J Obstet Gynecol.* 146(1):73–79.

Stovall TG, Elder RF, Ling FW. (1989). Predictors of pelvic adhesions. *J Reprod Med.* 34(5):345–348.

Surrey MW, Friedman S. (1982). Second-look laparoscopy after reconstructive pelvic surgery for infertility. *J Reprod Med.* 27:658–660.

Sutton C, MacDonald R. (1990). Laser laparoscopic adhesiolysis. *J Gynecol Surg.* 6:155–159.

Swanwick RA, Stockdale PH, Milne FJ. (1973). Healing of parietal peritoneum in the horse. *Brit Vet J.* 129:29–35.

Swolin K. (1966). Experimentelle studien zur prophylaxe von intraabdominalen verwachsungen: versuche an der ratte mit einer emulsion auslipid und prednisolon. *Acta Obstet Gynecol Scand.* 45:473–498.

Szigetvari I, Feinman M, Barad D, Bartfai G, Kaali SG. (1989). Association of previous abdominal surgery and significant adhesions in laparoscopic sterilization patients. *J Reprod Med.* 34:465–466.

Thomas JW, Rhoads JE. (1950). Adhesions resulting from removal of serosa from an area of bowel: failure of "oversewing" to lower incidence in the rat and the guinea pig. *Arch Surg.* 61:565–576.

Toaff R, Toaff ME, Peyser MR. (1976). Infertility following wedge resection of the ovaries. *Am J Obstet Gynecol.* 124:92–96.

Trimbos-Kemper TCM, Trimbos JB, van Hall EV. (1985). Adhesion formation after tubal surgery: results of the eighth-day laparoscopy in 188 patients. *Fertil Steril.* 43:395–400.

Trimpi HD, Bacon HE. (1952). Clinical and experimental study of denuded surfaces in extensive surgery of the colon and rectum. *Am J Surg.* 34:596–602.

Trusler JK. (1931). Peritonitis: an experimental model of healing in the peritoneum and the therapeutic effort of amniotic fluid concentrate. *Arch Surg.* 22:983–992.

Tsimoyiannis EC, Sarros CJ, Tsimoyiannis JC, Moutesidou K, Akalestos G, Kotoulas OB. (1988). Ranitidine and oxygen-derived free radical scavengers in hemorrhagic shock-induced gastric lesions. *Gut.* 29:826–829.

Tsimoyiannis EC, Tsimoyiannis JC, Sarros CJ, Akalestos GC, Moutesidou KJ, Lekkas ET, Kotoulas OB. (1989). The role of oxygen-derived free radicals in peritoneal adhesions formation induced by ileal ischaemia/reperfusion. *Acta Chir Scand.* 155:171–174.

Tulandi T, Hum HS, Gelfand MM. (1988). Closure of laparotomy incisions with or without peritoneal suturing and second-look laparoscopy. *Am J Obstet Gynecol.* 158:536–537.

Turunen AOI. (1933). Ueber die postoperativen verwachs ungen und deren verhutung speziell im anschluss an gynakologische laparotomien. *Duodecim Ser B.* 18:1–9.

Ulfelder H, Quinby WC Jr. (1951). Small bowel obstruction following combined abdominoperitoneal resection of the rectum. *Surgery.* 30:174–177.

Verlinden M, Michels G, Boghaert A, De Coster M, Dehertog P. (1985). Postoperative gastrointestinal atony: Cisapride promotes recovery. In: *Janssen Pharmaceutica.* 5th ed., 5.3.3. Wantage, England: 16–23.

Warren S. (1928). The effects of amniotic fluid on serous surfaces. *Arch Pathol.* 6:860–866.

Weibel M-A, Majno G. (1973). Peritoneal adhesions and their relation to abdominal surgery. *Am J Surg.* 126:345–353.

Weinstein D, Polishuk WZ. (1975). The role of wedge resection of the ovary as a cause for mechanical sterility. *Surg Gynecol Obstet.* 141:417–418.

Wilkins BM, Spitz L. (1986). Incidence of postoperative adhesion obstruction following neonatal laparotomy. *Br J Surg.* 73:762–764.

Williams DC. (1955). The peritoneum. A plea for a change in attitude towards this membrane. *Br J Surg.* 42:401–405.

Withers HR, Mason KA. (1974). The kinetics of recovery in irradiated colonic mucosa of the mouse. *Cancer.* 34:896–903.

Withers HR, Mason KA, Reid BO, Dubravsky N, Barkley HT, Brown BW, Chu AM, Smathers JB. (1974). Response of mouse intestine to neutrons and gammarays in relation to dose fractionation and division cycle. *Cancer.* 34:39–47.

Withers HR, Romsdahl MM. (1977). Post-operative radiotherapy for adenocarcinoma of the rectum and rectosigmoid. *Int J Radiat Oncol Biol Phys.* 2:1069–1074.

Withers HR, Cuasay L, Mason KA, Romsdahl MM, Saxton J. (1981). Elective radiation therapy in the curative treatment of cancer of the rectum and rectosigmoid colon. In: Stroehlein JR, Romsdahl MM, eds. *Gastrointestinal Cancer.* New York: Raven Press; 351–362.

Zachariae L. (1954). Hydrocortisone acetate applied intraperitoneally. I. Inhibitory effect on adhesions produced by talc. *Acta Endocrinol.* 16:149–159.

10

Prevention of Postoperative Adhesions

AN EXTENSIVE LITERATURE DESCRIBES AGENTS USED TO PREVENT FORmation of peritoneal adhesions, (Ellis 1971; Holtz, 1980; Pfeffer, 1980; Stangel, Nisbet, & Settles, 1984; Diamond & DeCherney, 1987; Jansen, 1990; Tulandi, 1990). In general, these treatments fall into three categories: prevention of fibrin deposition, reduction of local tissue inflammation, and removal of fibrin deposits. To date, no single therapeutic approach has proven universally effective in preventing formation of postoperative intraperitoneal adhesions.

Peritoneal Lavage

Prolonged drying of the peritoneum was shown by Ryan, Grobety, and Majno (1973) to induce significant injury. Immediately after drying, intact mesothelial cells were found to be absent in a rat cecal preparation. Four hours later, no mesothelial cells were seen; most of the surface contained only an irregular, thin coating of fibrin without cells. Continuous irrigation minimizes tissue desiccation and either dilutes or washes away fibrinous exudates. However, the choice of irrigating solution is important. Kappas et al. (1988) demonstrated an increase in adhesion formation in rats when the temperature of saline solution exceeded 37 °C. Concern arises over the use of nonbuffered peritoneal irrigating solutions due to the relatively elevated level of hydrogen ions (i.e., acidic) that forms in peritoneal fluid after surgery. Serosal damage with swelling of the underlying tissue and cell damage can occur with hypotonic and many nonbuffered irrigating solutions. For this reason, many clinicians perform intraoperative irrigation with Ringer's lactate. Yaacobi and Goldberg (1991) recently reported that both saline and Ringer's lactate may not be ideal intraperitoneal irrigants and in some cases, may promote adhesions in animal models.

Although antibiotics are frequently added to intraperitoneal lavage solutions, their efficacy is unproven. The efficacy of antibiotic peritoneal lavage in the formation of postoperative adhesions is controversial. The role of intraperitoneal cefazolin and tetracycline in the formation of adhesions was studied in a rodent model (Rappaport, Holcomb, Valente, & Chvapil, 1989). Rats treated with antibiotics had significantly more adhesions than controls. Histologic appearance of the antibiotic-irrigated groups showed mesothelial thickening with presence of fibroblasts and collagen. Cefazolin and tetracycline irrigation of the abdominal cavity contributes to the formation of peritoneal adhesions in the rat. Clinical data are not available.

Agents Affecting Coagulation

Heparinized Solutions

Because of their effects on inhibiting thrombosis and fibrin formation, heparinized solutions are often used in an attempt to prevent postoperative adhesions. Adhesion formation was reported to be significantly reduced following addition of heparinized saline prior to peritoneal closure in rats and rabbits after uterine reanastomosis or surgical trauma (Al-Chalabi & Otubo, 1987; Fukasawa, Girgis & diZerega, 1988). Subcutaneous administration of heparinized saline 30 minutes prior to either surgical procedure had no significant effect on adhesion formation relative to saline-treated controls.

Cohen, Heyman, and Mast (1983) compared the effect of heparin in a fixed volume of various intraperitoneal solutions infused prior to tissue closure on reducing adhesion formation in the rat uterine horn model. They found significant reduction in adhesion formation after infusion of Ringer's lactate alone, with human albumin, with ampicillin, with heparin, with dexamethasone, and with the combination of dexamethasone, hydrocortisone, and ampicillin. The reduction in adhesion formation was similar following the first three solutions, whereas the greatest reduction was seen with the solution containing steroids and ampicillin.

Heparin per se actively reduced adhesions in human and animal studies. However, in the early studies utilizing heparin, the dose required to reduce adhesion formation resulted in hemorrhagic diathesis. Two recent studies used lower doses of heparin and noted benefical results; one utilized a single intraperitoneal instillation, whereas the other employed continuous infusion over the traumatized site (Holtz, 1980; Al-Chalabi & Otubo, 1987). There are many mechanisms by which heparin may exert its beneficial effects. First, heparin in combination with antithrombin III inhibits clotting by enhancing serine esterase activity (Lane, MacGregor, Michalski, & Kakkar, 1978), thus reducing the deposition of fibrin strands that form the scaffold for fibroblast ingrowth. Second, heparin directly stimulates plasminogen activator activity (Rosenberg, 1978;

Andrade-Gordon & Strickland, 1986), which in turn enhances fibrinolysis. Third, heparin binds to fibroblast growth factor, which stimulates
wound healing (Markwardt & Klocking, 1977).

In clinical studies, Fayez and Schneider (1987) and Jansen (1988b)
reported no significant reduction in adhesions by the use of heparinized
Ringer's lactate (2,500 to 5,000 IU/L) compared to Ringer's lactate alone
in patients undergoing infertility surgery. Jansen reported no adverse
effects of the heparin solution on blood loss or wound healing. High-dose
heparin given intraperitoneally was associated with hemorrhage and delayed wound healing (Tarvady, Anguli, & Pichappa, 1987). Diamond et
al. (1991a) evaluated the use of Interceed as a local delivery device for
heparin. They found that a significant reduction in adhesion formation
was observed with the combination of an oxidized cellulose fabric (Interceed) plus heparin. In additional studies, heparin delivery by intraperitoneal (IP) lavage, intravenous injection, or intra-abdominal instillation failed to demonstrate efficacy. Similarly, heparin delivery with
other IP instillates (carboxymethylcellulose or 32% dextran 70) failed to
reduce adhesion formation. A recent study of Interceed used as a delivery
device for heparin demonstrated clinical efficacy similar to that of Interceed alone in a preliminary report (Reid, 1992).

Procoagulants

Blood together with peritoneal trauma can facilitate adhesion formation
(Golan & Winston, 1989; Elkins, 1989). Lindenberg and Lauritsen (1984)
found a reduction in adhesion formation in the rat following use of a
fibrin sealant spray containing thrombin, fibrinogen, and aprotinin. This
study questioned the effect of procoagulants on adhesion formation, i.e.,
did procoagulants produce a barrier effect or an effect on hemostasis?
Recently, McGaw, Elkins, DeLancey, McNeeley, and Warren (1988) reported that a thrombin spray was ineffective in reducing adhesion formation in a rat peritoneal abrasion model. Since this spray contained
procoagulant activity but provided only a minimal barrier effect, these
results support the conclusion that the barrier activity is of primary importance to adhesion prevention. In addition, the results of large clinical
studies with an oxidized cellulose fabric, Interceed, strongly suggest that
the barrier effect of this substance is directly dependent upon hemostasis
in the underlying tissue (Linsky et al., 1987; Interceed [TC7] Adhesion
Barrier Study Group, 1989; Sekiba et al., 1992). Linsky, Diamond, Cunningham, DeCherney, and diZerega (1988) observed a significant attenuation of the efficacy of oxidized cellulose in preventing adhesion formation in a rabbit model in the presence of autologous blood. As Elkins
(1989) indicated, the use of procoagulants in areas of substantial bleeding
seems to promote adhesion formation.

Surgical Techniques to Minimize Ischemia

Current theory regarding adhesion formation hypothesizes that factors that suppress plasminogen activator should result in suppression of fibrinolysis with subsequent formation of adhesions (Buckman, Buckman, Hufnagel, & Gervin, 1976; Montz, Shimanuki, & diZerega, 1987). Tissue ischemia is one of the primary causes of plasminogen activator suppression. Tissue ischemia can arise intraoperatively from crush injury, interruption of vascular supply, undue tension from sutures or oversuturing during reperitonealization, peritoneal or omental grafts, and foreign body reaction. In general, the use of surgical techniques that limit trauma, ischemia, foreign body contamination, hemorrhage, raw surfaces, and infection are recommended for minimizing the risk of intraperitoneal adhesion formation.

Sutures

All sutures elicit an acute inflammatory response following their placement. Histological differences between suture types become readily apparent following resolution of acute tissue reaction. Because they are absorbed by phagocytosis, catgut sutures elicit a greater tissue reaction than absorbable synthetic sutures (e.g., Dexon and Vicryl), which are absorbed by enzymatic hydrolysis. Acute and chronic inflammatory reactions and adhesion formation were reportedly less when polydioxanone sutures (PDS) were used relative to polyglactin 910 (Vicryl) in a rat uterine horn model (DeCherney & Laufer, 1983; Laufer, Merino, Trietsch, & DeCherney, 1984). In contrast, Neff, Holtz, and Betsill (1985) reported similar adhesion formation and tissue reactivity to these two synthetic absorbable sutures in a rabbit uterine horn model. Delbeke, Gomel, McComb, and Jetha (1983) also found no difference in tissue reactivity between polydioxanone and polyglactin 910 sutures in a rabbit model. Because the tensile strength of absorbable synthetic sutures is greater than that of natural material sutures such as catgut or silk, a smaller caliber suture can be used. Smaller sutures are associated with less tissue reaction than larger ones (e.g., Beauchamp, Guzick, Held, & Schmidt, 1988). Indeed, suture size rather than tissue reactivity to the suture material may be of greater importance in adhesion formation (Holtz, 1982a). The specific suture of choice among the available absorbable synthetic varieties will likely be dictated by the specific surgical procedure; however, evidence to date indicates that restricting suture size should help minimize intraperitoneal adhesion formation.

Foreign Body Contamination

The introduction of foreign bodies into the peritoneum can result in a series of tissue reactions that culminates in adhesion formation (reviewed by Ellis, 1990). Various materials induce foreign body reactions and subsequent adhesion formation including talc, starch, suture, dust, lint, and fiber from paper drapes (Myllarniemi, 1967; Weibel & Majno, 1973). Myllarniemi (1967) examined the relationship of foreign body reaction (i.e., granuloma) to postoperative adhesion formation. He evaluated 309 patients who previously underwent abdominal surgery and were currently undergoing another surgical procedure in the peritoneal cavity. The presence and severity of adhesions were noted and specimens of the adhesions were obtained and evaluated microscopically for evidence of a foreign body reaction. Granulomas were observed in 61% of the adhesions studied. There was a significant positive relationship between the extent of the injured peritoneal area and the occurrence of granulomas; granulomas were observed in 66% of patients who previously underwent major surgery compared to 49% in those who previously underwent relatively minor surgery. The incidence of granulomas also increased with the number of previous operations. Granulomas were observed in 76% of the adhesions taken from patients who previously underwent three or more operations. The frequency of granulomas was positively related to the severity or extent of the adhesion, although granulomas were not observed in 25% of patients with "abundant" adhesions. There was no relationship between the occurrence of granulomas and age, sex, or history of infection.

Glove powder (talc, starch, magnesium silicate) is the substance most frequently implicated in foreign body reactions and adhesion formation. Although the inflammatory reaction to starch powder was originally thought to be minimal, adhesions related to intraperitoneal starch granulomas are reported (McNaught, 1964; Cox, 1970). Despite the well-known inflammatory reaction to talc, talc contamination of surgical gloves still exists (Tolbert & Brown, 1980; Khan, Brown, Logan, & Hayes, 1983). These investigators reported that talc is used as a glove-mold release agent by many manufacturers of surgical gloves. They also found that the process of washing and wiping the gloves removed very little of the talc. Of equal or greater concern, talc contamination was found on sutures following simulation of the act of suturing while wearing the gloves. Thus, there is a shedding hazard for talc that could play a contributory role in intraperitoneal adhesion formation. Although most surgeons attempt to wash off talc from their gloves prior to surgery, complete elimination of this foreign body is problematic.

Microsurgical Techniques

Microsurgical techniques offer significant advantages over macrosurgical techniques in limiting adhesion formation. Eddy, Asch, and Balmaceda (1980) reported a fivefold increase in the incidence of adhesion formation when ovarian wedge resection was performed using macrosurgical techniques compared to microsurgical techniques in the rhesus monkey. In a retrospective analysis of infertile patients following laparotomy for removal of moderate to severe bilateral periadnexal adhesions, Diamond (1979) showed that the success rate (i.e., pregnancy) was 61% in the 140 women who underwent surgery utilizing microsurgical techniques but only 34% in the 220 women who underwent surgery limited to macrosurgical techniques. The percentage of women who delivered healthy term babies was also twofold greater following microsurgery (57%) than following macrosurgery (25%). Key differences between the two surgical techniques included the use of electrocautery for tissue excision, rubberized surgical drapes, constant irrigation, fine suction of excess fluid from the surgical site and specialized instruments to minimize tissue trauma in the microsurgical group compared to gross tissue dissection, and the use of paper surgical drapes, gauze to remove excess fluid, and forceps for handling tissue in the macrosurgical group.

Laparoscopic Surgery and Adhesion Formation

Luciano, Maier, Kock, Nulsen, and Whitman (1989) and Luciano (1990) reported a significantly greater reduction in adhesion scores in rabbits when laser adhesiolysis was performed via laparoscopy compared to laparotomy (Figure 10.1). Accordingly, many clinicians hoped that similar findings would occur in humans. At second-look laparoscopy Jansen (1988a) noted the presence of de novo adnexal adhesions in 58% of 256 consecutive laparotomies for infertility. All adhesions were removed at second-look laparoscopy. At third look laparoscopy, adhesion scores were improved in 33 patients and no patient had a worse score, although few

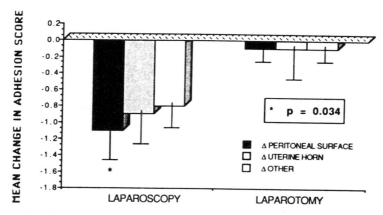

FIGURE 10.1. Changes in the mean (± SEM) postoperative adhesion scores at the surgical and incidental sites following laser adhesiolysis in rabbits by laparoscopy versus laparotomy (Luciano et al., 1990. Reproduced with the permission of John Wiley & Sons, Wiley-Liss, Inc.)

patients had no adhesions at third look (Figure 10.2). The reduced incidence in de novo adhesions following operative laparoscopic surgery was also noted by Nezhat, Nezhat, Metzger, and Luciano (1990). In a review of 500 nonselected, consecutive cases of laparoscopic surgery, Semm's group found a reduced incidence of adhesions compared to procedures performed by laparotomy (Tavmergen, Mecke, & Semm, 1990).

Although many clinicians assume that laparoscopic surgery will reduce and often eliminate postoperative adhesion formation, the data to support this assumption are not compelling. Diamond et al., (1987a) reported in 51 women only a 50% decrease in adhesion scores and a 96% incidence of adhesion in patients after laparoscopic adhesiolysis in a multicenter center study using early (8 to 79 days, mean 35 days after initial laparoscopic surgery) second-look laparoscopy (Figure 10.3; Operative Laparoscopy Study Group, 1991). Of the areas where adhesions were lysed, 67% contained adhesions at second-look. However, de novo adhesion formation was substantially reduced by laparoscopic surgery. In only 16% of the patients and in only 25% of the available sites in those patients were new adhesions noted. In only four patients did the adhesion score remain the same or increase. Thus, current laparoscopic surgical techniques appear to reduce de novo adhesion formation, whereas adhesion reformation continues to be a major concern.

Ovarian Surgery

Since the ovary is the most frequent site for postsurgical adhesion formation in the pelvis (Table 10.1), techniques for ovarian surgery are

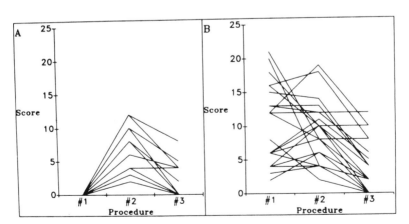

FIGURE 10.2. Effect of postoperative laparoscopy on adhesion scores in patients with no initial adhesions (A), and with initial adhesions (B). Procedures: initial infertility operation (#1), postoperative laparoscopy (#2), and subsequent evaluation (#3). (From Jansen, 1988a. Reproduced by permission of American Fertility Society.)

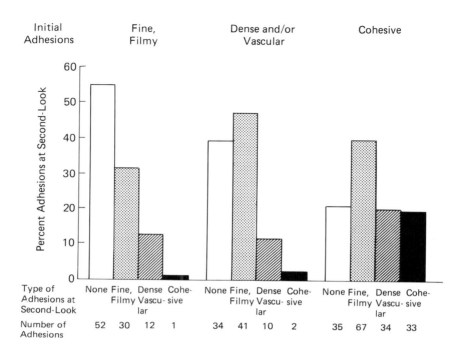

FIGURE 10.3. Frequency and type of adhesions observed at early second-look procedures after laparoscopic adhesiolysis of fine, filmy adhesions, dense and/or vascular adhesions, or cohesive adhesions. 45% of the fine/filmy, 62% of the dense and/or vascular, and 80% of the cohesive adhesions lysed at initial laparoscopic surgery reformed prior to second-look laparoscopy. (From Operative Laparoscopy Study Group, 1991. Reproduced by permission of American Fertility Society.)

important to pelvic surgeons. (Adashi et al., 1981; Butttram & Vaquero, 1975.) Gillett (1991) found that even minimal handling removed the surface epithelium of the human ovary (Figure 10.4). Lyles et al. (1989) treated four patients with polycystic ovarian disease who did not ovulate after receiving clomiphene citrate with ovarian electrocautery and two patients with ND:YAG laser photocoagulation. A second-look laparoscopy for evaluation of pelvic adhesions was performed 3 to 4 weeks later. All six second-look laparoscopies revealed ovarian adhesions, which were extensive in some cases.

Closure of the ovarian cortex is controversial. Dunn, Doody, Mohler, and Buttram (1988) evaluated ovarian surgical techniques in a primate model. Female baboons of reproductive age with no prior abdominal surgery underwent ovarian wedge resection using scalpel incision and closure versus cautery incision and closure. Influence of ovarian anatomical location was controlled by alternating the type of ovarian injury

TABLE 10.1. Incidence of adhesions at initial surgery and follow-up laparoscopy.

| Tissue | Adhesion rate | | | |
| | Initial surgery[a] | | Follow-up laparoscopy[b] | |
	No.	%	No.	%
Ovaries	303/387	78%	207/376	55%
Fimbria	244/384	64%	135/372	36%
Cul-de-sac	87/208	42%	42/208	20%
Omentum	32/208	15%	39/208	19%
Colon	63/208	30%	30/204	15%
Small intestine	30/208	14%	30/208	14%
Pelvic sidewall	124/208	60%	84/208	40%

[a]Initial surgery performed using CO_2 laser + 35% dextran 70 or nonlaser surgical technique with or without dextran. Results are pooled over three initial surgical procedure groups.
[b]Within 12 weeks of initial surgery.
Adapted from Diamond et al. (1984).

between animals. Adhesion scoring performed 2 weeks later via laparotomy showed no difference between the ovarian wedge resection techniques. Brumsted, Deaton, Lavigne, and Riddick (1990) performed wedge resections of rabbit ovaries with and without reapproximation of the ovarian cortex. In 17 of 19 rabbits adhesion scores were greater on the reapproximated ovary. Although outcome does not differ according to preliminary studies by this group, interpretation of these results is confounded by the fact that wedge resection was performed on the reapproximated ovary by scalpel and by ND:YAG laser on the nonreapproximated ovary. Wiskind, Toledo, Dudle, and Zusmanis (1990) showed that suturing of rabbit ovaries clearly enhanced postoperative adhesion formation to the ovary compared with a nonsutured control group (Figure 10.5).

Barrier Agents

Physical barriers are used to prevent adhesion formation by minimizing apposition of serosal surfaces. By limiting tissue apposition during the critical period of mesothelial repair, the development of a fibrin matrix between the tissue surfaces should be minimized. Barrier agents used for the prevention of postoperative adhesion formation include both mechanical barriers and viscous intraperitoneal solutions.

Limited success was reported with the use of the mechanical barrier, oxidized regenerated cellulose (Interceed), polytetrafluoroethylene (Gore-Tex) and with high molecular weight intraperitoneal solutions such as sodium carboxymethylcellulose and dextran. Although effective, these

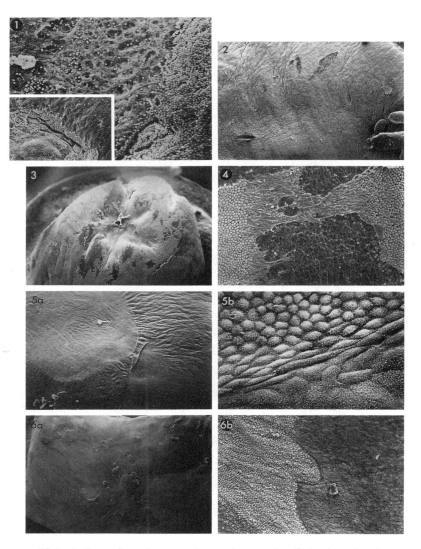

FIGURE 10.4. 1: Scanning electron photomicrograph of the junction between wiped and unwiped surfaces of a human ovary (×150). Inset: cells retained in a surface cleft (×55). 2: Scanning electron photomicrograph of the ovarian surface over a 20-mm follicle (×48). Note the small patch of lost cells. 3: Scanning electron photomicrograph of the ovarian surface over an old corpus luteum (×9). Note the bridges over the central healed stigma. Re-epithelialization is complete, but because of difficulty in retrieving this ovary at minilaparotomy, the surface around the healed stigma has lost cells. 4: Scanning electron photomicrograph of the surface of an ovarian capsule (×170). Note the lost cells and the migrating epithelial cells. 5: Scanning electron photomicrographs of the wall of a 16-mm follicle: (a) note the different cell zones—darker regions indicate flattened and larger cells (×25); (b) junction between the zones (×640). 6: Scanning electron photomicrographs of an ovarian capsule: (a) the whole surface is covered with an epithelial layer (×140); (b) junction between different cell zones (×90) (Gillett, 1991. Reproduced with the permission of CSIRO, Melbourne, Australia.)

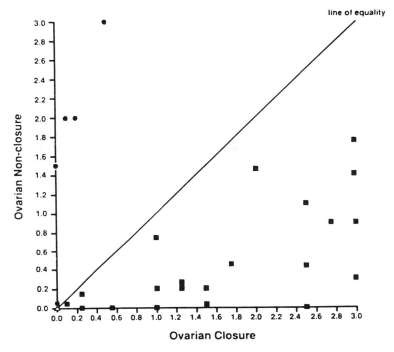

FIGURE 10.5. Graphic representation of adhesion scores that formed on rabbit ovaries with or without closure after surgical injury of the ovary. △ Represents four animals with adhesion score of zero on both ovaries. ■ Represents 21 animals with adhesion score of microsurgically closed ovary greater than adhesion score of nonclosure ovaries. ● Illustrates five animals with nonclosure ovary adhesion score greater than adhesion score of ovary microsurgically closed. Suturing of the ovaries enhanced postoperative adhesion formation compared to nonsutured controls. (From Wiskind et al., 1990. Reproduced by permission of C. V. Mosby.)

barrier agents do not totally prevent postoperative adhesion formation in animal models. In two large clinical studies Interceed was shown to be efficacious in adhesion reduction (Adhesion Barrier Study Group, 1983; Malinak, 1990; Sekiba et al., 1992).

Mechanical Barriers

Although many different mechanical barriers were tried in an attempt to prevent postoperative adhesion formation they have generally proven inadequate either because they cause ischemia, are nonabsorbable, or because they induce a foreign body reaction. The one exception to this is oxidized regenerated cellulose (ORC) barriers (see below). Two additional mechanical barriers warrant discussion—amniotic membrane grafts and Gore-Tex surgical membrane.

Amniotic Membrane Graft

Badawy, Baggish, ElBakry, and Baltoyannis (1989) reported a reduction in adhesion formation following the use of a human amniotic membrane graft applied to the deperitonealized surface in a rat sidewall abrasion model. These researchers failed to observe a benefit of the graft in a rat uterine horn anastomosis model or in a rat laser injury model. Young, Cota, Zund, Mason, and Wheeler (1991) reported less adhesion formation after application of a human amniotic membrane graft relative to suturing alone in a rabbit uterine horn incision model. Neither of these researchers observed rejection or infection at the graft site, although Soules, Dennis, Bosarge, and Moore (1982) observed amniotic membrane graft necrosis and the promotion of adhesion formation to the graft site in the rabbit.

Gore-Tex Surgical Membrane

Gore-Tex Surgical Membrane is a thin sheet of expanded polytetrafluoroethylene used successfully as a substitute for the pericardium. The Surgical Membrane has a very small pore size (≤ 1 micron) that reduces cellular penetration. The membrane must be anchored in place within the body and is nonabsorbable. Evaluations of its utility in reducing adhesion formation following intraperitoneal surgery are limited. Boyers, Diamond, and DeCherney (1988) reported significant reductions in the extent, type, and tenacity of adhesions with the use of Gore-Tex Surgical Membrane relative to the control-treated side in a rabbit uterine horn abrasion model. Furthermore, these researchers observed no adhesions to the Surgical Membrane itself 3 weeks after surgery in the 24 animals tested.

Conversely, Goldberg, Toledo, and Mitchell (1987) found no benefit of the Gore-Tex Surgical Membrane in another rabbit uterine horn abrasion model. Fifteen New Zealand white rabbits underwent laparotomy, with scrape and cut lesions created bilaterally on the uterine body and horns, respectively. On one side, the lesions were covered with Gore-Tex using 7-0 Gore-Tex suture; the contralateral side served as an internal control. After 4 weeks, the adhesions were graded and mean adhesion scores calculated. The Gore-Tex score was four times higher than the control for scrape lesions and two times higher for cut lesions. The Gore-Tex Surgical Membrane did not appear to be an effective adjuvant for postoperative adhesion prophylaxis in this animal model. However, these researchers observed minimal adhesion formation in their control animals, calling into question the sensitivity of their model to detect treatment-related reductions in adhesion formation.

A multicenter clinical study evaluated Gore-Tex Surgical Membrane in patients treated for one of the following: (1) moderate to severe pelvic adhesive disease, (2) significant deperitonealization, or (3) myomectomy (Surgical Membrane Study Group, 1992). Adhesiolysis sites were scored with a system that ranged from 0 to 11 for type, tenacity, and extent of the adhesions. Adhesions were lysed or the myoma removed and a Gore-Tex Surgical Membrane sutured into the site. Two to six weeks later, the Gore-Tex Surgical Membrane was removed laparoscopically and the adhesiolysis or myomectomy site was scored using the same system. The area covered by the Gore-Tex Surgical Membrane had significantly lower scores than prior to surgery (Figure 10.6). There was no morbidity (i.e., infection, inflammation) attributable to the use of the Gore-Tex Surgical Membrane. All Gore-Tex Surgical Membranes were removed at laparoscopy by cutting the sutures and withdrawing the membrane through an operating channel. Histological analysis of the retrieved Gore-Tex Surgical Membranes showed no tissue adherence to the material and mild

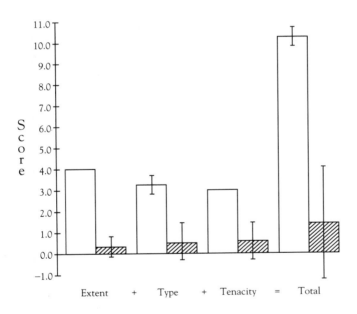

FIGURE 10.6. The efficacy of Gore-Tex Surgical Membrane in the reduction of peritoneal adhesion reformation in a clinical setting was examined. The initial scores for extent, type, tenacity, and total of these three are shown in the open bars. In the hatched bars these same parameters were evaluated at second look after placement of the Gore-Tex Surgical Membrane. These data are mean ± SEM for 12 sites (Surgical Membrane Study Group, 1992).

to no foreign body response. Third-look laparoscopy of a single sidewall site showed no adhesion formation subsequent to removal of the Gore-Tex Surgical Membrane.

Oxidized Regenerated Cellulose Barrier

Ideally, a physical barrier for adhesion prevention should be completely absorbable and nonreactive; furthermore, it should stay in place within the body without the use of sutures or staples. Oxidized regenerated cellulose (ORC) barriers appear to satisfy these criteria. This material is completely absorbable and has been shown to be nonreactive. It does not support bacterial growth; rather this material has antibacterial properties in vivo (Queralt, Laguens, Lozano, & Morandeira, 1987). Lastly it maintains its position within the peritoneum without the use of sutures when residual peritoneal fluid is minimized.

Initial studies with ORC evaluated the use of Surgicel, an absorbable material that is used extensively in maintaining hemostasis. When left in the body, Surgicel is converted into a gelatinous mass and absorbed within a few days in the majority of animals (rabbits; Nishimura, Bieniarz, Nakamura, & diZerega, 1983a). Many evaluations of Surgicel in animal models of adhesion formation show it reduces the severity and/or the incidence of adhesion formation. A significant reduction in adhesion formation was demonstrated in the rat cecal trauma model (Larsson, Nisell, & Granberg, 1978), rat multiple peritoneal trauma and ischemic peritoneal models (Raftery, 1980), rabbit uterine horn trauma model (Galan, Leader, Malkinson, & Taylor, 1983; Nishimura et al., 1983a; Shimanuki, Nishimura, & diZerega, 1987) and rabbit bowel reanastomosis model (Shimanuki, Nishimura, & diZerega, 1987).

However, not all studies demonstrated efficacy of Surgicel in preventing adhesions. Schroder, Willumsen, Hart Hansen, and Hart Hansen (1982) and Yemini, Meshorer, Katz, Rozeman, and Lancet (1984) evaluated Surgicel among other modalities and failed to demonstrate a reduction in cecal adhesions in rats. Soules et al. (1982) found that Surgicel offered no advantage over no treatment after a standardized cut or scrape of the rabbit uterine horn. Hixson, Swanson, and Friedman (1986) studied the ability of Surgicel to prevent postsurgical adhesions to the fimbria and ovaries; Surgicel did not reduce adnexal adhesions.

Recently, a modification of Surgicel was found to be more effective in preventing adhesion formation in the rabbit (Diamond et al., 1987a; Linsky et al., 1987). This new material (Interceed) is also an oxidized regenerated cellulose. The difference is that the knitted pattern was changed so that Interceed has a longer intraperitoneal residence time than Surgicel. A significant reduction in adhesion formation was observed following use of Interceed after uterine or peritoneal sidewall trauma in the rabbit (Diamond et al., 1987; Linsky et al., 1987, 1988).

A prospective, multicenter, randomized clinical evaluation of Interceed was conducted to evaluate clinical efficacy (Interceed [TC7] Adhesion Barrier Study Group, 1989; Malinak, 1990). Infertility patients ($n = 134$) in 13 investigational centers underwent lysis of bilateral pelvic sidewall adhesions. Following adhesiolysis, the area of the deperitonealized surface was measured. Interceed was applied in an amount sufficient to completely cover deperitonealized surfaces on the sidewall; the contralateral sidewall was left uncovered, thereby serving as control. A second-look laparoscopy was performed between 10 days and 14 weeks after the laparotomy. Interceed barrier was found to significantly reduce the incidence, extent, and severity of postoperative adhesions (Table 10.2). Interceed also significantly reduced adhesion formation between ovaries and the peritoneal sidewall (Figure 10.7) and prevented the reformation of adhesions in over twice as many patients as did the control. These observations were recently confirmed by a similar multicenter study performed in Japan (Table 10.3; Figure 10.8; Sekiba et al., 1992). In September 1989 Interceed received approval by the Food and Drug Administration (FDA) as the first adjuvant indicated for the reduction of postsurgical adhesions.

Larsson et al. (1978) suggested that oxidized regenerated cellulose prevents adhesion formation by its transformation into a gelatinous mass that covers the damaged peritoneum and thereby protects it from involvement in adhesion formation. This gelatinous "cocoon" seems to provide a protective coating over healing tissue during the initial postoperative interval (Diamond et al., 1987b; Linsky et al., 1987). During

TABLE 10.2. Clinical evaluation of Interceed following adhesiolysis among infertile patients[a]

| | Treatment group | |
Adhesion parameter	TC7 ($n = 134$)	Control ($n = 134$)
Adhesions at second-look		
Present	66 (49%)	102 (76%)
Absent	68 (50%)	32 (23%)
Mean area of adhesions (cm³)		
At laparotomy	10.8	8.8
At laparoscopy	1.6	3.1
Adhesion severity at second-look		
None	66%	45%
Filmy	18%	25%
Severe	16%	30%

[a]Patients underwent laparotomy for adhesiolysis of bilateral pelvic sidewall adhesions. Following surgery Interceed barrier was applied over deperitonealized surfaces on one sidewall; other left untreated. Second-look laparoscopy was performed 10 days to 14 weeks later for assessment of adhesions (Malinak, 1990).

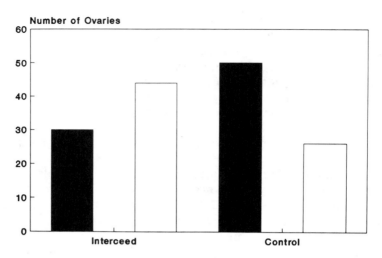

FIGURE 10.7. Interceed significantly reduced the reformation of ovarian-sidewall adhesions when the pelvic sidewall was covered with Interceed after adhesiolysis. The number of ovaries with adhesions is represented by the closed bars and the number of ovaries without adhesions is represented by open bars (Malinak, 1990).

this time, re-epithelialization of damaged peritoneal surfaces is completed (7 to 10 days, see Chapter 9). In preclinical studies, the presence of blood significantly reduced the efficacy of ORC barriers such as Interceed (Linsky et al., 1988). To obtain maximum benefit, it is essential to achieve hemostasis prior to applying the Interceed. This means that the barrier should not turn brown or black after application. This color change is indicative of inadequate hemostasis.

TABLE 10.3. Adhesions present (+) or absent (−) on sidewall of women at second-look laparoscopy.

Interceed treated	−	+	−	+	
Control sidewall	+	−	−	+	
North American study (Malinak 1990)	34%	7%	16%	41%	$n = 134$
Japanese study (Sekiba et al., 1992)	39%	4%	19%	36%	$n = 63$
Combined	36%	6%	17%	40%	$n = 197$

Matched pair comparison of treatment effect sidewalls with no adhesions.

Study	Interceed	Control	Interceed benefit
North American	46 (82%)	10 (17%)	4.6×
Japanese	25 (89%)	3 (10%)	8.3×
Combined	71 (84%)	13 (15%)	5.5×

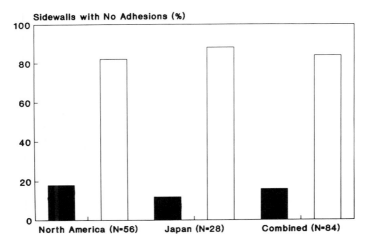

FIGURE 10.8. Interceed (closed bar) was found to significantly reduce adhesion reformation to the pelvic sidewall compared to state-of-the-art surgery alone (open bar) as determined by multicenter clinical studies in North America (Malinak, 1990) and Japan (Sekiba et al., 1992).

Intraperitoneal Barrier Solutions

Many years ago, Kajihara (1960) reported that chondroitin is useful in adhesion prevention. Elkins et al. (1984a, 1984b) and Fredericks, Kotry, Holtz, Askalani, and Serour (1986) showed that carboxymethylcellulose prevented formation of adhesions in animal models. Chondroitin sulfate and carboxymethylcellulose both show promise in animal studies as liquid barriers to prevent adhesions. Oelsner et al. (1987) compared the two regimens in an animal model and found chondroitin sulfate superior to either carboxymethyl sulfate or Hyskon in preventing postsurgical adhesions. However, in comparing the regimens in a standardized rat model, Graebe et al. (1989) found carboxymethylcellulose to be as effective as chondroitin sulfate, and significantly better than Hyskon, in preventing adhesions. Elkins et al. (1984a, 1984b) found carboxymethylcellulose effective in preventing adhesions in the rat. The clinical utility of these "liquid barriers" awaits the scrutiny of toxicity studies and clinical trials.

Dextran

Dextran is a water-soluble glucose polymer that was originally investigated as a plasma expander. Of all the intraperitoneal agents evaluated for prevention of adhesion formation, it has received the most attention. Although dextran can be manufactured in a variety of molecular weights, most of the research in adhesion prevention focused on 32% dextran 70 (Hyskon, Pharmacia; molecular weight 70,000).

The basis for dextran's effects on adhesion formation hypothetically relates to a variety of activities (see Stangel et al., 1984). Dextran may cause a mechanical separation of serosal surfaces. Tissues are held apart by the heavy fluid in the peritoneal cavity, resulting in "hydroflotation." This effect is further enhanced by the osmotic gradient created by dextran that draws fluid into the peritoneal cavity. The osmotic gradient caused by application of 32% dextran 70 into the peritoneal cavity can draw in 2.5 to 3 times the volume instilled from the vascular space (Krinsky, Haseltine, & DeCherney, 1984). Dextran may have a "siliconizing" effect and coats raw serosal surfaces, thus preventing tissue apposition. Dextran may have antithrombotic activity, which retards adherence of blood clot and deposition of fibrin matrix. Furthermore, dextran can modify the fibrin network and thereby facilitate fibrinolysis.

A recent study suggests that 32% dextran 70 may have immunosuppressant activity. In cells isolated from patients undergoing laparoscopy, lymphocyte proliferation and macrophage phagocytosis were reduced in vitro following incubation with 32% dextran 70 (Rein & Hill, 1989). In addition, 32% dextran 70 was shown to reduce the ability of severe intraperitoneal trauma to depress plasminogen activator activity; dextran can cause plasminogen activation in vitro (Wagaman, Ingram, Rao, & Saba, 1986).

Flessner, Dedrick, and Schultz (1985) demonstrated a positive relationship between dextran molecular weight and prolonged absorption rate. The greater the molecular weight, the longer the intraperitoneal residence. Thus, higher molecular weight dextrans should provide a greater and longer-lasting "hydroflotation" effect than lower molecular weight dextran, and should result in a greater reduction in adhesion formation. In general, lower molecular weight dextrans have less of an effect on adhesion prevention than do higher molecular weight compounds. For example, Ruiz Navas, Lopez, Flores, and Romeroz (1988) reported that dextran 70 was significantly more effective than dextran 40 in reducing the incidence of adhesion formation in a rat uterine horn model. Beneficial effects of dextran 70 (either 6% or 32%) on the incidence and/ or severity of adhesion formation are usually observed in animal models (see review by Dlugi & DeCherney, 1984). Failures to observe any beneficial effect with dextran 70 in animals studies were also reported (e.g., Holtz, Baker & Tsai, 1980; ten Kate-Booij, van Geldorp, & Drogenijk, 1985).

Two prospective, controlled, clinical studies in patients undergoing infertility surgery reported a significant beneficial effect of 32% dextran 70 on adhesion formation. In one study, a total of 102 patients undergoing surgery for distal tubal disease, endometriosis, or pelvic adhesions had 250 mL of 32% dextran 70 ($n = 55$) or 250 mL saline ($n = 47$) instilled intraperitoneally prior to closure of the abdomen (Adhesion Study Group, 1983). Although prophylactic antibiotics were given to all patients, no other therapeutic adjuvants were used. The extent and severity of adhesions were evaluated at the time of the initial laparotomy and at a second-look laparoscopy performed 8 to 12 weeks later. Patients with severe adnexal adhesions at the time of the initial laparotomy had a greater reduction in adhesions if they received 32% dextran 70 than if they received saline. Furthermore, a marked reduction in adhesion formation was observed in more of the 32% dextran 70 treated patients (50%) than in saline treated patients (30%). Adhesions were found to occur significantly more frequently at the time of the second-look laparoscopy in control patients than in 32% dextran 70 patients at the ovary, cul-de-sac, and pelvic sidewall.

In the second prospective study, patients undergoing infertility surgery were randomized to receive 200 mL 32% dextran 70 ($n = 23$) or 200 mL Ringer's lactate ($n = 21$) intraperitoneally prior to closure (Rosenberg & Board, 1984). Four to 12 weeks after the initial surgery, a second-look laparoscopy was performed. There was a significant difference between the two groups with respect to the net change in patients' adhesion scores at the time of the initial surgery and at laparoscopy. Adhesion scores tended to worsen after receiving Ringer's lactate, whereas they improved after receiving 32% dextran 70. Thirty-nine of the patients underwent lysis of adhesions at the time of the original surgery. The same pattern of results was evident in these patients: no improvement or worsening in the control group but improvement in the 32% dextran 70 group.

Although not a direct assessment of adhesion prevention, Smith (1983) reported a higher pregnancy rate among 25 patients who received 32% dextran 70 intraperitoneally at the time of infertility surgery than among 25 patients who received an instillation of saline into the peritoneal cavity.

Not all clinical evaluations reported a therapeutic benefit of 32% dextran 70 on adhesion formation. In a prospective, controlled evaluation of 250 mL of 32% dextran 70 versus saline in 39 patients undergoing salpingoneostomy, fimbrioplasty, or adhesiolysis, Larsson et al. (1985) reported no difference between the two treatments in reducing the adhesions at follow-up laparoscopy 4 to 10 weeks later. Jansen (1985) also reported no benefit from the addition of 100 to 200 mL 32% dextran 70 on adhesion scores at follow-up laparoscopy performed 12 days later in patients after infertility surgery (Figure 10.9).

Dextran Side Effects

The clinical use of 32% dextran 70 is associated with side effects. Ascites is commonly observed following administration of 32% dextran 70. Cleary, Howard, and diZerega (1985) reported that serum dextran levels gradually increase during the initial days after surgery and that clinical ascites was resolved by the 4-week follow-up visit in each of the five

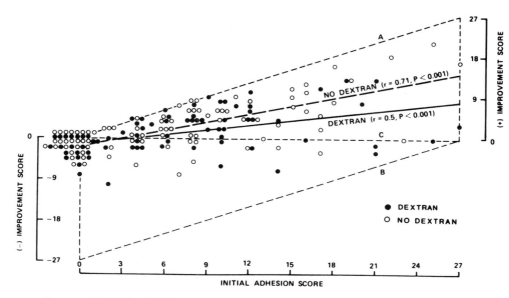

FIGURE 10.9. Distribution of adhesion improvement scores (●, 32% dextran 70; ○, no dextran) in relationship to initial adhesion scores. The permissible area of distribution of adhesion improvement scores is a parallelogram, the inclined boundaries of which represent the best (line A) and the worst (line B) possible outcomes (line C represents no change in adhesion scores). Because a positive relationship between higher initial adhesion scores and better improvement scores is inevitable, the initial adhesion score is an important covariate that must be controlled for accurate between-treatment comparisons. With this type of analysis, 32% dextran 70 was found not to be associated with a reduction in postsurgical adhesion formation compared to untreated controls. (From Jansen, 1985. Reproduced by permission of C. V. Mosby.)

patients. A transient weight gain is usually observed with 32% dextran 70 (Magyar, Hayes, Spirtos, Hull, & Moghissi, 1985). Perhaps the most common clinical complication after intraperitoneal instillation of 32% dextran 70 is vulvar edema, which may occur in 2% of cases (Magyar et al., 1985; Adhesion Study Group, 1983). In addition to vulvar edema, Tulandi (1987) reported edema of the leg and pleural effusion. Pleural effusion (Adoni, Adatto-Levy, Mogle, & Palti, 1980; Rose, 1987) and coagulopathy (Rose, 1987) are less frequent in patients receiving intraperitoneal 32% dextran 70; all of these side effects resolve either spontaneously or with supportive therapy. Anaphylactic shock or allergic symptoms occur in a small percentage of patients given 32% dextran 70 intraperitoneally (Bailey, Strub, Klein, & Salvaggio, 1967; Borten, Seibert, & Taymor, 1983; Trimbos-Kemper & Veering, 1989) or as a hysteroscopic distention media (Ahmed, Falcone, Tulandi, & Houle, 1991). Stangel et al. (1984) reported that two patients treated with intraperitoneal 6% dextran 70 developed disseminated intravascular coagulation and anaphylactoid shock.

Gauwerky, Heinrich, and Kubli (1986) performed a prospective evaluation of complications that occur after repeated use of intraperitoneal dextran. In 47 patients (dextran group: 32 patients, control group: 15 patients) undergoing laparotomy for microsurgical removal of adhesions and tuboplasty, the complications of a repeated postoperative intraperitoneal instillation of 6% dextran 70 (5 days) were monitored. In the dextran-treated group, abdominal pain and dyspnea occurred significantly more frequently than in the control group. In six cases, edema of the vulva and in two cases edema of the thigh developed. During intraperitoneal irrigation with dextran, a significant increase of body weight (Figure 10.10) and central venous pressure (Figure 10.11) were noted. Bradycardia was observed between the 3rd and 6th postoperative days. Blood pressure remained unchanged. Seventy-five percent of the patients in the dextran group had pleural effusions containing dextran when sampled on the 5th postoperative day.

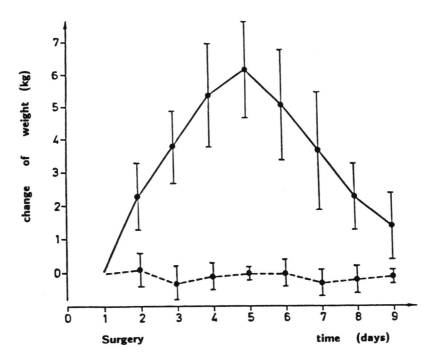

FIGURE 10.10. Postoperative changes in weight in relation to the patient's original weight. Values are given as mean ± standard error. Dextran group: ●———●; control group ●------● (From Gauwerky et al., 1986. Reproduced by permission of Georg Thieme Verlag.)

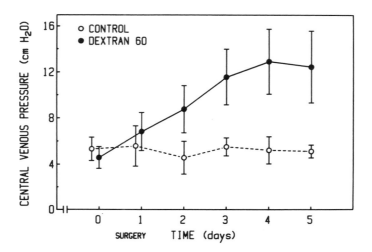

FIGURE 10.11. Postoperative change of central venous pressure. Mean values ± standard error. (●———●: dextran group, ○------○ control group). (From Gauwerky et al., 1986. Reproduced by permission of Georg Thieme Verlag.)

Administration of 32% dextran 70 into the peritoneal cavity may produce an increase in the postoperative SGOT and SGPT values (Weinans, Kauer, Klompmaker, & Wijma, 1990). The use of 32% dextran 70 in combination with corticosteroids or halothane (or halogenated drugs) was reported to increase the risk of liver function disturbances. The increase in serum transaminase levels appears to be self-limited and transient. In a group of 31 patients in whom it was possible to follow the SGOT and SGPT values after hospital discharge, in 29 patients the values were normal within 6 months (Weinans et al., 1990).

There appears to be a disparity between in vitro data and clinical experience with dextran in cases of pelvic infection; 32% dextran 70 was reported to support bacterial and fungal growth in vitro (Bernstein, Mattox, & Ulrich, 1982; King, 1989). We partially confirmed this report in that gram (+) anaerobic cocci were found to proliferate in dextran (Hammil & diZerega, unpublished observation). However, infectious complications of dextran use are very uncommon in clinical practice. King (1989) reported the case history of a patient who developed a *C. albicans* pelvic infection after intraperitoneal administration of 32% dextran 70. Although infection-related complications of 32% dextran 70 are uncommon, its use in the presence of pelvic infection is unwarrented.

Sodium Carboxymethylcellulose

Sodium carboxymethylcellulose (CMC) is a heat-stable, high molecular weight (approximately 350,000 d), substitute polysaccharide that is used as a thickener in many foods. Most solutions of CMC tested for adhesion prevention are clear and semigelatinous with a viscosity greater than 32% dextran 70 (Hyskon, Pharmacia; 220 cps). The viscosity of 1 wt% and 2 wt% CMC solution are approximately 5,300 and 36,000 cps, respectively (Diamond, Linsky, Cunningham, Constantine, & DeCherney, 1988). Compared to untreated controls, CMC (1%, 7 ml/kg) prevented adhesion formation (Moll, Schumacher, Wright, & Spano, 1990). A study was designed to test various high molecular weight solutions in the prevention of postoperative intra-abdominal adhesions. The bicornuate rat uterus was used as the surgical model; 80 rats were randomly divided into groups of five that received intraperitoneally 5 ml of chondroitin sulfate, sodium carboxymethylcellulose, and 32% dextran 70, respectively; one group underwent microsurgical repair, and another group received no therapy (control). Significantly better results in adhesion prevention were demonstrated in the sodium carboxymethylcellulose group versus the other groups.

In both rat and rabbit adhesion formation models, CMC was shown to significantly reduce adhesion formation relative to control-treated animals when placed in the peritoneal cavity prior to closure (Diamond et al., 1988; Elkins et al., 1984a, 1984b; Fredericks et al., 1986). CMC was also significantly more effective in reducing adhesion formation than either low molecular weight (10% dextran 40) or high molecular weight dextran (32% dextran 70) (Elkins et al., 1984a, 1984b; Fredericks et al., 1986). CMC was also significantly more effective in preventing adhesion reformation than 32% dextran 70 in a rat cecum adhesion model (Elkins et al., 1984b); 2 weeks following adhesiolysis, significant adhesions were observed in 90% of the rats treated with 32% dextran 70 but in only 50% of the animals treated with 1% CMC.

The reduction in adhesion formation with CMC is concentration-dependent; significantly greater reductions were apparent following administration of 3% CMC compared to 1% CMC (Figure 10.12; Diamond et al., 1988; Fredericks et al., 1986). Increased viscosity with increasing concentrations of CMC may contribute to the enhanced efficacy of the higher concentrations. In support of the hypothesis that CMC prevents adhesion formation by "siliconizing" the tissue and hence preventing tissue apposition, Diamond et al. (1988) reported that the reduction in adhesion formation with CMC was volume-dependent. The degree of adhesion formation was less following administration of 50 mL compared to 20 mL of 2% CMC. Elkins et al. (1984a, 1984b) observed large amounts (>3 mL) of CMC in the peritoneal cavity 24 and 48 hours postoperatively; even at 14 days postoperatively, some free-floating CMC was apparent in a minority of the animals they evaluated.

In some of the studies with CMC, infection and peritonitis were observed in a few of the animals (Elkins et al., 1984a, 1984b). In some instances the infection was fatal. No increase in infection rates was ob-

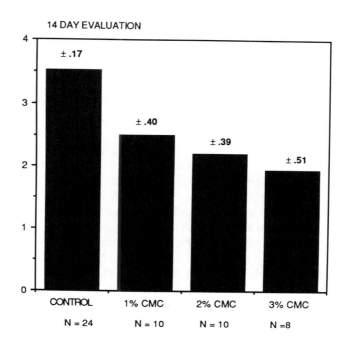

FIGURE 10.12. Adhesion scores in the rabbit uterine horn model in control rabbits and following intraperitoneal instillation of 20 mL of 1%, 2%, or 3% carboxymethylcellulose (Diamond et al., 1988).

served after instillation of CMC in joints or the eye (Homsey, Stanky, & King, 1973) and a preliminary study found that CMC is less likely to support bacterial growth in vitro than 32% dextran 70 (Elkins et al., 1985). Nevertheless, further studies are needed to address whether CMC supports bacterial growth in a clinically relevant setting.

Neither 32% dextran 70 nor sodium carboxymethylcellulose activated in vitro oxygen free radical production in phorbol myristate acetate (PMA)-stimulated neutrophils, caseinate-elicited peritoneal macrophages, or alveolar macrophages, (Elkins, Warren & Portz, 1991; Portz et al., 1991). In addition, neither of these high molecular weight substances altered the capacity of neutrophils to secrete the lysosomal enzyme, β-glucuronidase. The results of these in vitro experiments support the hypothesis that these substances exert their effects on adhesion formation by imposing a temporary barrier to prevent tissue apposition of serosal surfaces during reperitonealization rather than by interfering with the inflammatory process.

Other Barrier Solutions

Other high molecular weight solutions were administered intraperitoneally in an attempt to prevent tissue apposition and thus minimize adhesion formation. These include chondroitin sulfate, hyaluronic acid, silicon, and polymer solutions. The results of animal studies conducted with these intraperitoneal solutions are encouraging and a number of health care companies are pursuing clinical evaluation of these solutions in adhesion prevention. To date, however, controlled clinical studies of these intraperitoneal barrier solutions are lacking.

Oelsner et al. (1987) demonstrated that a 25% chondroitin sulfate solution (viscosity of 232 cps) was significantly more effective than 32% dextran 70, 1% CMC, or normal saline when administered intraperitoneally prior to closure in preventing adhesion formation in the rabbit uterine horn model. In this study, 88% of uterine horns from animals treated with chondroitin sulfate were adhesion-free compared to 33%, 40%, 47%, and 35% of uterine horns from animals treated with CMC, dextran, saline, or no solution, respectively. A 5% chondroitin sulfate solution was less effective than either CMC and not different than 32% dextran 70 or control treatment in another study (DeCherney & Mezer, 1984).

The adhesion prevention properties of chondroitin sulfate are thought to be related to its ability to coat epithelial surfaces and prevent tissue apposition by emitting repelling negative charges. Like chondroitin sulfate, sodium hyaluronate is also a member of the glycosaminoglycan family and shares a similar proposed mechanism of action in preventing adhesion formation. To date, however, published reports of sodium hyaluronate in preventing adhesion formation are primarily limited to models of tendon adhesion formation (e.g., St. Onge, Weiss, Denlinger, & Balazs, 1980; Thomas, Jones, & Hungerford, 1982; Weiss, Levy, Denlinger, Suros, & Weiss, 1986; Weiss et al., 1987). A initial report of hyaluronic acid in a rat cecal abrasion model indicates that this agent is more efficacious than CMC, polyvinylpyrrolidone (PVP) or Ringer's lactate in preventing adhesion formation in this model (Yaacobi & Goldberg, 1991).

The beneficial effect of Poloxamer 407 solution, a commercially available copolymer of polyoxyethylene and polyoxypropylene, on intraperitoneal adhesion formation was reported in a rat uterine horn model (Leach & Henry, 1990). In this study, adhesions were evident in 95% of untreated uterine horns but in only 40% of Poloxamer 407–treated uterine horns. Leach and Henry hypothesized that Poloxamer 407 acted as a mechanical barrier for deperitonealized surfaces until reperitonealization occurred; in their study, there was no evidence of residual material 21 days after surgery. Steinleitner, Lambert, Kazensky, and Cantor (1991) confirmed and extended these observations. They found that a 30% to

35% solution of Poloxamer 407 effectively reduced both adhesion formation and reformation.

Studies applying liquid silicone intraperitoneally prior to closure yielded mixed results with respect to effects on adhesion formation. O'Leary (1985) reported a significant beneficial effect of liquid silicone on adhesion formation in a dog peritoneal abrasion model. Ballantyne, Hawthorne, Ben-Hur, Seidman, and Rees (1971) also reported a reduction in adhesion formation following intraperitoneal administration of 16 mL liquid silicone in a rat peritoneal abrasion model; smaller volume of silicone (2 to 3 mL) had no effect in this study. In contrast, Brody and Frey (1968), Frey, Thorpe, and Brody (1967) and O'Leary, Turner, and Feldman (1969) reported an enhancement in the incidence and severity of adhesion formation following administration of liquid silicone intraperitoneally in rat and rabbit abrasion models.

Perspective

Systemic administration of medicaments requires adequate blood supply to the site of potential adhesion formation in order that sufficient tissue levels of medicament are available to achieve pharmacological effects. Many postsurgical sites become devoid of blood supply during the course of surgery. These ischemic areas, which are likely candidates for adhesion formation, are also not available to systemically administered pharmaceuticals. Accordingly, one of the major challenges to the pharmacotherapy of adhesion prevention is the development of appropriate drug delivery systems.

The multifactorial nature of infertility and pain necessarily limit the utility of trials designed to assess the clinical efficacy of adhesion prevention agents. Accordingly, the clinical problems associated with adhesion formation were not evaluated in any of the aforementioned studies. Studies of "clinical efficacy" have only assessed the presence or absence of adhesions and not the clinical benefits of adhesion prevention per se.

What constitutes sufficient benefit from an adhesion prevention adjuvant or regimen to justify its use in clinical practice? What clinical response to a new device or drug is necessary and sufficient to justify FDA approval for an adhesion prevention indication? The outcome of the adhesion(s) that is responsible for the patient's symptomatology, whether it is prevented from reforming or persists, will determine the clinical benefit or failure. Adhesion formation to the rest of the peritoneum may have no clinical significance and as a result be irrelevant to the patient's well-being. Unfortunately, clinical problems caused by adhesions are multifactorial in nature and consequently necessitate large patient studies to address clinical benefits.

Inhibition of Fibroblast Proliferation and Local Inflammatory Response

Anti-inflammatory drugs were evaluated for their effects on postoperative adhesion formation since they may limit the release of fibrinous exudate in response to inflammation at the surgical site. Two general classes of these drugs were tested: corticosteroids and nonsteroidal anti-inflammatory drugs. The results of corticosteroid use in experimental models of intraperitoneal adhesion formation generally have not been encouraging; furthermore, clinical use of these drugs in a postoperative situation is limited by their other pharmacologic properties, such as immunosuppression and delayed wound healing.

Experimental evaluations of nonsteroidal anti-inflammatory drugs in postoperative adhesion formation shows more promise; however, clinical evaluation of these drugs for this indication is not available.

Corticosteroids

Although Cohen et al. (1983) reported significant reductions in adhesion formation following the use of intraperitoneal solutions containing steroids, others have not observed any reduction of adhesion formation after intraperitoneal administration of glucocorticoids in animal models (Liao, Suehiro, & McNamara, 1973; Gomel, 1978; diZerega & Hodgen, 1980; Tschoepe, Wright, & Gizang, 1980). Sustained release of dexamethasone in the peritoneal cavity by use of biodegradable microparticles (polylactide-glycolide) reduced both the incidence and severity of adhesions in a rat model (Höckel, Ott, Siemann, & Kissell, 1987). Clinical use of glucocorticoids in intraperitoneal surgery also yielded mixed results (Replogle, Johnson, & Gross, 1966; Swolin, 1967, 1975; Grosfield, Berman, Schiller, & Morse, 1973; Horne, Clyman, Debrovner, & Griggs, 1973; Querleu, Vankeerberghen, Deffense, Boutteville, 1989). In some of these studies, the antihistamine promethazine was added to the treatment regimen, thereby obscuring the specific effect of the glucocorticoid.

Why has the use of corticosteroids not proven as beneficial in adhesion prevention as the pharmacological properties of these drugs would suggest? Peritoneal surgery initiates an inflammatory process that may simply overwhelm the therapeutic response to corticosteroids at doses usually studied. When higher doses of corticosteroids are used, their effects on organ systems not involved with adhesion formation per se become a clinical concern. Perhaps development of a glucocorticoid class of compounds with more specific effects on fibrin deposition will be more useful.

Because of the potential for high-dose glucocorticoids to cause immunosuppression and poor wound healing, these agents should be used with caution in surgical patients. Additionally, Magyar, Hayes, Moghissi, and Subramanian (1984) reported that two of their 25 patients undergoing surgical correction of tubal or peritoneal abnormalities expressed short-term suppression of the hypothalamic-pituitary-adrenal axis as demonstrated by failure to achieve a normal rise in serum cortisol despite adequate hypoglycemia upon insulin hypoglycemia testing on postoperative day 6. All patients had received dexamethasone (20 mg) and promethazine (25 mg) preoperatively, intraoperatively, and postoperatively.

Many clinician have considered the use of corticosteroids in patients with ongoing pelvic infection. Kolmorgen and Akkermann (1988) reported 59 patients with acute pelvic inflammatory disease verified by laparoscopy who were treated with two kinds of therapies. Twenty-seven patients were given ampicillin and metronidazol for 10 days, 32 patients were additionally given prednisolone. The results of both groups during hospital treatment and during second-look laparoscopy carried out 2 months later were compared. In the group treated with prednisolone fever was reduced more rapidly and a normalization of erythrocyte sedimentation rate was achieved. However, leukocytosis persisted for a longer time and no difference in tubal patency was found. Of the women treated with prednisolone, 70% did not have any pelvic adhesions compared with 53% of the controls.

Calcium Channel Blockers

The mechanism or mechanisms by which calcium channel blockers act to reduce adhesion formation is a matter of speculation (Steinleitner, Lambert, Montoro, Swanson, & Sueldo, 1988). Calcium channel blockade was shown to reduce ischemic cellular injury in a number of animal models. Release of vasoactive mediators associated with the acute inflammatory response (e.g., histamine and prostaglandin E and F) is reduced by calcium channel blockade, whereas the release of prostacyclin, a potent vasodilator, is stimulated. The effect of pentoxifylline on prevention of adhesion reformation was assessed in a rabbit uterine horn model (Steinleitner, Lambert, Kazensky, Danks, & Roy, 1990). Rabbits received a standardized lesion to the left uterine horn. One week later a laparotomy was performed for evaluation (prescore) and subsequent lysis of adhesions. After closure, the animals were randomized to treatment with vehicle or subcutaneous pentoxifylline, 2.5 mg/kg, administered at 12-hour intervals for six doses. Seven days later, the rabbits were sacrificed and evaluated in a blinded manner to quantify adhesion reformation. The adhesion scores were significantly reduced by pentoxifylline compared to control. These data demonstrate an inhibition of adhesion reformation after lysis of pelvic adhesions with the use of pentoxifylline in rabbits.

Recently, Dunn, Steinleitner, and Lambert (1991) evaluated the combined effects of verapamil and tissue plasminogen activator (tPA) on the prevention of adhesion formation in rabbits when administered intraperitoneally. Verapamil by itself reduced the adhesion score of the saline-treated controls by 57%; tPA alone reduced the score 75%; verapamil together with tPA reduced the score 94%. All eight of the verapamil-tPA treated rabbits had minimal adhesions. The synergistic benefits of these drugs indicate that they prevent adhesion formation by different mechanisms. Approval for clinical use of medicament combinations is confounded by requirements of regulatory agencies to demonstrate respective effects of each medicament and vehicle alone as well as in the preferred formulation. Clinical studies evaluating surgical patients are especially difficult to perform using these criteria.

Nonsteroidal Anti-inflammatory Drugs

Nonsteroidal anti-inflammatory drugs (NSAIDs) are a class of compounds that alter the metabolism of arachidonic acid in a variety of tissues and thereby alter the endogenous balance of the cyclooxygenase, lipoxygenase, and epoxygenase enzyme systems and formation of their end products. Arachidonic acid metabolites are produced by the polymorphonuclear leukocytes (PMNs) and macrophages present at the site of inflammation or may result from platelet aggregation and thereby mediate inflammatory events. Labeled arachidonic acid metabolized by peritoneal exudate cells (PEC; see Chapter 6) form metabolites by the lipoxygenase and cyclooxygenase pathways including prostaglandins, thromboxane, and hydroxyeicosatetraenoic acid (HETE) (Shimanuki, Nakamura, & diZerega, 1986). An increase in 15-HETE and di-HETE and a decrease in 5-HETE formation beginning 24 hours after surgical injury was observed in rabbits. In addition, there was an increase in thromboxane B_2 and prostaglandin E_2 (PGE_2) throughout the study interval (2 to 10 days postoperatively). These arachidonic acid metabolites mediate some aspects of the postsurgical inflammatory response. PGs are involved in events that occur during the generation of inflammation including leukocyte infiltration, edema formation, and endothelial cell procoagulant activities (Randall, Eakins, & Higgs, 1980). Golan et al. (1990; 1991) found that addition of prostaglandins $F_{2\alpha}$ and E_2 into the peritoneal cavity of rats enhanced the formation of adhesions to the injury site. NSAIDs inhibit the formation of arachidonic acid metabolites through suppression of cyclooxygenase and lipoxygenase pathways and thus lead to a reduction in inflammation mediated by these metabolites (Vane, 1971; Flower, Gryglewski, Herbaczynska-Cedro, & Vane, 1972).

NSAIDs in Reduction of Adhesion Formation

NSAIDs were shown to reduce formation of peritoneal adhesions in a variety of animal models (Table 10.4). However, not all studies dem-

TABLE 10.4. Summary of representative experimental studies of nonsteroidal anti-inflammatory drugs (NSAIDs) on postoperative adhesion formation.

Experimental model	NSAID (dose)	Treatment regimen	Results[a]	Study reference
Rabbit ileum trauma	Piroxicam (PIR) (10 mg/kg/day IM)	2 h or immediately presurgery and daily postop for 7 days	PIR > Control	Malvendez (1987)
Rat uterine horn reanastomosis	Ibuprofen (IBU) (12.5 mg/kg IP)	30 min presurgery and q8h postop for 2 days	IBU = Control IBU < Dexamethasone	Luciano (1983)
Rabbit uterine horn reanastomosis	Ibuprofen (IBU) (7 mg/kg IV)	30 min presurgery and q8h postop for 2 days	IBU > Control IBU = Dexamethasone	Siegler (1980)
Rabbit uterine horn reanastomosis	Ibuprofen (IBU) (75 mg IV) Flurbiprofen (FLUR) (12.5 mg IV)	Immediately presurgery and q6h postop for 2 days	IBU > Control FLUR > Control	Jarrett & Dawood (1986)
Rabbit uterine horn trauma	Ibuprofen (IBU) (10 mg/kg IM)	30 min presurgery and q8h postop for 4 days	IBU > Control	Bateman et al. (1982)
Rabbit uterine adhesiolysis	Ibuprofen (IBU) (12.5 mg/kg IM)	15 min presurgery and q12h postop for 3 days	IBU = Control	Holtz (1982)
Guinea pig uterine horn reanastomosis	Ibuprofen (IBU) (12.5 mg/kg IM) Indomethacin (INDO) (1 mg/kg IM)	30 min presurgery and q8h postop for 3 days	IBU > Control INDO > Control	DeLeon (1984)
Rabbit cecum trauma	Oxyphenbutazone (OXY; 10 mg/kg)[b]	Six days[b]	OXY > Control	Kapur et al. (1972)

[a]Results of statistical analysis of treated versus control groups.
[b]Unspecified route of administration and dosing frequency.

onstrated adhesion reduction with NSAID (Holtz, 1982). Most studies were conducted using systemic administration of these agents. Oxyphenbutazone, administered perioperatively in rats and monkeys, reduced postoperative adhesion formation (Kapur, Talwar, & Gulati, 1969; Kapur, Gulati, & Talwar, 1972; Larsson, Svanberg, & Swolin, 1977). Siegler, Kontopoulos, and Wang (1980) and Bateman, Nunley, and Kitchen (1982) observed a marked reduction in adhesions formation following systemic administration of 7 and 10 mg/kg of ibuprofen, respectively, during the perioperative interval. Nishimura, Shimanuki, and diZerega (1984a) found that administration of two doses of ibuprofen after the completion of surgery did not affect adhesion formation. However, a significant reduction in adhesion formation was noted after five doses (including preoperative dosing) of ibuprofen (70 mg/kg) when administered systemically (Nishimura, Nakamura, & diZerega, 1983b, 1984b). Further studies were conducted with NSAIDs administered intraperitoneally in an attempt to reduce adhesion formation. However, not all studies demonstrated adhesion reduction with NSAIDs (Holtz, 1982). Intraperitoneal administration of ibuprofen through a miniosmotic pump, in hydron polymer or in a liposome carrier, reduced adhesion formation following abrasion of the parietal peritoneum and serosal surface of the colon (Shimanuki, Nishimura, & diZerega, 1985; Rodgers, Bracken, Richer, Girgis, & diZerega, 1990a). Tolmetin, another NSAID, reduced adhesion formation after low concentrations of tolmetin, administered in miniosmotic pumps, were utilized in the surgical model described above (Rodgers, Girgis, Johns, & diZerega, 1990b). Tolmetin, in a series of micellar (5% Tween 80) and vesicle (multilaminar liposomes) preparations, significantly reduced adhesion formation in a variety of animal models (Rodgers et al., 1990a, 1990b). Tolmetin reduced adhesion formation in animals models when placed in a high molecular weight carrier, which may act as a viscoelastic barrier in conjunction with the pharmacological effects of tolmetin (Rodgers, 1990). These data suggest that inhibitors of arachidonic acid metabolism, such as ibuprofen and tolmetin, effectively reduce postoperative adhesion formation. The question remains as to clinical efficacy, which may be dependent upon identification of an appropriate delivery vehicle.

NSAID Mechanisms of Action

There are several possible mechanisms by which NSAIDs reduce adhesion formation following peritoneal surgery. First, adhesion formation may be reduced through diminished PG synthesis, which would subsequently reduce inflammatory events mediated by PGs (Randall et al., 1980). A decrease in leukocyte infiltration and coagulation (which follows platelet aggregation) may decrease the formation of matrix (see Chapter 5) necessary for fibroblast organization. Although PGs are cytostatic agents (Plescia, Smith & Greenwich, 1975), and hence a reduction in PG synthesis may increase fibroblast proliferation; without a fibrin-supporting matrix to allow fibroblast organization, no adhesion formation would occur. Alternatively, macrophages secrete plasminogen activator (PA) (Unkeless, Gordon, & Reich, 1974; Chapman, Vavrin, & Hibbs, 1982; Orita, Gale, Campeau, Nakamura, & diZerega, 1986), which activates the fibrinolytic enzyme, plasmin. Tolmetin-enhanced secretion of PA by postsurgical macrophages would lyse clots and reduce the formation of fibrinous bands that would support fibroblast organization.

A decrease in PA synthesis coincides with the initiation of inflammation-induced differentiation of macrophages (Bonney & Davies, 1984). Many macrophage functions that are modulated during inflammation are suppressed in resident macrophages by PG (Bonney & Davies, 1984). Therefore, a decrease in PG synthesis through chemical intervention could allow a more rapid differentiation of resident and infiltrating leukocytes in response to inflammatory signals such as complement and bacterial endotoxin following surgery. If stimulation of differentiation by NSAIDs occurred, any potential infection present would be cleared more rapidly and would therefore be less stimulatory to leukocytes.

Macrophages and PMNs are centrally involved in the initial clearance of bacteria and damaged tissue. Macrophages and PMNs increase capacities including phagocytosis (Ratzan, Musher, Keusch, & Weinstein, 1972), superoxide anion (O_2^-) release (Johnston, Godzik, & Cohn, 1978), and tumoricidal/microbiocidal (Hibbs, Chapman, & Weinberg, 1978) activity following inflammatory and other stimuli, which, in turn, allows for the rapid clearance of infectious agents. Since many of these functions that are enhanced during inflammation may be regulated by PGs, administration of an NSAID, which inhibits PG synthesis (Taylor & Salata, 1976), may modulate these enhanced leukocytic cell functions.

Modulation of Macrophage Function by Tolmetin

After rat surgery, administration of tolmetin significantly elevates O_2^- release at postoperative days 3 and 5, phagocytic capability at days 7 and 14, and tumoricidal activity at day 3 (Figure 10.13). Differential staining and microscopic analysis revealed increases in PMN numbers with tolmetin doses of 3 and 10 mg (Rodgers, Ellefson, Girgis, Scott, & diZerega, 1988). PGs modulate PMN chemotaxis during inflammation. PG synthesis and release initially decrease during inflammation followed by a concomitant increase in neutral protease secretion by macrophages (Unkeless et al., 1974; Humes et al., 1980). These findings suggest that PG synthesis by macrophages is necessary to maintain the resident differentiative state of the macrophage. As a result, inhibition of PG synthesis by NSAIDs may provide the necessary signal(s) to initiate macrophage (and perhaps PMN) differentiation.

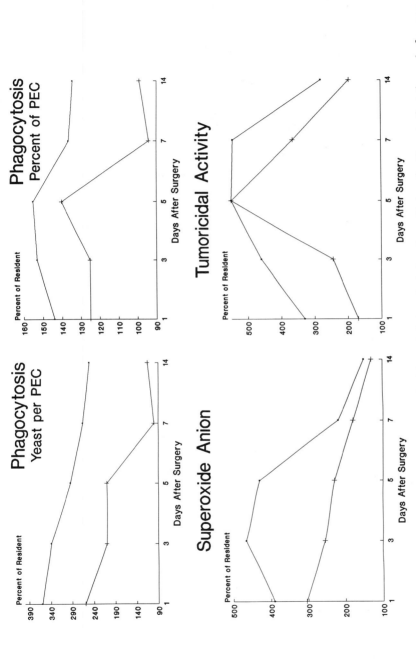

FIGURE 10.13. The effect of peritoneal trauma with (■) and without (+) the administration of tolmetin (3 mg/rat) at the end of surgery on peritoneal exudative cell (PEC) function. The functions that were examined include phagocytosis, respiratory burst, and tumoricidal activities, which are important in the clearance of bacteria. These data are presented as the percentage of resident peritoneal cell function. As can be seen, all parameters examined were increased at early postoperative time points and further elevated by the acute administration of tolmetin (Rodgers et al., 1988).

Following surgery, there is an increase in the functional activity of PEC (peritoneal exudative cells, see Chapter 6; Rodgers et al., 1988). The enhanced phagocytic capability of peritoneal leukocytes allows for a more rapid removal of damaged tissue. By postsurgical day 7, the activities of the PEC from control animals return to resident cell levels. Administration of tolmetin lengthens the time after surgery during which peritoneal leukocyte functions are elevated (Rodgers et al., 1988). Microscopic examination of PEC indicates that the influx of macrophages into the peritoneum after surgery is delayed by tolmetin administration. In control and treated animals, the infiltration of macrophages into the peritoneum corresponds to the time point at which the early elevations in peritoneal leukocyte phagocytic and respiratory burst activities begin to return to control levels (Rodgers et al., 1988). PMN activity alone may be responsible for the increase in peritoneal cell functions, and/or indirect PMN interaction with macrophages is necessary for these elevated functions.

Protease Activity

NSAIDs may reduce adhesion formation through increasing the expression of fibrinolytic activity either through modulation of protease and protease inhibitor secretion or reduction of protease inhibitor activity in wound fluid (Rodgers, 1990; Rodgers, Ellefson, Girgis, & diZerega, 1992). Following peritoneal surgery, the level of neutral proteases secreted by peritoneal macrophages increases (see Chapter 8). Exposure of postsurgical rabbit macrophages to tolmetin in vitro suppresses collagenase and elevates elastase activities at early time points after surgery (Table 10.5).

TABLE 10.5. Modulation of protease activity in macrophage conditioned media by tolmetin.

Hours after Surgery	Collagenase	Elastase	PAI
0	71 ± 6*	272 ± 4[+]	45 ± 4*
6	49 ± 9*	129 ± 1[+]	83 ± 2*
12	50 ± 10*	113 ± 4	65 ± 3*
24	68 ± 4*	95 ± 6	78 ± 3*
48	60 ± 12*	101 ± 4	81 ± 2*
72	74 ± 21	99 ± 7	98 ± 10
96	141 ± 17[+]	94 ± 1	106 ± 4

Macrophages were harvested from rabbits at various times after surgery, placed in culture for 4 days with 2 mg/ml tolmetin, and the protease or protease inhibitor activity in the supernatant measured. Data are presented as percent of surgical control (Rodgers, 1990).
*Significantly ($p \leq .05$) suppressed compared to control.
[+]Significantly ($p \leq .05$) elevated compared to control.

In contrast, the level of PA inhibitory (PAI) activity in cultures of postsurgical macrophages harvested within 48 hours after surgery is reduced by in vitro exposure of postsurgical macrophages to tolmetin. These data suggest that NSAIDs modify the ability of postsurgical macrophages to remodel and clear debris from the site of trauma.

Collagenase activity is reduced in macrophage-conditioned media up to 48 hours after surgery after exposure to tolmetin (Table 10.5). Wahl and Lampel (1987) found that indomethacin (a PG synthesis inhibitor) decreased the level of collagenase secreted by human monocytes. They proposed that collagenase secretion contains a PG-dependent step (Wahl & Winter, 1984). Up to 48 hours after surgery peritoneal macrophages appear to be susceptible to modulation by tolmetin (Rodgers, 1990; Rodgers et al., 1992).

Elastase secretion by postsurgical macrophages is also elevated by in vitro exposure to tolmetin (Table 10.5). Previous studies by Werb, Banda, and Jones (1980) showed that purified macrophage elastase could cleave elastin as well as fibronectin, laminin, fibrinogen, proteoglycan, and matrix secreted by rat smooth muscles. In the peritoneal cavity, elastase may be important for the clearance of fibrin clots and tissue debris after surgery. The increase in elastase secretion observed after in vitro exposure to tolmetin suggests an additional mechanism by which tolmetin reduces adhesion formation.

A decrease in the level of plasminogen activator inhibitor (PAI) activity found in postsurgical macrophage-conditioned media may increase fibrinolytic activity in the peritoneal cavity after surgery. In vitro exposure of peritoneal macrophages to tolmetin for up to 48 hours after surgery reduces the amount of PAI activity in macrophage-conditioned media (Rodgers et al., 1990b, 1992). Since adhesion formation may be dependent upon fibrin deposition to support fibroblast organization, an increase in fibrinolysis would decrease adhesion formation.

Conclusion

NSAIDs may act to reduce adhesions after abdominal surgery through a reduction in PG synthesis, which in turn reduces inflammation and stimulates macrophage functions. In vivo or in vitro exposure to tolmetin modulates the secretion of neutral proteases and PAI activity. These changes increase the fibrinolytic potential of the peritoneal cavity, thereby reducing the amount of fibrin available to support the ingrowth of fibroblast and subsequent adhesion formation.

Progesterone

Some clinicians find that adhesion formation may be less when patients undergo pelvic surgery in the luteal phase of the menstrual cycle. In addition, adhesion formation after Cesarean section even when complicated by endometritis may appear to be less than after other uterine surgery (myomectomy or metroplasty) performed in the nongravid state. Initial studies with progesterone suggested that it might reduce intraperitoneal adhesion formation (Eddy et al., 1980; Maurer & Bonaventura, 1983). Later studies, however, demonstrated an increase in postoperative adhesion formation after intraperitoneal administration of progesterone in either an aqueous or oil suspension (Beauchamp, Quigley, & Held, 1984; Blauer & Collins, 1988).

Removal of Fibrin Deposits

Since fibrin deposition begins during surgery and continues through the immediate postoperative interval, adhesion prevention strategies based on removal of fibrin must begin soon after peritoneal injury and continue during the period of fibrin deposition. These requirements limit the types of medicaments that may be efficacious and underscore the importance of delivery systems for adhesion prevention. Proteolytic enzymes such as pepsin, trypsin, and papain augment the local fibrinolytic system and theoretically should limit postoperative adhesion formation. Unfortunately these enzymes are rapidly neutralized by peritoneal exudates rendering them virtually useless for adhesion prophylaxis. Fibrinolytics, such as fibrinolysin, streptokinase, and urokinase, were also advocated for adhesion prophylaxis (Bryant, 1963; Ellis, 1971; Gervin, Puckett, & Silver, 1973). One potential complication to the clinical use of these enzymes in postoperative adhesion prevention is excessive bleeding resulting from their administration.

Tissue Plasminogen Activator

The recent development of recombinant technology allows for the large scale production of highly purified proteins for clinical use. Tissue plasminogen activator (tPA), the enzyme that converts plasminogen into plasmin, is now in use as a drug to treat cardiovascular disease. The first study to demonstrate the benefit of tPA in preventing postsurgical adhesion formation utilized a miniosmotic pump to deliver tPA to the specific site of surgical injury (Orita, Fukasawa, Girgis, & diZerega, 1991). To determine the time period in which locally delivered tPA must be given to prevent adhesions, the pumps were disconnected from the catheters at various days after surgery. It was found that effective adhesion prevention occurred with only 2 days of treatment, beginning the day of surgery. Menzies and Ellis (1989) also evaluated the effect of tPA on adhesion reformation in rabbits. Adhesions were produced by stripping peritoneum from corresponding parietal and visceral areas. One week later the adhesions were divided. Either tPA or placebo was applied to the divided adhesion. After a further week the adhesions were assessed. Sixty strips were performed; 55 adhesions were produced (92%). Placebo gel was applied to 28 sides and tPA applied to 27. Adhesions recurred in 22 of the placebo group (79%); two of the recombinant tissue plasminogen activator (rtPA) group reformed (7%). To further define the benefit of tPA as an agent for reducing postoperative adhesions, a rabbit uterine horn model was studied. Fifty-five rabbits underwent laparotomy, at which time the uterus was abraded with a scalpel and a thermal injury was induced with electrocautery (Doody, Dunn, & Buttram, 1989). Before abdominal closure, tPA was applied topically in various dosages. Adhesions were evaluated at a second laparotomy performed 2 weeks later. Treatment significantly reduced both adhesion quantity and adhesion density (Figure 10.14). No wound healing or bleeding complications were seen.

The dose-response relationships observed in these studies demonstrate that tPA in pharmacologic amounts may supplement the depressed endogenous fibrinolytic system and significantly decrease adhesion formation after laparotomy. Accordingly, tPA may prove a valuable adjuvant to surgical therapy in the prevention of adhesions once an appropriate intraperitoneal delivery system is available. Importantly, no complications of tPA therapy such as systemic fibrinolysis, fibrinogen consumption, or abnormal wound healing were encountered. These studies both underscore the importance of fibrin deposition in adhesion formation as well as identify the postoperative time when adhesion pre-

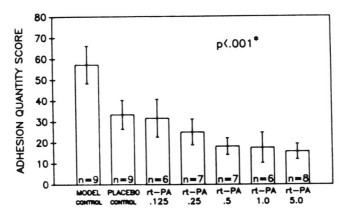

FIGURE 10.14. Effect of recombinant tPA (rt-PA) on postoperative adhesion prevention. Dosage shown is concentration in mg/g of vehicle. The bars represent the mean ± SEM quantitative adhesion score. *Significant treatment effect determined by ANOVA. (From Doody et al., 1989. Reproduced by permission of Americal Fertility Society.)

vention by these medicaments is feasible. Ongoing efforts are focused on the development of delivery systems designed to provide drug to the surgical site.

Adhesion Lysis

In addition to removing fibrin deposition by augmenting or stimulating the endogenous fibrinolytic system, adhesions can also be surgically removed. Adhesiolysis or resection often reduces complications (i.e., infertility) from adhesion formation. Where the existence of adhesions is thought to play a role in infertility, adhesiolysis has been used to restore fertility (Table 10.6). Gomel (1983) and Bronson and Wallach (1977) reported an overall pregnancy rate of approximately 60% following adhesiolysis by laparoscopy and laparotomy, respectively. Tulandi, Falcone, and Kafka (1989) found that the pregnancy rate was significantly higher among infertile patients who underwent salpingo-ovariolysis for periadnexal adhesions (45% at 24 months) than among those who received no treatment for their adhesions (15% at 24 months) (Figure 10.15).

Second-Look Laparoscopy

Although the effect on pregnancy rates of "second-look" laparoscopy to lyse adhesions that form after reproductive surgery was examined, generalized use of second-look laparoscopy remains controversial. Tables 10.7 and 10.8 summarize the overall pregnancy rates and rates of ectopic pregnancy in five studies employing second-look laparoscopy during which adhesions were separated and/or lysed. Daniell, Pittaway, and

TABLE 10.6. Results of adhesiolysis: representative literature reports.

	No. of patients	% Live births	% Ectopic pregnancies	ESLL
Conventional technique				
Wallach et al. (1983)	94	45.7	2.1	No
Young et al. (1970)	47	32.0	4.0	No
Trimbos-Kemper et al. (1985)	N/A	48.0	N/A	Yes
Microsurgical technique				
Frantzen Schlösser (1982)	49	38.8	4.1	No
Diamond (1979)	140	57.1	0.7	No
Luber et al. (1986)	13	62.0	7.7	Yes
Hulka (1982)	47	25.5	2.1	No
Laparoscopic lysis only				
Gomel (1983)	92	58.7	5.4	—

ESLL, early second-look laparoscopy; N/A = not available.
From Luber et al., 1986.

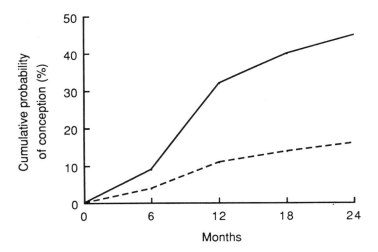

FIGURE 10.15. Cumulative probability of conception among women with periadnexal adhesions who were treated by salpingo-ovariolysis (solid line) and women who were not treated (broken line). (From Tulandi et al., 1990b. Reproduced by permission of C. V. Mosby.)

Maxson (1983) described intrauterine pregnancy in 9 of 25 infertility patients within 6 months after adhesiolysis performed at second look laparoscopy 4 to 6 weeks after the initial laparotomy. Trimbos-Kemper, Trimbos, and van Hall (1985) and Jansen (1988a) reported success with second-look laparoscopy as early as 8 days after surgery. After second-look laparoscopy, intrauterine pregnancy rates (40%) were the same in both groups although a decrease in ectopic pregnancies was noted (Figure 10.16; Trimbos-Kemper et al., 1985).

Many studies directly evaluated the rate of adhesion reformation after adhesiolysis. Adhesiolysis by second-look laparoscopy was effective in preventing adhesion reformation in 52% of 64 patients who underwent a second follow-up laparoscopy (e.g., third-look procedure; Trimbos-Kemper et al., 1985). Furthermore, in this study, significantly more of the adnexa evaluated at the time of the third-look laparoscopy had no adhesions present when adhesiolysis was performed at the second-look procedure (63%) than when no adhesiolysis via second-look laparoscopy was performed (39%). Similar findings using third-look laparoscopy were reported by Jansen (1988a) (Figure 10.2) and Osada (personal communication). Diamond et al. (1984) reported significant reductions in the incidence of adhesions involving the ovaries, fimbria, cul-de-sac, colon, and pelvic sidewall at the time of second-look laparoscopy following reproductive surgery. The overall reduction in adhesions involving these tissues at the time of the second-look procedure ranged from 30% to 50%

TABLE 10.7. Postoperative pregnancy rates, by procedure.[a]

Procedure	No. of patients	Outcome of first pregnancy				Eventual outcome	
		% IUP	% SAB	% Term	% Ectopic pregnancies	% EIUP	% E Term
Adhesiolysis[*]	13	62 (8)	8 (1)	54 (7)	8 (1)	69 (9)	62 (8)
Fimbrioplasty[*]	20	30 (6)	15 (3)	15 (3)	10 (2)	35 (7)	25 (5)
Salpingostomy[†]	17	12 (2)	0	12 (2)	12 (2)	18 (3)	18 (3)
Cornual resection[†]	10	30 (3)	0	30 (3)	20 (2)	50 (5)	40 (4)
Total	60	32 (19)	7 (4)	25 (15)	12 (7)	40 (24)	33 (20)

IUP, Intrauterine pregnancy; SAB, spontaneous abortion; EIUP, eventual intrauterine pregnancy; E term, eventual term pregnancy.
[a]Numerals in parentheses represent number of patients.
[*]Adhesiolysis versus fimbrioplasty significant at 0.05; adhesiolysis versus salpingostomy significant at 0.01.
[†]Cornual resection versus salpingostomy significant at 0.05. Other pairings do not achieve statistical significance.
From Luber et al., 1985.

TABLE 10.8. Summary of pregnancy rates following second-look laparoscopy (SLL).

Reference	Interval between original surgery and SLL	No. of patients	Percent of patients	
			Pregnant	Ectopic Pregnancy
Raj & Hulka (1982)[a]	4–8 weeks	51	20%	14%
Surrey & Friedman (1982)	6–8 weeks	31	52%	0%
	≥6 months	6	17%	17%
Trimbos-Kemper et al. (1985)	8 days	188	30%	10%
Tulandi et al. (1989)[b]	12 months	19	67%[b]	47%[b]

[a]Originally 60 patients were evaluated, 9 of whom had no postoperative adhesions and were excluded. Majority of the 60 patients (83%) had SLL after 4 to 8 weeks; three patients had SLL ≤2 weeks and seven patients had SLL > 12 weeks postoperatively.
[b]Cumulative probability at 36 months using life-table analysis.

(see Table 10.1). Swolin (1967), Osada (personal communication), Trimbos-Kemper et al. (1985), Jansen (1988a), and Serour, Badraoui, El-Agizi, Hamed, and Abdel-Aziz (1989) all reported success with early second-look laparoscopy. Not all reports are as favorable. Mecke, Semm, Freys, Argiriou, and Gent (1989) found that 50% of the ipsilateral adnexa still contained adhesions at third-look after their resection following laparoscopic removal of an ectopic pregnancy (Table 10.9).

Table 10.10 summarizes studies employing second-look laparoscopy during which adhesions were separated and/or lysed (Tulandi, 1991). Serour et al. (1989) demonstrated that second-look laparoscopy performed 9 to 12 months after the initial procedure in infertility cases eliminated adhesion reformation in 10 of 22 cases. Thirty patients with secondary infertility underwent laparoscopic adhesiolysis; 45% showed no recurrence of adhesions at second-look laparoscopy performed 9 to 12 months later. This study suggests that laparoscopy has a role in adhesiolysis of mild and moderate adhesions and second-look laparoscopy provides further opportunity to relyse reformed adhesions.

The interval between the initial surgery and the second-look laparoscopy varied in these studies. In those studies where either a control group that did not receive second-look laparoscopy was included (Tulandi et al., 1989) or where the interval between the initial surgery and second-look laparoscopy varied among patients (Raj & Hulka, 1982; Surrey & Friedman, 1982), the benefits of second-look laparoscopy appear to be greater the shorter the postoperative interval prior to the procedure. This clinical impression is not clearly supported by studies. Many clinicians believe that adhesion density and organization increase as the duration of the postoperative interval increases (DeCherney & Mezer, 1984; Raj & Hulka, 1982; Surrey & Friedman, 1982). DeCherney and Mezer (1984)

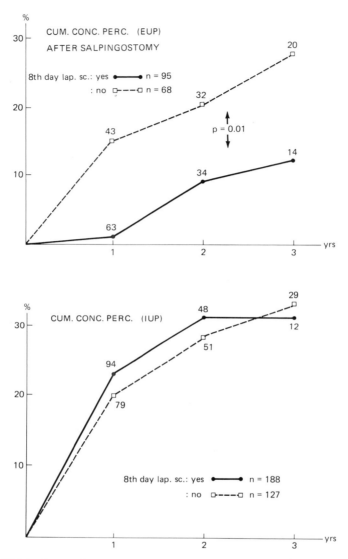

FIGURE 10.16. Above: Cumulative conception percentages of ectopic pregnancies in patients with and without second-look laparoscopy on the 8th day after salpingostomy. Below: Cumulative conception percentage of intrauterine pregnancies in patients with and without second-look laparoscopy on the 8th day after salpingostomy, fimbrioplasty, or adhesiolysis. (From Trimbos-Kemper et al., 1985. Reproduced by permission of American Fertility Society.)

TABLE 10.9. Degree of pelvic adhesions postpelviscopic organ-preserving therapy of tubal pregnancy and adhesiolysis, dependent upon the presence of previously existing adhesions ($n = 33$).

	Adhesions diagnosed at the initial treatment of the tubal pregnancy			Adhesions diagnosed at the follow-up of the intra-abdominal site		
	Ipsilateral	Contralateral	Adhesion-free	Ipsilateral	Contalateral	Adhesion-free
n	11	10	18 (55%)	15	6	16 (48%)
Grade I	5	3		11	3	
Grade II	6	5		3	2	
Grade III	0	2		1	1	

From Mecke et al., 1989.

found a 75% incidence of adhesion formation at the time of second-look laparoscopy at both 4 to 16 weeks and 16 to 19 months after laparotomy in infertility patients (Figure 10.17). There was, however, a relative enhancement in the adhesion grades that were present between the two groups.

Laser Surgery

The laser is used via laparoscopy in an attempt to reduce adhesion formation. The first multicenter study of laser laparoscopy and adhesion formation confirmed by early second-look laparoscopy (<12 weeks postoperative) studied 106 women (Diamond et al., 1984). The CO_2 laser was used to vaporize adhesions and endometriosis, resect ovarian tissue, or perform neosalpingostomies. No difference in adhesion formation between laser and nonlaser was found with respect to postoperative adhesion formation using historical controls. Daniell, Miller, and Tosh (1986) reported a tubal patency rate of 92% and a postoperative pregnancy rate of 21% following the use of the CO_2 laser for neosalpingostomy. Using historic controls, they concluded that the postoperative pregnancy rates were similar between laser and nonlaser techniques. In a study by Donnez (1987) of 124 patients, laser was used to vaporize endometriotic implants or adnexal adhesions. Half of the patients became pregnant. Donnez indicated that postoperative adhesion formation was minimal. Because of the absence of a control group, these reports cannot effectively compare the use of laser to that of scissors or microelectrocautery (Keye, 1991).

Controlled Human Studies

Tulandi (1986) randomized 63 infertile women with adnexal adhesions into either a CO_2 laser-treated group ($n = 30$) or an electrocautery-treated

TABLE 10.10. Results of early and late second-look laparoscopy (SLL) following reproductive surgery.

Authors	SLL (No. of patients)		Study design	Results
	Early	Late		
Swolin (1967)	—		Cohort	Introduction to the use of SLL.
Raj and Hulka (1982)	1–8 weeks (53)	1 year (7)	Cohort	Optimal time of SLL appears to be 4 to 8 weeks after a reproductive surgery.
Surrey & Friedman (1982)	6 weeks (31)	6 mos (6)	Cohort	Pregnancy rate after early SLL (52%) was higher than after late SLL (16.67%).
Daniell & Pittaway (1983)	4–6 weeks (25)	—	Cohort	Early SLL may improve pregnancy rates.
DeCherney & Mezer (1984)	4–6 weeks (20)	16–19 mos (41)	Cohort	60% of early SLL patients had filmy adhesions; 63% of the late SLL patients had thicker adhesions.
Trimbos-Kemper et al. (1985)	8 days (188)	—	Historical control	SLL reduces the occurrence of ectopic pregnancy.
Diamond et al. (1987a)	1–12 weeks (161)	—	Cohort	Reproductive surgery by laparotomy is frequently complicated by de novo adhesions formation.
Jansen (1988a)	8–21 days (256)	—	Cohort	Early SLL is safe and effective in reducing adhesions formation.
Tulandi et al. (1989)	—	1 year (74)	Randomized control	Late SLL does not increase the pregnancy rate or decrease the incidence of ectopic pregnancy.

From Tulandi, 1991.

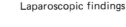

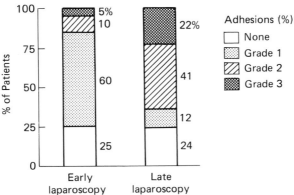

FIGURE 10.17. Type of adhesion at post–tubal-surgery laparoscopy. A relative enhancement in the grade of adhesions was noted between early (4 to 16 weeks) and late (16 to 19 months after surgery) laparoscopy (DeCherney & Mezer, 1984).

group ($n = 33$). All procedures were performed at laparotomy. The laser was used at power densities of 2,000 to 10,000 W/cm². Pregnancy rates were the same. Since second-look laparoscopies were not performed, no conclusions could be drawn regarding postoperative adhesion formation (Keye, 1991).

Tulandi (1987) also compared postoperative adhesion formation and tubal patency following neosalpingostomy using the CO_2 laser or microelectrocautery. Thirty-nine women with hydrosalpinx were treated at laparotomy and a relatively late second-look laparoscopy was performed (11 and 9 months, respectively). No differences were found in postoperative adhesions, in the rate of reocclusion of the hydrosalpinx, or in the rate of fimbrial phimosis (Keye, 1991).

Barbot, Parent, Pibursson, and Aubiot (1987) compared adhesiolysis with the CO_2 laser ($n = 158$) with microelectrocautery ($n = 136$) at laparotomy. At second-look laparoscopy performed 8 days postoperatively, no significant difference in postoperative adhesion formation was found between the two groups. Unfortunately, the patients were not randomized into two groups, thus limiting the strength of the conclusions drawn by the authors (Keye, 1991).

Although application of laser technology may facilitate the performance of surgery in some cases, adhesion formation remains a clinically significant problem. Filmar, Jetha, McComb, and Gomel (1989a) found that cutting with a carbon dioxide laser in animal models may produce less carbon deposits and less foreign body reaction than electromicrosurgery. However, in the same study the carbon dioxide laser was reported to produce more necrosis and more extensive foreign body reaction than cutting with microscissors (Filmar, Jetha, McComb, & Gomel, 1989b).

Surgical Treatment of Ectopic Pregnancy and Adhesion Formation

Lundorff, Thorburn, and Lindblom (1990) reported that 48% and 68% of 102 patients formed adhesions to the site of ectopic pregnancy removed via laparoscopy by salpingostomy or to the contralateral side, respectively (Table 10.11). During the 4-year period of 1984 to 1987, 102 women with ectopic pregnancy underwent second-look laparoscopy 6 to 10 weeks after surgery. Almost 40% of the patients presented with adhesions on the affected side compared with the status at the time of ectopic pregnancy surgery (Figure 10.18). Lysis of adhesions was performed during the second-look laparoscopy in 42 patients (41%). Bruhat, Manhes, Mage, and Povly (1980), Mecke et al. (1989), and Lundorff, Hahlin, Kallfelt, Thorburn, and Lindblom (1991) found reduced adhesion formation when patients with ectopic gestations were treated by laparoscopic surgery. Of their patients with tubal pregnancy, 44% were found to have adhesions on the ipsilateral tube on follow-up examination after laparoscopic resection. Thus, adhesion formation to the ipsilateral tube commonly occurs after removal of an ectopic pregnancy by both laparotomy and laparoscopic techniques. Accordingly, second-look laparoscopy may be useful after surgical treatment of ectopic pregnancy in patients desirous of subsequent pregnancy.

Adhesion Classification

Although numerous schemes for classifying adhesions are used, no single classification scheme is universally adopted. The need for a consensus among researchers with respect to adopting a classification scheme is important if comparisons of treatment regimens for adhesions are to have widespread utility.

The most frequently used systems for classifying adhesions are those developed by the American Fertility Society (1988) (Figure 10.19) and Hulka (1990) (Table 10.12). These classification systems were developed for adnexal adhesions. The classification system for adnexal adhesions proposed by the American Fertility Society (AFS) is a modification of the system developed by the AFS Endometriosis Committee. The AFS system for adnexal adhesions records the extent of ovarian and tubal involvement with adhesions, the nature of the adhesions, and the prognostic classification for adnexal adhesions; the left and right adnexa are described separately. In addition the surgeon records the prognosis es-

TABLE 10.11. Adhesion and tubal scores in 31 patients operated on by laparoscopy and in 42 patients operated on by laparotomy at time for ectopic pregnancy (EP) surgery and second-look laparoscopy.

	EP Surgery								Second-look laparoscopy							
	Ipsilateral side				Contralateral side				Ipsilateral side				Contralateral side			
	1[a]	2	3	4	1	2	3	4	1	2	3	4	1	2	3	4
Laparoscopy (n = 31) Adhesions score	21	6	4	0	20	7	0	4	18	8	4	1	16	8	5	2
Laparotomy (n = 42) Adhesions score	26	11	4	1	32	7	3	0	10	19	11	2	21	14	5	2

[a]Grade 1, no adhesions; grade 4, most severe adhesions.
From Lundorff et al., 1991.

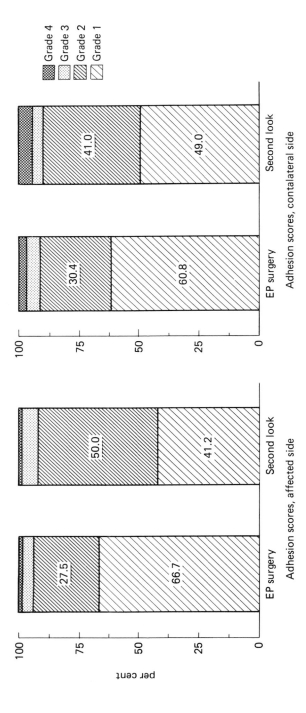

FIGURE 10.18. Adhesion score change on the affected side and the contralateral side in 102 patients between ectopic pregnancy (EP) surgery and second-look laparoscopy. (From Lundorff et al., 1990. Reproduced by permission of American Fertility Society.)

TABLE 1
THE AMERICAN FERTILITY SOCIETY CLASSIFICATION OF ADNEXAL ADHESIONS

Patient's Name ______________________ Date ________ Chart # ________

Age ____ G ____ P ____ Sp Ab ____ VTP ____ Ectopic ____ Infertile Yes ____ No ____

Other Significant History (i.e. surgery, infection, etc.) ______________________

____

HSG ______ Sonography ______ Photography ______ Laparoscopy ______ Laparotomy ______

	ADHESIONS	<1/3 Enclosure	1/3 - 2/3 Enclosure	>2/3 Enclosure
OVARY	R Filmy	1	2	4
	Dense	4	8	16
	L Filmy	1	2	4
	Dense	4	8	16
TUBE	R Filmy	1	2	4
	Dense	4*	8*	16
	L Filmy	1	2	4
	Dense	4*	8*	16

* If the fimbriated end of the fallopian tube is completely enclosed, change the point assignment to 16.

Prognostic Classification for Adnexal Adhesions

	LEFT		RIGHT
A. Minimal	______	0-5	______
B. Mild	______	6-10	______
C. Moderate	______	11-20	______
D. Severe	______	21-32	______

Treatment (Surgical Procedures): ______________________

____

____

____

____

Prognosis for Conception & Subsequent Viable Infant**

______ Excellent (> 75%)

______ Good (50-75%)

______ Fair (25%-50%)

______ Poor (< 25%)

**Physician's judgment based upon adnexa with least amount of pathology.

Recommended Followup Treatment: ______________________

____

____

Additional Findings: ______________________

____

____

____

____

____

DRAWING

L R

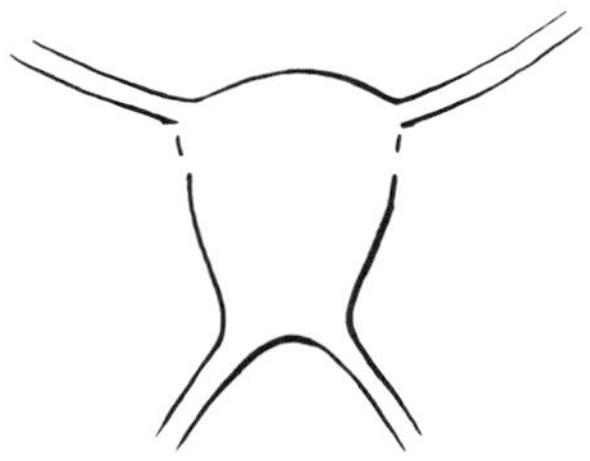

Property of
The American Fertility Society

For additional supply write to:
The American Fertility Society
2140 11th Avenue, South
Suite 200
Birmingham, Alabama 35205

FIGURE 10.19. American Fertility Society classification system for adnexal adhesions. (From American Fertility Society, 1988. Reproduced by permission of American Fertility Society.)

TABLE 10.12. Simplified classification scheme for
adnexal adhesions.[a]

| | Nature of adhesion | |
Extent of ovarian involvement	Filmy	Dense
<50% enclosed	I[b]	II
>50% enclosed	III	IV

Prognosis estimates (based on best adnexum)
   I: 50–75%
   II: 25–50%
   III: 12–25%
   IV: 0–12%.
[a]As proposed by Hulka, 1990.
[b]Classification assignment. Each adnexum classified separately.

timate for conception and delivery of a subsequent viable infant based
on the adnexa with the least amount of pathology.

Hulka's classification scheme (1982) for adnexal adhesions is a simplified system that considers only the extent of ovarian involvement (less
than versus more than 50% of ovary enclosed by adhesions) and the
nature of the adhesions (filmy versus dense). Hulka's system assigns different prognostic estimates for conception and subsequent delivery of a
viable infant to each of the four possible classifications. Although this
classification system is easy to use, it does not take into account tubal
pathology or other fertility factors.

Conclusion

Adhesions are not required for peritoneal repair. They are a major cause
of postoperative morbidity and failure of surgical therapy and cannot be
prevented by surgical technique alone. The development of adjuvants to
prevent postsurgical adhesion formation is encumbered by differences
between the process of skin and peritoneal healing, access to the peritoneal
cavity, interspecies differences in peritoneal physiology, limitations of
animal models, and the complexities of intraperitoneal circulation and
transperitoneal transport. Clinical utilization of adhesion prevention regimens is slowed by the ambiguities of efficacy assessment. Clinical benefits
of adhesion prevention are only a part of the multifactorial problems of
pain, bowel obstruction, and infertility. A direct cause-and-effect relationship between adhesion prevention and amelioration of disease is difficult to establish.

To date no treatment has proven uniformly effective in preventing
postoperative adhesion formation. The use of surgical techniques that
limit tissue ischemia, as well as the use of absorbable, nonreactive, me-

chanical barriers provide clinical benefits to patients today. Ongoing evaluations of liquid and nonabsorbable barriers, drugs that modify the local inflammatory response (e.g., nonsteroidal anti-inflammatory drugs), and agents that promote plasminogen activator activity (e.g., recombinant tissue plasminogen activator) show promise for limiting adhesion formation in the future.

References

Adashi Ey, Rock JA, Guzick D, Wentz AC, Jones GS, Jones HW Jr. (1981). Fertility following bilateral ovarian wedge resection: a critical analysis of 90 consecutive cases of the polycystic ovary syndrome. *Fertil Steril.* 36:320–328.

Adhesion Study Group. (1983). Reduction of postoperative pelvic adhesions with intraperitoneal 32% dextran 70: a prospective, randomized clinical trial. *Fertil Steril.* 40:612–619.

Adoni A, Adatto-Levy R, Mogle P, Palti Z. (1980). Postoperative pleural effusion caused by dextran. *Int J Gynecol Obstet.* 18:243–247.

Ahmed N, Falcone T, Tulandi T, Houle G. (1991). Anaphylactic reaction because of intrauterine 32% dextran-70 instillation. *Fertil Steril.* 55:1014–1016.

Al-Chalabi HA, Otubo JAM. (1987). Value of a single intraperitoneal dose of heparin in prevention of adhesion formation: an experimental evaluation in rats. *Int J Fertil.* 32(4):332–335.

American Fertility Society. (1988). The American Fertility Society classifications of adnexal adhesions, distal tubal occlusion, tubal occlusion secondary to tubal ligation, tubal pregnancies, Mullerian anomalies and intrauterine adhesions. *Fertil Steril.* 49:944–955.

Andrade-Gordon P, Strickland S. (1986). Interaction of heparin with plasminogen activators and plasminogen: effects on the activations of plasminogen. *Biochemistry.* 25:4033–4040.

Badawy SZA, Baggish MS, ElBakry MM, Baltoyannis P. (1989). Evaluation of tissue healing and adhesion formation after an intraabdominal amniotic membrane graft in the rat. *J Reprod Med.* 34:198–202.

Bailey G, Strub R, Klein RC, Salvaggio F. (1967). Dextran-induced anaphylaxis. *JAMA.* 200:185–189.

Ballantyne DL Jr, Howthorne G, Ben-Hur N, Seidman I, Rees TD. (1971). Effect of silicone fluid on experimentally induced peritoneal adhesions. *Isr J Med Sci.* 7:1046–1049.

Barbot J, Parent B, Pibursson JB, Aubiot FX. (1987). A clinical study of the CO_2 laser and electro surgery for adhesion lysis in 172 cases followed by early second-look laparoscopy. *Fertil Steril.* 48:140–142.

Bateman BG, Nunley WC, Kitchen JD. (1982). Prevention of postoperative peritoneal adhesion: an assessment of ibuprofen. *Fertil Steril.* 38:107–115.

Beauchamp PJ, Quigley MM, Held B. (1984). Evaluation of progestogens for postoperative adhesion prevention. *Fertil Steril.* 42:538–542.

Beauchamp PJ, Guzick DS, Held B, Schmidt WA. (1988). Histologic response to microsuture materials. *J Reprod Med.* 33:615–623.

Bernstein J, Mattox J, Ulrich J. (1982). The potential for bacterial growth with dextran. *J Reprod Med.* 27:77–79.

Blauer KL, Collins RL. (1988). The effect of intraperitoneal progesterone on postoperative adhesion formation in rabbits. *Fertil Steril.* 49:144–149.

Bonney RJ, Davies P. (1984). Possible autoregulatory functions of the secretory products of mononuclear phagocytes. *Contemp Top Immunol.* 10:199–223.

Borten M, Seibert CP, Taymor ML. (1983). Recurrent anaphylactic reaction to intraperitoneal dextran 75 used for prevention of postsurgical adhesions. *Obstet Gynecol.* 61:755–757.

Boyers SP, Diamond MP, DeCherney AH. (1988). Reduction of postoperative pelvic adhesions in the rabbit with Gore-Tex surgical membrane. *Fertil Steril.* 49:1066–1070.

Brody GL, Frey CF. (1968). Peritoneal response to silicone fluid. A histologic study. *Arch Surg.* 96:237–241.

Bronson RA, Wallach EE. (1977). Lysis of periadnexal adhesions for correction of infertility. *Fertil Steril.* 28:613–619.

Bruhat MA, Manhes H, Mage G, Povly JL. (1980). Treatment of ectopic pregnancy by means of laparoscopy. *Fertil Steril.* 33:411–414.

Brumsted JR, Deaton J, Lavigne E, Riddick DH. (1990). Postoperative adhesion formation after ovarian wedge resection with and without ovarian reconstruction in the rabbit. *Fertil Steril.* 53:723–726.

Bryant LR. (1963). An evaluation of the effect of fibrinolysin on intraperitoneal adhesion formation. *Am J Surg.* 106:892–897.

Buckman RF, Buckman PD, Hufnagel HV, Gervin AS. (1976). A physiologic basis for the adhesion-free healing of deperitonealized surfaces. *J Surg Res.* 21:67–76.

Buttram VC Jr, Vaquero C. (1975). Postovarian wedge resection adhesive disease. *Fertil Steril.* 26:874–876.

Chapman HA, Vavrin Z, Hibbs JB. (1982). Macrophage fibrinolytic activity: identification of two pathways of plasmin formation by intact cells and of a plasminogen activator inhibitor. *Cell.* 28:653–662.

Cleary RE, Howard T, diZerega GS. (1985). Plasma dextran levels after abdominal instillation of 32% dextran 70: evidence for prolonged intraperitoneal retention. *Am J Obstet Gynecol.* 152:78–79.

Cohen BM, Heyman T, Mast D. (1983). Use of intraperitoneal solutions for preventing pelvic adhesions in the rat. *J Reprod Med.* 28:649–653.

Cox KR. (1970). Starch granuloma (pseudo-malignant seedings). *Br J Surg.* 57:650–653.

Daniell JF, Pittaway DE. (1983). Short interval second-look laparoscopy after infertility surgery: a preliminary report. *J Reprod Med.* 28:281–283.

Daniell JF, Pittaway DE, Maxson WE. (1983). The role of laparoscopic adhesion lysis in an in vitro fertilization program. *Fertil Steril.* 40:49–52.

Daniell JF, Miller W, Tosh R. (1986). Initial evaluation of the use of the potassium-titanyl-phosphate (KTP/532) laser in gynecologic laparoscopy. *Fertil Steril.* 46:373–377.

DeCherney A, Laufer N. (1983). The use of a new synthetic absorbable monofilament suture, polydioxanone (PDS), for surgery [Abstract]. *Fertil Steril.* 39:401.

DeCherney AH, Mezer HC. (1984). The nature of posttuboplasty pelvic adhesions as determined by early and late laparoscopy. *Fertil Steril.* 41:643–646.

Delbeke L, Gomel V, McComb P, Jetha N. (1983). Histologic reaction to four synthetic microsutures in the rabbit. *Fertil Steril.* 40:248–252.

DeLeon FD, Toledo AA, Sanfilippo JS, Yussman MA. (1984) The prevention of adhesion formation by nonsteroidal antiinflammatory drugs: An animal study comparing ibuprofen and indomethacin. *Fertil Steril.* 41:639–642.

Diamond E. (1979). Lysis of postoperative pelvic adhesions in infertility. *Fertil Steril.* 31:287–295.

Diamond MP, Daniell JF, Martin DC, Feste J, Vaughn WK, McLaughlin DS. (1984). Tubal patency and pelvic adhesions at early second-look laparoscopy following intraabdominal use of the carbon dioxide laser: initial report of the intraabdominal laser study group. *Fertil Steril.* 42:717–723.

Diamond MP, DeCherney AH. (1987). Pathogenesis of adhesion formation/reformation: application to reproductive pelvic surgery. *Microsurgery.* 8:103–107.

Diamond MP, Daniell JF, Feste J, Surrey MW, McLaughin DS, Friedman S, Vaughn WK, Martin DC. (1987a). Adhesion formation and de novo adhesion formation after reproductive pelvic surgery. *Fertil Steril.* 47:864–866.

Diamond MP, Linsky CB, Cunningham T, Constantine B, diZerega GS, DeCherney AH. (1987b). A model for sidewall adhesions in the rabbit: reduction by an absorbable barrier. *Microsurgery.* 8:197–200.

Diamond MP, Linksy CB, Cunningham T, Constantine B, DeCherney AH. (1988). Assessment of carboxymethylcellulose and 32% dextran 70 for prevention of adhesions in a rabbit uterine horn model. *Int J Fertil.* 33:278–282.

Diamond MP, Linsky CB, Cunningham T, Kamp L, Pines E, DeCherney AH, diZerega GS. (1991a). Adhesions reformation reduction by the use of Interceed TC7 plus heparin. *J Gynecol Surg.* 7:1–6.

Diamond MP, Pines E, Linsky CB, DeCherney AH, Cunningham T, diZerega GS, Kamp L. (1991b). Synergistic effects of Interceed TC7 and heparin in reducing adhesion formation in the rabbit uterine horn model. *Fertil Steril.* 55:389–394..

diZerega GS, Hodgen GD. (1980). Prevention of postsurgical tubal adhesions: comparative study of commonly used agents. *Am J Obstet Gynecol.* 136:173–178.

Dlugi AM, DeCherney AH. (1984). Prevention of postoperative adhesion formation. *Semin Reprod Endocrinol.* 2:125–129.

Donnez J. (1987). CO_2 laser laparoscopy in infertile women with endometriosis and women with adnexal adhesions. *Fertil Steril.* 48:390–394.

Doody KJ, Dunn RC, Buttram VC Jr. (1989). Recombinant tissue plasminogen activator reduces adhesion formation in a rabbit uterine horn model. *Fertil Steril.* 51:509–512.

Dunn R, Doody K, Mohler M, Buttram VC Jr. (1988). Development of a reproducible pelvic model for postsurgical adhesion formation in a primate species. Atlanta, GA. AFS Abstract #089.

Dunn R, Steinleitner AJ, Lambert H. (1991). Synergistic effect of intraperitoneally administered calcium channel blockade and recombinant tissue plasminogen activator to prevent adhesion formation in an animal model. *Am J Obstet Gynecol.* 164:1327–1330.

Eddy CA, Asch RH, Balmaceda JP. (1980). Pelvic adhesions following microsurgical and macrosurgical wedge resection of the ovaries. *Fertil Steril.* 33:557–561.

Elkins TE, Bury RJ, Ritter JL, Ling FW, Ahokas RA, Homsey CA, Malinak LR. (1984a). Adhesion prevention by solutions of sodium carboxymethylcellulose in the rat. I. *Fertil Steril.* 41:926–928.

Elkins TE, Ling FW, Ahokas RA, Abdella TN, Homsey CA, Malinak LR. (1984b). Adhesion prevention by solutions of sodium carboxymethylcellulose in the rat. II. *Fertil Steril.* 41:929–932.

Elkins TE, Trenthem L, McNeeley SG Jr, Ling FW, Preu HJ, Homsey CA, Malinak LR. (1985). Potential for in vitro growth of common bacteria in solutions of 32% dextran 70 and 1.0% sodium carboxymethylcellulose. *Fertil Steril.* 43:477–478.

Elkins TE. (1989). Can a pro-coagulant substance prevent adhesions? In: GS diZerega, Malinak LR, Diamond MP, Linsky CB, eds. *Treatment of Post Surgical Adhesion.* New York: Wiley-Liss; 358:103–112.

Elkins TE, Warren J, Portz DM. (1991). Oxygen free radicals and pelvic adhesion formation: II. The interaction of oxygen free radicals and adhesion preventing solutions. *Int J Infert.* 36:231–237.

Ellis H. (1971). The cause and prevention of postoperative intraperitoneal adhesions. *Surg Gynecol.* 133:497–511.

Ellis H. (1990). The hazards of surgical glove dusting powders. *Surg Gynecol Obstet.* 171:521–527.

Fayez JA, Schneider PJ. (1987). Prevention of pelvic adhesion formation by different modalities of treatment. *Am J Obstet Gynecol.* 157:1184–1188.

Filmar S, Jetha N, McComb P, Gomel V. (1989a). A comparative histologic study on the healing process after tissue transection. I. Carbon dioxide laser and electromicrosurgery. *Am J Obstet Gynecol.* 160:1062–1067.

Filmar S, Jetha N, McComb P, Gomel V. (1989b). A comparative histologic study on the healing process after tissue transection. II. Carbon dioxide laser and surgical microscissors. *Am J Obstet Gynecol.* 160:1068–1072.

Flessner M, Dedrick R, & Schultz J. (1985). Exchange of macromolecules between peritoneal cavity and plasma. *Am J Physiol.* 248: H15–25.

Flower R, Gryglewski R, Herbaczynska-Cedro K, Vane JR. (1972). Effects of anti-inflammatory drugs on prostaglandin biosynthesis. *Nature New Biol.* 238:104–106.

Frantzen C, Schlösser HW. (1982). Microsurgery and postinfectious tubal infertility. *Fertil Steril.* 38:397–420.

Fredericks CM, Kotry I, Holtz G, Askalani AH, Serour GI. (1986). Adhesion prevention in the rabbit with sodium carboxymethylcellulose solutions. *Am J Obstet Gynecol.* 155:667–670.

Frey CF, Thorpe C, Brody G. (1967). Silicone fluid in the prevention of intestinal adhesions. *Arch Surg.* 95:253–256.

Fukasawa M, Girgis W, diZerega GS. (1988). Inhibition of postsurgical adhesion formation in a standardized rabbit model. II. Intraperitoneal treatment with heparin. *Int J Fertil.* 45:460–466.

Galan N, Leader A, Malkinson T, Taylor PJ. (1983). Adhesion prophylaxis in rabbits with Surgicel and two absorbable microsurgical sutures. *J Reprod Med.* 28:662–664.

Gauwerky JF, Heinrich D, Kubli F. (1986). Complications of intraperitoneal dextran application for prevention of adhesions. *Biol Res Pregnancy Perinatol.* 7:93–97.

Gervin AS, Puckett GL, Silver D. (1973). Serosal hypofibrinolysis: a cause of postoperative adhesions. *Am J Surg.* 125:80–87.

Gillett WR. (1991). Artefactual loss of human ovarian surface epithelium: potential clinical significance. *Reprod Fertil Dev.* 3:93–98.

Golan A, Winston RML. (1989). Blood and intraperitoneal adhesion formation in the rat. *J Obstet Gynecol.* 9:248–252.

Golan A, Stolik O, Wexler S, Langer R, Ber A, David MP. (1990). Prostaglandins—a role in adhesion formation. An experimental study. *Acta Obstet Gynecol Scand.* 69:339–341.

Golan A, Bernstein T, Wexler S, Neuman M, Bukovsky I, David MP. (1991). The effect of prostaglandins and aspirin: an inhibitor of prostaglandin synthesis on adhesion formation in rats. *Hum Reprod (Eynsham).* 6:251–254.

Goldberg JM, Toledo AA, Mitchell DE. (1987). An evaluation of the Gore-Tex surgical membrane for the prevention of postoperative peritoneal adhesions. *Obstet Gynecol.* 70:846–848.

Gomel V. (1978). Recent advances in surgical correlation of tubal disease producing infertility. *Curr Probl Obstet Gynecol.* 1:10–17.

Gomel V. (1983). *Microsurgery in Female Infertility.* 1st ed. Boston: Little, Brown; Chapter 20.

Graebe RA, Oelsner G, Cornelison TL, Pan S-B, Haseltine FP, DeCherney AH. (1989). An animal study of different treatments to prevent postoperative pelvic adhesions. *Microsurgery.* 10:53–55.

Grosfield JL, Berman IR, Schiller M, Morse TS. (1973). Excessive morbidity resulting from the prevention of intestinal adhesions with steroids and antihistamines. *J Pediatr Surg.* 8:221–226.

Hibbs JB, Chapman HA, Weinberg JB. (1978). The macrophage as an antineoplastic surveillance cell: biological perspective. *J Reticuloendothel Soc.* 24:549–556.

Hixson C, Swanson LA, Friedman CI. (1986). Oxidized cellulose for preventing adnexal adhesions. *J Reprod Med.* 31:58–60.

Höckel M, Ott S, Siemann U, Kissell T. (1987). Prevention of peritoneal adhesions in the rat with sustained intraperitoneal dexamethasone delivered by a novel therapeutic system. *Ann Chir Gynaecol.* 76:306–313.

Holtz G. (1980). Prevention of postoperative adhesions. *J Reprod Med.* 24:141–146.

Holtz G, Baker E, Tsai C. (1980). Effect of thirty-two per cent dextran 70 on peritoneal adhesion formation and re-formation after lysis. *Fertil Steril.* 33:660–662.

Holtz G. (1982a). Adhesion induction by suture of varying tissue reactivity and caliber. *Int J Fertil.* 27:134–135.

Holtz G. (1982b). Failure of a non-steroidal anti-inflammatory agent (ibuprofen) to inhibit peritoneal adhesion reformation after lysis. *Fertil Steril.* 37:582–583.

Homsey CA, Stanley RF, King JW. (1973). Pseudo-synovial fluids based on sodium carboxymethyl cellulose. In: Gabelnick HL, Litt M, eds. *Rheology of Biological System.* Springfield, IL: Charles C. Thomas; 278–295.

Horne HW Jr, Clyman M, Debrovner C, Griggs G. (1973). The prevention of postoperative pelvic adhesions following conservative operative treatment for human infertility. *Int J Fertil.* 18:109–115.

Hulka JF. (1982). Adnexal adhesions: a prognostic staging and classification system based on a five-year survey of fertility surgery results at Chapel Hill, North Carolina. *Am J Obstet Gynecol.* 144:141–148.

Hulka JF. (1990). Staging of adnexal adhesions: a brief review. *Prog Clin Biol Res.* 358:13–21.

Humes JL, Burger G, Galavage M, Keuhl FA, Wightman PD, Dahlgren ME, Davies P, Bonney RJ. (1980). The diminished production of arachidonic acid oxygenation products by elicited mouse peritoneal macrophages: possible mechanisms. *J Immunol.* 124:2110–2116.

Interceed (TC7). Adhesion Barrier Study Group. (1989). Prevention of postsurgical adhesions by Interceed (TC7), an absorbable adhesion barrier: a prospective, randomized multicenter clinical study. *Fertil Steril.* 51:933–938.

Jansen RPS. (1985). Failure of intraperitoneal adjuncts to improve the outcome of pelvic operations in young women. *Am J Obstet Gynecol.* 153:363–371.

Jansen RPS. (1988a). Early laparoscopy after pelvic operations to prevent adhesions safety and efficacy. *Fertil Steril.* 49:26–31.

Jansen RPS. (1988b). Failure of peritoneal irrigation with heparin during pelvic operations upon young women to reduce adhesions. *Surg Gynecol Obstet.* 166:154–160.

Jansen RPS. (1990). Prevention and treatment of postsurgical adhesions. *Med J Aust.* 152:305–307.

Jarrett J & Dawood M. (1986) Adhesion formation and uterine tube healing in the rabbit: A controlled study of the effects of ibuprofen and flurbiprofen. *Am. J Obstet Gynecol.* 115:1186–1192.

Johnston RB, Godzik CA, Cohn ZA. (1978). Increased superoxide anion production by immunologically activated and chemically elicited macrophages. *J Exp Med.* 142:115–122.

Kajihara Y. (1960). The use of chondroitin sulfuric acid for the prevention of peritoneal adhesions. *J Kurume Med Assoc.* 23:4641–4649.

Kappas AM, Fatouros M, Papadimitriou K, Katsouyannopoulos V, Cassioumis D. (1988). Effect of intraperitoneal saline irrigation at different temperatures on adhesion formation. *Br J Surg.* 75:854–856.

Kapur BML, Gulati SM, Talwar JR. (1972). Prevention of reformation of peritoneal adhesions: effect of oxyphenbutazone, proteolytic enzymes for carcia papaya and dextran 40. *Arch Surg.* 105:761–764.

Kapur BML, Talwar JR, Gulati SM. (1969). Oxyphenbutazone: anti-inflammatory agent in prevention of peritoneal adhesions. *Arch Surg.* 98:301–302.

Keye WR Jr. (1991). Laser surgery and adhesion formation. In: diZerega G, Malinak LR, Diamond MP, Linsky CB, eds. *Treatment of Post Surgical Adhesions.* New York: Wiley-Liss; 358:67–76.

Khan MA, Brown JL, Logan KV, Hayes RI. (1983). Suture contamination by surface powders on surgical gloves. *Arch Surg.* 118:738–739.

King IR. (1989). Candida albicans pelvic abscess associated with the use of 32% dextran-70 in conservative pelvic surgery. *Fertil Steril.* 51:1050–1052.

Kolmorgen K, Akkermann N. (1988). Adjuvant prednisolone therapy for the prevention of adhesions after acute adnexitis. *Zentralbl Gynakol.* 110:1433–1436.

Krinsky AH, Haseltine FP, DeCherney A. (1984). Peritoneal fluid accumulation with dextran 70 instilled at time of laparoscopy. *Fertil Steril.* 41:647–649.

Lane DA, MacGregor JR, Michalski R, Kakkar VV. (1978). Anticoagulant activities of four unfractionated and fractionated heparins. *Thromb Res.* 12:257–271.

Larsson B, Svanberg SG, Swolin K. (1977). Oxyphenbutazone—an adjuvant to be used in prevention of adhesions in operations for fertility. *Fertil Steril.* 28:807–808.

Larsson B, Nisell H, Granberg I. (1978). Surgicel—an absorbable hemostatic material—in prevention of peritoneal adhesions in rats. *Acta Chir Scand.* 144:375–378.

Larsson B, Lalos O, Marsk L, Tronstad SE, Bygdeman M, Pehrson S, Joelson I. (1985). Effect of intraperitoneal instillation of 32% dextran 70 on postoperative adhesion formation after tubal surgery. *Acta Obstet Gynecol Scand.* 64:437–441.

Laufer N, Merino M, Trietsch HG, DeCherney AH. (1984). Macroscopic and histologic tissue reaction to polydioxanone, a new, synthetic, monofilament microsuture. *J Reprod Med.* 24:307–310.

Leach RE, Henry RL. (1990). Reduction of postoperative adhesions in the rat uterine horn model with poloxamer. *Am J Obstet Gynecol.* 162:1317–1319.

Liao S-K, Suehiro GT, McNamara JJ. (1973). Prevention of postoperative intestinal adhesions in primates. *Surg Gynecol Obstet.* 137:816–818.

Lindenberg S, Lauritsen JG. (1984). Prevention of peritoneal adhesion formation by fibrin sealant. *Ann Chir Gynaecol.* 73:11–13.

Linsky CB, Diamond MP, Cunningham T, Constantine B, DeCherney AH, diZerega GS. (1987). Adhesion reduction in the rabbit uterine horn model using an absorbable barrier, TC-7. *J Reprod Med.* 32:17–20.

Linsky CB, Diamond MP, Cunningham, T, DeCherney AH, diZerega GS. (1988). Effect of blood on the efficacy of barrier adhesion reduction in the rabbit uterine horn model. *Infertility.* 11:273–280.

Luber K, Beeson CC, Kennedy JF, Villanueva B, Young PE. (1986). Results of microsurgical treatment of tubal infertility and early second-look laparoscopy in the post-pelvic inflammatory disease patient: implications for in vitro fertilization. *Am J Obstet Gynecol.* 154:1264–1270.

Luciano A, Hauser K, Benda J. (1983). Evaluation of community used adjuvants in the prevention of postoperative adhesions. *Am J Obstet Gynecol.* 146:88–92.

Luciano AA, Maier DB, Kock EI, Nulsen JC, Whitman GF. (1989). A comparative study of postoperative adhesions following laser surgery by laparoscopy versus laparotomy in the rabbit model. *Obstet Gynecol.* 74:220–224..

Luciano AA. (1990). Laparotomy vs laparoscopy. In: diZerega GS, Malinak LR, Diamond MP, Linsky CB, eds. *Treatment of Postoperative Surgical Adhesions.* New York: Wiley Liss; 35–44.

Lundorff P, Thorburn J, Lindblom B. (1990). Second-look laparoscopy after ectopic pregnancy. *Fertil Steril.* 53:604–609..

Lundorff P, Hahlin M, Kallfelt B, Thorburn J, Lindblom B. (1991). Adhesion formation after laparoscopic surgery in tubal pregnancy: a randomized trial versus laparotomy. *Fertil Steril.* 55:911–915..

Lyles R, Goldzieher JW, Betts JW, Franklin RR, Buttram VC, Feste JR, Malinak LR. (1989). Early second look laparoscopy after the treatment of polycystic ovarian disease with laparoscopic ovarian electrocautery and/or ND:YAG laser photocoagulation. Abstract O-061.

Magyar DM, Hayes MF, Moghissi KS, Subramanian MG. (1984). Hypothalamic-pituitary-adrenocortical function after dexamethasone-promethazine adhesion regimen. *Obstet Gynecol.* 63:182–185.

Magyar DM, Hayes MF, Spirtos NJ, Hull ME, Moghissi KS. (1985). Is intraperitoneal dextran 70 safe for routine gynecologic use? *Am J Obstet Gynecol.* 152:198–204.

Malinak LR. (1990). Interceed (TC7) as an adjuvant for adhesion reduction: clinical studies. In: diZerega GS, Malinak LR, Diamond M, Linsky C, eds. *Treatment of Postoperative Surgical Adhesion.* New York: Wiley-Liss; 193–206.

Markwardt F, Klocking HP. (1977). Heparin induced release of plasminogen activator. *Haemostasis.* 6:370–374.

Maurer JH, Bonaventura LM. (1983). The effect of aqueous progesterone on operative adhesion formation. *Fertil Steril.* 39:485–489.

McGaw T, Elkins TE, DeLancey JOL, McNeeley SG, Warren J. (1988). Assessment of intraperitoneal adhesion formation in a rat model: can a procoagulant substance prevent adhesions? *Obstet Gynecol.* 71:774–778.

McNaught GHD. (1964). Starch granuloma: a present day surgical hazard. *Br J Surg.* 51:845–849.

Mecke H, Semm K, Freys I, Argiriou C, Gent H-J. (1989). Incidence of adhesions in the true pelvis after pelviscopic operative treatment of tubal pregnancy. *Gynecol Obstet Invest.* 28:202–204.

Menzies D, Ellis H. (1989). Intra-abdominal adhesions and their prevention by topical tissue plasminogen activator. *J Soc Med.* 82:534–535.

Moll HD, Schumacher J, Wright JC, Spano JS. (1990). Evaluation of sodium carboxymethylcellulose for prevention of experimentally induced abdominal adhesions in ponies. *Am J Vet Res.* 52:88–91.

Montz FJ, Shimanuki T, diZerega GS. (1987). Postsurgical mesothelial re-epithelialization. In: DeCherney AH, Polan ML, eds. *Reproductive Surgery.* New York: Year Book Medical Publishers; 31–47.

Murphy AA, Schlaff WD, Hassiakos D, Durmusoglu F, Damewood MD, Rock JA. (1991). Laparoscopic cautery in the treatment of endometriosis-related infertility. *Fertil Steril.* 55:246–251.

Myllarniemi H. (1967). Foreign material in adhesion formation after abdominal surgery. *Acta Chir Scand.* 377:1–48.

Neff MR, Holtz GL, Betsill WL Jr. (1985). Adhesion formation and histologic reaction with polydioxanone and polyglactin suture. *Am J Obstet Gynecol.* 151:20–23.

Nezhat CR, Nezhat FR, Metzger DA, Luciano AA. (1990). Adhesion reformation after reproductive surgery by videolaseroscopy. *Fertil Steril.* 53:1008–1011.

Nishimura K, Bieniarz A, Nakamura RM, diZerega GS. (1983a). Evaluation of oxidized regenerated cellulose for prevention of postoperative intraperitoneal adhesions. *Jpn J Surg.* 13:159–163.

Nishimura K, Nakamura RM, diZerega GS. (1983b). Biochemical evaluation of postsurgical wound repair: prevention of intraperitoneal adhesion formation with ibuprofen. *J Surg Res.* 34:219–226.

Nishimura K, Shimanuki T, diZerega GS. (1984a). Ibuprofen in the prevention of experimentally induced postoperative adhesions. *Am J Med.* 77:102–106.

Nishimura K, Nakamura RM, diZerega GS. (1984b). Ibuprofen inhibition of postsurgical adhesion formation: a time and dose response biochemical evaluation in rabbits. *J Surg Res.* 36:115–124.

O'Leary J, Turner A, Feldman A. (1969). Silicone in the prevention of pelvic adhesions. *Am Surg.* 35:622–623.

O'Leary JA. (1985). Liquid silicone for the prevention of pelvic adhesions. *J Reprod Med.* 30:761–763.

Oelsner G, Graebe RA, Pan S-B, Haseltine FP, Barnea ER, Fakih H, DeCherney

AH. (1987). Chondroitin sulphate. A new intraperitoneal treatment for post-operative adhesion prevention in the rabbit. *J Reprod Med.* 32:812–814.

Operative Laparoscopy Study Group. (1991). Postoperative adhesion development after operative laparoscopy: evaluations at early second look procedures. *Fertil Steril.* 55:700–704.

Orita H, Gale J, Campeau JD, Nakamura RM, diZerega GS. (1986). Differential secretion of plasminogen activator by post-surgical activated macrophages. *J Surg Res.* 41:569–573.

Orita H, Fukasawa M, Girgis W, diZerega GS. (1991). Inhibition of postsurgical adhesions in a standardized rabbit model: intraperitoneal treatment with tissue plasminogen activator. *Int J Fertil.* 36:172–177.

Pfeffer WH. (1980). Adjuvants in pelvic surgery. *Fertil Steril.* 33:245–256.

Pfeffer WH. (1980). The effect of dexamethasone and promethazine administration on adhesion formation, tubal function and ultrastructure following microsurgical anastomosis of rabbit oviducts. *Fertil Steril.* 34:162–180.

Plescia OJ, Smith AH, Greenwich K. (1975). Subversion of immune system by tumor cells and the role of prostaglandins. *Proc Natl Acad Sci USA.* 72:1848–1853.

Portz DM, Elkins TE, White R, Warren J, Adadevoh S, Randolph J. (1991). Oxygen free radicals and pelvic adhesion formation: I. Blocking oxygen free radical toxicity to prevent adhesion formation in an endometriosis model. *Int J Fertil.* 36:39–42.

Queralt CB, Laguens G, Lozano R, Morandeira JR. (1987). Prevention of peritonitis with oxidized regenerated cellulose. *Infect Surg.* Dec.:659–660.

Querleu D, Vankeerberghen DF, Deffense F, Boutteville C. (1989). The effect of noxytiolin and systemic corticosteroids in infertility surgery a prospective randomized study. *So J Gynecol Obstet Biol Reprod.* 18:935–940.

Raftery AT. (1980). Absorbable haemostatic materials and intraperitoneal adhesion formation. *Br J Surg.* 67:57–58.

Raj SG, Hulka JF. (1982). Second-look laparoscopy in infertility surgery: therapeutic and prognostic value. *Fertil Steril.* 38:325–329.

Randall RW, Eakins KE, Higgs GA. (1980). Inhibition of arachidonic acid cyclo-oxygenase and lipo-oxygenase activities by indomethacin and compound BW755. *Agents Actions.* 10:553–555.

Rappaport WD, Holcomb M, Valente J, Chvapil M. (1989). Antibiotic irrigation and the formation of intraabdominal adhesions. *Am J Surg.* 158:435–437.

Ratzan KR, Musher DM, Keusch GT, Weinstein L. (1972). Correlation of increased metabolic activities resistance to infection, enhanced phagocytosis and inhibition of bacterial growth by macrophages from listeria and BCG-infected mice. *Infect Immunol.* 5:499–503.

Reid R. (1992). Clinical experience of Interceed and heparin. In: Diamond MP, diZerega GS, Reid R, Linsky CB, eds. *Gynecologic Surgery and Adhesion Prevention.* New York: Wiley-Liss. (in press).

Rein MS, Hill JA. (1989). 32% dextran 70 (hyskon) inhibits lymphocyte and macrophage function in vitro: a potential new mechanism for adhesion prevention. *Fertil Steril.* 52:953–957.

Replogle RL, Johnson R, Gross RE. (1966). Prevention of postoperative intestinal adhesions with combined promethazine and dexamethasone therapy: experimental and clinical studies. *Ann Surg.* 163:580–588.

Rodgers K, Ellefson D, Girgis W, Scott L, diZerega GS. (1988). Effects of tolmetin sodium dihydrate on normal and postsurgical peritoneal cell function. *Int J Immunopharmacol.* 10:111–120.

Rodgers KE. (1990). Nonsteroidal anti-inflammatory drugs (NSAIDs) in the treatment of postsurgical adhesion. In: diZerega GS, Malinak LR, Diamond MD, Linsky CP, eds. *Treatment of Adhesions.* New York: Wiley-Liss; 119–130 .

Rodgers KE, Bracken K, Richer L, Girgis W, diZerega GS. (1990a). Inhibition of postsurgical adhesions by liposomes containing nonsteroidal anti-inflammatory drugs. *Int J Infertil.* 35:315–320.

Rodgers K, Girgis W, Johns D, diZerega GS. (1990b). Intraperitoneal tolmetin prevents postsurgical adhesion formation in rabbits. *Int J Infertil.* 35:40–45.

Rodgers KE, Ellefson D, Girgis W, diZerega GS. (1992). Protease and protease inhibitor secretion by post-surgical macrophages following in vitro exposure to tolmetin. *Agents Actions.* (in press).

Rose BI. (1987). Safety of hyskon for routine gynecologic surgery. A case report. *J Reprod Med.* 32:134–136.

Rosenberg RD. (1978). Heparin antithrombin and abnormal clotting. *Annu Rev Med.* 29:367–378.

Rosenberg SM, Board JA. (1984). High-molecular weight dextran in human infertility surgery. *Am J Obstet Gynecol.* 148:380–385.

Ruiz Navas MT, Lopez E, Flores DP, Romeroz JA. (1988). Comparative experimental study of the effectiveness of different types of macromolecules carboxymethylcellulose dextran 40 and dextran 70 in the prevention of adhesions. *Rev Esp Obstet Gynecol.* 47:43–50.

Ryan GB, Grobety J, Majno G. (1973). Mesothelial injury and recovery. *Am J Pathol.* 71:93–112.

Schroder M, Willumsen H, Hart Hansen JP, Hart Hansen O. (1982). Peritoneal adhesion formation after the use of oxidized cellulose (Surgicel) and gelatin sponge (Spongostan) in rats. *Acta Chir. Scand* 148:595–596.

Sekiba K, and the Obstetrics and Gynecology Adhesion Prevention Committee. (1992). Use of Interceed (TC7) absorbable adhesions barrier to reduce postoperative adhesion reformation in infertility and endometriosis surgery. *Obstet Gynecol.* 79:518–522.

Serour GI, Badraoui MH, El-Agizi HM, Hamed AF, Abdel-Aziz F. (1989). Laparoscopic adhesionlysis for infertile patients with pelvic adhesive desease. *Int J Gynaecol Obstet.* 30:249–252.

Shimanuki T, Nishimura K, diZerega GS. (1985). Prevention of postoperative peritoneal adhesions in rabbits with ibuprofen. *Sem Reprod Endocrinol.* 3:295–300.

Shimanuki T, Nakamura RM, diZerega GS. (1986). A kinetic analysis of peritoneal fluid cytology and arachidonic acid metabolism after abrasion and reabrasion of rabbit peritoneum. *J Surg Res.* 41:245–251.

Shimanuki T, Nishimura K, diZerega GS. (1987). Localized prevention of postsurgical adhesion formation and reformation with oxidized regenerated cellulose. *J Biomed Mater Res.* 21:173–185.

Siegler AM, Kontopoulos V, Wang CF. (1980). Prevention of postoperative adhesions in rabbits with ibuprofen, a nonsteroidal anti-inflammatory agent. *Fertil Steril.* 34:46–49.

Smith DC. (1983). Comparison of irrigation solutions used in infertility surgery.

Presented at the 50th Annual Meeting Pacific Coast Obstetrical & Gynecological Society, Vancouver, BC, September 6-11, 1983.

Soules MR, Dennis L, Bosarge A, Moore DE. (1982). The prevention of postoperative pelvic adhesions: an animal study comparing barrier methods with dextran 70. *Am J Obstet Gynecol.* 143:829–834.

St. Onge R, Weiss C, Denlinger JL, Balazs EA. (1980). A preliminary assessment of Na-hyaluronate injection into "No Man's Land" for primary flexor tendon repair. *Clin Orthop.* 146:269–275..

Stangel JJ, Nisbet JD II, Settles H. (1984). Formation and prevention of postoperative abdominal adhesions. *J Reprod Med.* 29:143–156.

Steinleitner A, Lambert H, Montoro L, Swanson J, Sueldo CE. (1988). Use of diltiazem for preventing postoperative adhesions. *J Reprod Med.* 38:891–894.

Steinleitner A, Lambert H, Kazensky C, Danks P, Roy S. (1990). Pentoxifylline, a methylxanthine derivative, prevents postsurgical adhesion reformation in rabbits. *Obstet Gynecol.* 75:926–928.

Steinleitner A, Lambert H, Kazensky, Cantor B. (1991). Poloxamer 407 as an intraperitoneal barrier material for the prevention of postsurgical adhesion formation and reformation in rodent models for reproductive surgery. *Obstet Gynecol.* 77:48–52.

Surgical Membrane Study Group. (1992). Prophylaxis of pelvic sidewall adhesions with Gore-Tex surgical membrane: a multicenter clinical investigation. *Fertil Steril.* 57:921–923.

Surrey MW, Friedman S. (1982). Second-look laparoscopy after reconstructive pelvic surgery for infertility. *J Reprod Med.* 27:658–660.

Swolin K. (1967). Die einwwirkung von grossen, intraperitoneal en dusen glukokortikoid auf die bildung von postoperative adhasionen. *Acta Obstet Gynecol Scand.* 46:204–209.

Swolin K. (1975). Electromicrosurgery and salpingostomy: long term results. *Am J Obstet Gynecol.* 121:418–422.

Tarvady S, Anguli VC, Pichappa CV. (1987). Effect of heparin on wound healing. *J Biosci.* 12:33–40.

Tavmergen EN, Mecke H, Semm K. (1990). Frequency of intraabdominal adhesions following pelviscopy and laparotomy. *Zentralbl Gynaekol.* 112:1163–1169.

Taylor RJ, Salata JJ. (1976). Inhibition of prostaglandin synthetase by tolmetin (Tolectin, McN-2559), a new non-steroidal anti-inflammatory agent. *Biochem Pharmacol.* 25:2479–2484.

ten Kate-Booij MJ, van Geldorp HJ, Drogendijk AC. (1985). Dextran and adhesions in guinea-pigs. *J Reprod Fertil.* 75:183–188.

Thomas SC, Jones LC, Hungerford DS. (1982). Hyaluronic acid and its effect on postoperative adhesions in the rabbit flexor tendon. *Clin Orthop Relat Res.* 206:281–289.

Tolbert TW, Brown JL. (1980). Surface powders on surgical gloves. *Arch Surg.* 115:729–732.

Trimbos-Kemper TCM, Trimbos JB, van Hall EV. (1985). Adhesion formation after tubal surgery: results of the eighth-day laparoscopy in 188 patients. *Fertil Steril.* 43:395–400.

Trimbos-Kemper TC, Veering BT. (1989). Anaphylactic shock from intracavitary 32% Dextran-70 during hysterectomy. *Fertil Steril.* 51:1053–1054.

Tschoepe R, Wright KKH, Gizang E. (1980). The effect of dexamethasone and promethazine administration on adhesion formation, tubal function and ultrastructure following microsurgical anastomosis in rabbit oviducts. *Fertil Steril.* 34:162–168.

Tulandi T. (1986). Salpingo-ovariolysis: a comparison between laser surgery and electrosurgery. *Fertil Steril.* 45:489–491.

Tulandi T. (1987). Adhesion formation after reproductive surgery with and without the carbon dioxide laser. *Fertil Steril.* 47:704–706.

Tulandi T, Falcone T, Kafka I. (1989). Second-look operative laparoscopy 1 year following reproductive surgery. *Fertil Steril.* 52:421–424.

Tulandi T. (1990). Prevention of postoperative intra-abdominal adhesions. *Curr Opinion Obstet Gynecol.* 2:287–290.

Tulandi T. (1991). Clinical and scientific implications of second-look laparoscopy. In: diZerega GS, Malinak LR, Diamond MP, Linsky CB, eds. *Treatment of Post Surgical Adhesions.* New York: Wiley-Liss; 358:85–92.

Unkeless JC, Gordon S, Reich S. (1974). Secretion of plasminogen activator by stimulated macrophages. *J Exp Med.* 139:834–850.

Vane JR. (1971). Inhibition of prostaglandin synthesis as a mechanism of action for aspirin-like drugs. *Nature New Biol.* 231:232–235.

Wagaman R, Ingram JM, Rao PS, Saba HI. (1986). Intravenous versus intraperitoneal administration of dextran in the rabbit: effects on fibrinolysis. *Am J Obstet Gynecol.* 155:464–470.

Wahl LM, Winter CC. (1984). Regulation of guinea pig macrophage collagenase by dexamethasome and colchicine. *Arch Biochem Biophys.* 230:661–667.

Wahl LM, Lampel LL. (1987). Regulation of human peripherial blood monocyte collagenase by prostaglandins and anti-inflammatory drugs. *Cell Immunol.* 105:411–422.

Wallach EE, Manara LR, Eisenberg E. (1983). Experience with 143 cases of tubal surgery. *Fertil Steril.* 39:609–617.

Weibel M-A, Majno G. (1973). Peritoneal adhesions and their relation to abdominal surgery. *Am J Surg.* 126:345–353.

Weinans MJN, Kauer FM, Klompmaker IJ, Wijma J. (1990). Transient liver function disturbances after the intraperitoneal use of 32% dextran 70 as adhesion prophylaxis in infertility surgery. *Fertil Steril.* 53:159–161.

Weiss C, Levy HJ, Denlinger J, Suros JM, Weiss HE. (1986). The role of Na-hylan in reducing postsurgical tendon adhesions. *Bull Hosp Jt Dis Orthop Inst.* 45:9–15.

Weiss C, Suros JM, Michalow A, Denlinger J, Moore M, Tejeiro W. (1987). The role of Na-hylan in reducing postsurgical tendon adhesions: Part 2. *Bull Hosp Jt Dis Orthop Inst.* 47(1):31–39.

Werb Z, Banda MJ, Jones PA. (1980). Degradation of connective tissue by macrophages: I. Proteolysis of elastin, glycoproteins and collagen by proteinases isolated from macrophages. *J Exp Med.* 152:1340–1357.

Wiskind AK, Toledo AA, Dudle AG, Zusmanis K. (1990). Adhesion formation after ovarian wound repair in New Zealand white rabbits: a comparison or ovarian microsurgical closure with ovarian nonclosure. *Am J Obstet Gynecol.* 163:1674–1678.

Yaacobi Y, Goldberg EP. (1991). Effect of Ringer's lactate irrigation on the formation of postoperative abdominal adhesions. *J Invest Surg.* 4:31–36.

Yemini M, Meshorer A, Katz Z, Rozenman D, Lancet M. (1984). Prevention of reformation of pelvic adhesions by "barrier" methods. *Int J Fertil.* 29:194–196.

Young PE, Egan JE, Barlow JJ, Mulligan WJ. (1970). Reconstructive surgery for infertility at the Boston Hospital for Women. *Am J Obstet Gynecol.* 108:1092–1097.

Young RL, Cota J, Zund G, Mason BA, Wheeler JM. (1991). The use of an amniotic membrane graft to prevent postoperative adhesions. *Fertil Steril.* 55:624–628.

Index